VULNERABLE POPULATIONS
IN THE UNITED STATES

VULNERABLE POPULATIONS IN THE UNITED STATES

Leiyu Shi
Gregory D. Stevens

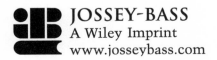

JOSSEY-BASS
A Wiley Imprint
www.josseybass.com

Library of Congress Cataloging-in-Publication Data

Shi, Leiyu.
  Vulnerable populations in the United States / Leiyu Shi and Gregory D. Stevens.
    p. cm.
  Includes bibliographical references and index.
  ISBN 0-7879-6958-3 (alk. paper)
    1. Poor—Medical care—United States. 2. People with social disabilities—Medical care—United
  States. 3. Health services accessibility—United States. I. Stevens, Gregory D., 1973-   . II. Title.
    [DNLM: 1. Vulnerable Populations—United States. 2. Health Services Accessibility—United States.
  WA 300 S555v 2004]
  RA418.5.P6S54 2004
  362.1'086'9420973—dc22   2004014537

Printed in the United States of America
FIRST EDITION
HB Printing 10 9 8 7 6 5 4 3 2 1

CONTENTS

FIGURES, TABLES, AND EXHIBITS

Figures

Tables

Exhibits

PREFACE

We have written this book to call attention among policymakers, health care providers, social scientists, public health researchers, and students of these fields to the inequitable health and health care experiences of vulnerable populations in the United States. Having a high level of population health is commensurate with the worldwide leadership position of the United States. Without attention to reducing these disparities within the nation, the United States will continue to spend more and have far poorer health across many indicators when compared with other industrialized nations. By providing this up-to-date account of disparities in access, quality, and health status of the nation's vulnerable populations, this book heightens awareness of the challenges we face and measures progress that has been made toward reducing disparities.

The scientific and theoretical literature lacks a coherent, well-integrated, general framework to study vulnerable populations. Typically, vulnerable populations are studied as discrete population subgroups, but this method is problematic for developing and implementing truly effective health policy because these vulnerable subgroups are not mutually exclusive. This book contributes to the literature by introducing an integrated framework to study vulnerable populations. Operationalizing vulnerability as a combination or convergence of risk factors is preferred to studying risk factors separately because vulnerability, when defined as a convergence of risks, can best capture reality. This approach not only reflects the co-occurrence of risk factors but underscores our belief that it is difficult to address disparities in one risk factor without addressing others.

Furthermore, the focus on vulnerable populations as a national health policy priority should be enhanced for political, social, economic, and moral reasons. Unfortunately, today's health care delivery system is not designed to address the health care needs of vulnerable populations adequately. National policies and programs are at best patchworks of fragmented, uncoordinated, categorical initiatives. This book reviews existing programs, identifies their limitations, and proposes a new course of action that aims to improve the health services system and addresses the multifaceted health needs of vulnerable populations.

As national, state, and local policies have gained momentum in addressing the needs of vulnerable populations, there has also been an increasing demand for knowledge about these populations. Not only is there interest in documenting the health and health care experiences of vulnerable populations, there is also growing interest in the mechanisms underlying these disparities. This book provides in-depth data on access to care, quality of care, and health status to meet this demand for data, and it tracks progress made toward reducing or eliminating disparities as identified in *Healthy People 2010*. It also updates and summarizes what is currently known and unknown regarding the pathways and mechanisms linking vulnerability with poor health and health care outcomes.

Finally, we intend for this book to provide a new perspective on a complex and important subject area. We hope that readers will gain a clear and sophisticated knowledge of the issues related to the health of vulnerable populations, and draw inspiration for making significant improvements to the health care and social systems in the United States and other nations. For current practitioners, program administrators, and policymakers, we hope the book provides a practical guide to addressing the plight of vulnerable populations. For academics, social scientists, and health care researchers, we hope the book and the conceptual framework we propose will assist and guide their research on vulnerable populations and that the up-to-date literature review provides a comprehensive and substantive foundation on which to build future work.

Organization of This Book

The book is organized into six chapters (see Figure P.1). The first chapter discusses the definition and measures of a general conceptual framework used to study vulnerable populations. Chapter Two examines the determinants of vulnerability using a broad conceptual framework that includes both social and individual determinants, and portrays the mechanisms whereby vulnerability affects access,

FIGURE P.1. ORGANIZATION OF THIS BOOK

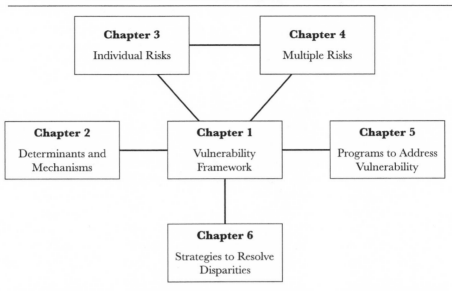

quality, and health status. In Chapters Three and Four, we summarize the literature and provide empirical evidence of disparities in health care access, quality, and outcome for vulnerable populations, with particular emphasis on socioeconomic status, health insurance, and racial/ethnic disparities. Chapter Three focuses on influences of individual risk factors and Chapter Four on influences of multiple risk factors. Chapter Five reviews programs currently in place for vulnerable populations, discusses the mechanisms of vulnerability addressed by these programs, and systematically critiques their potential to improve access, quality, and health of vulnerable populations. In Chapter Six, we review strategies and propose a course of action to address the needs of vulnerable populations and reduce or eliminate disparities. The course of action reflects the framework of determinants of vulnerability and takes into account the barriers and feasibility in its implementation.

Throughout the book, we present front-line experiences from health care practitioners who have had interesting and illustrative experiences in serving vulnerable populations. These experiences provide a practical sense of the theories and ideas we present. Commonly encountered terminology is compiled in a

Glossary at the end of the book. We also provide discussion questions and assignments at the end of each chapter. There is a designated Web site for the book with PowerPoint slides, exam and essay questions, and a discussion board for feedback. We hope that our integrated approach to writing about vulnerable populations will make this book particularly useful to students.

Acknowledgments

We gratefully acknowledge the contributions of Jane Marks, Lynda Burton, Jane Lyon, Liz Mercer, Lorraine Lemus, Lila Guirguis, Kynna Wright, Lily Quiette, and Phinney Ahn to the Front-Line Experiences sections of this book. We also acknowledge the extensive assistance of the following research and administrative assistants at Johns Hopkins University for helping put this book together: Lisa Green, Margaret Connor, Samantha Gottlieb, Normalie Barton, and Tanisha Carino. We acknowledge as well the valuable contributions by the following reviewers: Aram Dobalian, Charl du Plessis, Gail D. Hughes, and Bridget K. Gorman.

We greatly appreciate the assistance of numerous friends and readers in assembling the Glossary: Yerado Abrahamian, Phinney Ahn, Aloka Kloppenburg, Linda Lange, Alexi Saldamando, Harvinder Sareen, and Matthew Zerden.

Feedback and Suggestions

We welcome comments and suggestions from our readers, including instructors and students in particular. We will carefully study suggestions with an eye to incorporating them into a future edition of the book. Communications can be directed to both of the authors:

Leiyu Shi, Department of Health Policy and Management, School of Public Health, Johns Hopkins University, 624 North Broadway, Room 409, Baltimore, MD 21205–1996; lshi@jhsph.edu.

Gregory D. Stevens, Center for Healthier Children, Families, and Communities. University of California, Los Angeles, Department of Pediatrics, 1100 Glendon Ave, Suite 850, Los Angeles, CA 90024; gregory@ucla.edu.

August, 2004   Leiyu Shi
                                                                           Gregory D. Stevens

ABOUT THE AUTHORS

Leiyu Shi is an associate professor in the Department of Health Policy and Management at the Johns Hopkins University Bloomberg School of Public Health and codirector of Johns Hopkins Primary Care Policy Center for the Underserved Populations. He received both a master's in business administration and doctorate of public health from the University of California, Berkeley. His research focuses on primary care, health disparities, and vulnerable populations. He has conducted extensive studies on the association between primary care and health outcomes, particularly on the role of primary care in mediating the adverse impact of income inequality on health outcomes. He is well known for his extensive research on the nation's vulnerable populations, in particular community health centers that serve vulnerable populations, including their sustainability; provider recruitment and retention experiences; financial performance; experience under managed care; quality of primary care; and disparities in care and health. He has published numerous textbooks and over a hundred peer-reviewed journal articles.

Gregory D. Stevens is a senior researcher with the UCLA Center for Healthier Children, Families, and Communities. He completed both a master's degree and doctorate in health policy at the Johns Hopkins University Bloomberg School of Public Health. He has focused his research and consultation efforts on health insurance programs and policy for children and families, primary health care quality for vulnerable children, racial/ethnic and socioeconomic disparities in health care, and patient-provider relationship issues. Stevens has contributed to the development, design, and analysis of several statewide and local community-based studies of quality and satisfaction for both adults and children. He is well versed in national health policy issues for children and in conducting research on health care relating to pediatric primary care systems.

VULNERABLE POPULATIONS IN THE UNITED STATES

CHAPTER ONE

A GENERAL FRAMEWORK TO STUDY VULNERABLE POPULATIONS

Despite extensive research on vulnerable populations and national efforts at reducing disparity in **health** and health care between them and the general public, there is no explicit consensus as to what constitutes vulnerability. *Webster's* dictionary defines *vulnerable* as "capable of being physically wounded" or "open to attack or damage." In a broad medical sense, **vulnerability** denotes susceptibility to poor health. Based on the epidemiological notion of risk—the probability that a person will become ill over a given period of time—everyone is potentially vulnerable over an extended period of time. Yet researchers and policymakers obviously do not have everyone in mind when they address vulnerable populations.

Rather, research and policy regarding vulnerable populations typically focus on distinct subpopulations (Aday, 2001): racial or ethnic **minorities,** the uninsured, children, the elderly, the poor, the chronically ill, the physically disabled or handicapped, the terminally ill, the mentally ill, persons with acquired immunodeficiency syndrome (AIDS), alcohol or substance abusers, homeless individuals, residents of rural areas, individuals who do not speak English or have other difficulties in communicating, and those who are poorly educated or illiterate, to name just a few. For example, in *Healthy People 2000* (U.S. Department of Health and Human Services, 1991), a U.S. national prevention strategy for significantly improving the health of the American people, vulnerable populations were identified as those with low income, disabilities, and minority groups. The

U.S. federal government recently launched an initiative to eliminate racial and ethnic disparities in health, specifically, infant mortality, cancer screening and management, cardiovascular disease, diabetes, AIDS, and immunizations (U.S. Department of Health and Human Services, 1999, 2000). Various terms have been used to describe these subpopulations, including *disadvantaged,* **under-privileged,** *medically underserved, poverty stricken, distressed populations,* and the *American underclasses.*

A closer examination reveals that these subpopulations share many common traits and typically experience a convergence or interaction of multiple vulnerable characteristics or risk factors. For example, racial/ethnic minorities are disproportionately distributed at the lower end of the socioeconomic ladder, are more likely to be uninsured, and have poorer health than white Americans (AMA Council on Ethical and Judicial Affairs, 1990; AMA Council on Scientific Affairs, 1991; Kramarow, Lentzner, et al., 1999). The subpopulations identified as vulnerable often lack the necessary physical capabilities, educational backgrounds, communicative skills, or financial resources to safeguard their own health adequately. They have also been shown to bear increased burdens of illness, have poorer access to health care, and receive health care of poorer quality. These commonalities call for a renewed conceptualization of vulnerability.

This chapter introduces a new **framework** to study vulnerable populations that reflects this convergence of vulnerable characteristics. The framework will serve as the core organizing principle for the literature reviews, studies and analyses, discussions of health and social programs, and suggested solutions that are discussed in this book.

Why Study Vulnerable Populations

This book is about vulnerable populations, and we have chosen to highlight those with minority racial/ethnic backgrounds, with low socioeconomic status (SES), and those lacking health insurance coverage. There are many reasons to focus national attention on the needs of vulnerable populations and reducing health and health care disparities experienced by these groups. We offer five reasons for enhancing the national focus on vulnerable populations: (1) vulnerable populations have greater health needs; (2) the prevalence of vulnerable groups in the population is increasing; (3) vulnerability is primarily a social issue that is created through social forces and resolved through social (as opposed to individual) means; (4) vulnerability is intertwined with the nation's health and resources; and (5) there is a growing emphasis on **equity** in health.

Vulnerable Populations Have Greater Health Needs

Vulnerable populations are at substantially greater risk of poor physical, mental, and social health and have much higher rates of morbidity and mortality. They experience much higher rates of asthma and higher rates of depression, and report more social exclusion than other groups. Despite these greater health needs, they also typically face greater barriers to accessing timely and needed care and, even when receiving care, have worse **health outcomes** than others. The magnitude and multifaceted nature of their health needs places a greater demand on medical care, public health, and related social and human services delivery sectors.

There Is an Increasing Prevalence of Vulnerability in the United States

The United States has become increasingly multiethnic. By the middle of the twenty-first century, the minority population is estimated to nearly equal the size of the non-Hispanic white population (DeVita and Pollard, 1996). The national poverty rate too has only increased since reaching its low in the early 1970s, and the number of individuals in poverty continues to increase steadily, with a particularly sharp spike in the past four years, from about 31 million individuals in the United States to nearly 35 million since 1999 (Proctor and Dalaker, 2003). Demographic and immigration shifts and socioeconomic trends in both the United States and other nations will likely result in vulnerable groups' becoming the majority population within this century. The health needs of these vulnerable populations will place an incredible strain on the capacity and resources of medical and social services to ensure a national population with a high level of health and well-being.

Vulnerability Is Influenced and Remedied by Social Forces

Vulnerability to poor health does not represent a specific personal deficiency but, rather, as described in Chapter Two, the interaction effects of many individual, community, and social or political factors, some of which individuals have little or no control over. This aspect of how vulnerability is created implies that society as a whole has a responsibility to assist these populations and actively promote the health of these individuals. Many programs are in place to address specific health disparities. The most effective approaches to mitigating the consequences of vulnerability and reducing levels of vulnerability in the first place must include broader health and social policies that address these social forces and ecological contexts.

Vulnerability Is Fundamentally Linked with National Resources

The well-being of vulnerable populations is closely intertwined with the overall health and resources of the nation. The United States continues to rank poorly compared to other nations on key national health indicators, including infant mortality, mortality rates, and life expectancy. Poor health not only has an impact on individual families and lives but detracts from national productivity and economic prosperity. The poor health that vulnerable populations experience further subsumes national resources for social progress, when health and social conditions (such as violence), which could have effectively been prevented, are left untreated, are exacerbated by neglect, and end up costing society billions more dollars in treatment than in prevention. Fundamental improvement of the nation's health and resources cannot be accomplished without very specific efforts aimed at improving the health of vulnerable populations.

Vulnerability and Equity Cannot Coexist

Perhaps the most important reason for focusing on vulnerable populations is the guiding principle of equity. *Equity* is defined by *Webster's* dictionary as "the quality of being fair." There are various ways in which fairness is conceptualized. For example, in terms of medical care, policies that ensure equal access to health services, such as universal health insurance or health care programs such as the promotion of an AIDS surveillance system, may benefit the public equally. Fairness, however, could also be defined in a relative way, such that the degree of access to health services is determined proportionately by the health needs of an individual or a population. Therefore, by this definition, an equitable health care system is one in which the health need of an individual is the sole determinant of his or her health care utilization. By either definition, if equity is a guiding principle for the United States, then vulnerability cannot be allowed to persist.

Documents from the founding of the nation, in fact, identify equality as a governing principle. The Declaration of Independence states, "We hold these truths to be self-evident, that all men are created *equal,* that they are endowed by their Creator with certain unalienable Rights, that among these are Life, Liberty and the pursuit of Happiness." These principles of equity, while pursued and interpreted in ways that are sometimes inconceivable today (for example, slavery was looked at as an exception, declaring those who were slaves to be counted in the U.S. census for purposes of representation as "three-fifths of a human"), have at critical points in history been markedly important for vulnerable groups.

The abolition of slavery in 1865 marked what was perhaps the first national legislation reflecting the guiding principles of equality and directly, changing the immediate status of this vulnerable population. Perhaps the second landmark legislation for vulnerable groups was the winning of women's suffrage in 1920, giving women more, but still not fully equal opportunity for, political control in guiding the nation. While earlier public policy focused on equality in freedoms and political power, progressive policies in the 1960s enhanced racial, gender, and SES equality in social and educational opportunities for U.S. citizens.

The Civil Rights Act of 1964, for example, made **discrimination** based on race, color, religion, and national origin illegal and has been updated several times to include other specific discriminatory factors, such as gender and sexual preference. The Johnson administration's War on Poverty during the 1960s further shifted public attention and social policies toward issues of social, educational, and health **inequalities.**

The past two decades have evolved to see a national and political interest in equality of results attained rather than just opportunity (Moss, 2000). In the social and medical realms, the *Healthy People 2010* report explicitly identifies health and health care equity as a public health objective and has called for a reduction in **health disparities** in the United States. The Institute of Medicine (1988), in its landmark report, *The Future of Public Health,* asserted that "the ultimate responsibility for assuring equitable access to health care for all, through a combination of public and private sector action, rests with the federal government" (IOM, 1988, p. 13). Finally, a presidential initiative has also called for eliminating health disparities by the year 2010 (U.S. Department of Health and Human Services, 1999).

Front-Line Experience: Dependence Is the Tip of the Iceberg for Vulnerable Seniors

Jane Marks, associate director of the Johns Hopkins Geriatrics Education Center, and Lynda Burton, associate professor of the Johns Hopkins Bloomberg School of Public Health, remind us that many of the difficulties created by the vulnerabilities discussed in this book are compounded for older patients due to a lack of mobility and transportation, unavailable family support, and a complex array of health conditions that require vigilant monitoring.

When caring for older patients, health care professionals are aware that a relatively small change in a person's health can trigger a major cascade of changes in his or her life. Nurses in our geriatrics practice, located in a primarily low-income, urban community, are trained to closely monitor these changes in health and work closely with patients and family members, if present, to address their health needs early.

In our geriatrics practice, we have recognized the need to make house calls as a strategy to serve our vulnerable older patients better. House calls are convenient for homebound patients who have limited physical mobility or transportation problems. They also help us to assess living arrangements and how they may support or hinder our patients' continued independence.

Physicians and nurses make home visits to our patients frequently. Nurses visit the homes first to assess the situation, involve the physician when necessary, and then follow up with regular phone calls. Even with this frequent follow-up, nurses still cannot reduce all of the risks that the most vulnerable patients encounter. The effect of even minor events on health and independence is enormous and is often compounded by mobility problems, lack of family support, and co-occurring health conditions, including such problems as depression. One patient served by our practice provides an example of the compounding influence of these overlapping health and social risk factors.

Helen (this is a pseudonym) is eighty-seven years old and was widowed fifteen years ago, but she has been able to care for herself while living alone in her small apartment. She has no family living in the area but does have friends in the neighborhood. Over the past five years, her congestive heart failure, hypertension, and arthritis have gradually worsened, making it difficult for her to get around. She also has macular degeneration and with her worsening eyesight was forced to give up driving, an important avenue of independence for her. She now depends entirely on her friends to help her with groceries, shopping, other errands, and, most important for her, getting to church.

Helen developed a rather serious cough, and during one of our phone conversations we recommended that she get a chest x-ray at the local hospital. She asked a friend to drive her, and while she was getting into the car, her feet got tangled and she had a minor fall. Her very worried friend helped her up and into her home, and then called us for help. Our nurses went out to the home to examine her that day and found that she did not seem to have a fracture. She was bruised but not in discomfort, and she could walk without pain. When the nurses phoned her each of the next two days, she said she was still doing fine.

Later that week, however, Helen developed some stiffness and began to have difficulty walking. Nurses made another home visit after receiving a phone call and found her near tears because she had become so stiff that she had extreme difficulty getting up from her bed. Her friends were not around enough to be able to help her move to the bathroom in time, so she chose to stop taking her diuretic (used to treat congestive heart failure) to prevent incontinence. Because she had stopped the medication, her congestive heart failure had worsened, and a hospital stay was required to get this back in control. Her evaluation showed only soft tissue injury in addition to the congestive heart failure. But her immobility had the cumulative effect of deconditioning her muscles, making it more and more difficult for her to get around.

Helen did not have sufficient income to hire a caregiver to assist her full time during her recovery once she returned home. She also had difficulty affording and maintaining her ongoing and new medications. Without physical or financial assistance, we determined that she could not independently maintain herself at home. She was admitted to a rehabilitation center, where professionals worked to help restore her mobility. Even with this rehabilitation, the minor fall that she had and the cascade of events that followed prevented her from returning to her home and living an independent life.

Since cases like Helen's are not uncommon, comprehensive assistance programs have been developed to intervene in the cascade of health deterioration. The Program for All Inclusive Care of the Elderly (PACE), for example, is available to certain older patients who are eligible for nursing home care but instead provides nursing assistance at home or in adult day care centers. PACE services would have greatly helped Helen during her recovery by providing her with a nursing assistant at home for a few days, keeping her moving to prevent immobilization, and maintaining her prescribed medications. However, PACE eligibility required that she be a Medicaid recipient and that she meet criteria for nursing home admission. Her income was above the Medicaid eligibility level, and prior to her fall, she would not have met criteria for nursing home admission. Given that the population of older patients is increasing, programs like PACE or others that afford home visits by health professionals can have a dramatic effect on reducing the burden of illness and, ultimately, the costs of care for vulnerable populations.

Models for Studying Vulnerability

Over the years, studies of vulnerable populations have used many different paradigms or models to examine why vulnerable groups experience poorer access to health care and poorer health status. Most of these models have focused on single explanations but increasingly have begun to acknowledge the multifaceted nature of vulnerability. Many have examined individual-level explanations for why vulnerability has negative influences on health. They highlight characteristics of individuals, their health-related behaviors, and their personal socioeconomic circumstances and health care access. Other models have suggested a broader community-level conceptualization of vulnerability, whereby individuals have poorer health due to community or social forces. Here, we summarize the major relevant models that have helped define and shape our understanding of vulnerable populations.

Individual Determinants Model

Perhaps the most foundational, and most common, model for understanding vulnerability is one that identifies specific population groups (based on individual characteristics) as inherently more vulnerable than others. The model focuses on characteristics such as age, gender, race and ethnicity, education, income, and life changes (Rogers, 1997). Rogers considered three stages of life as inherently vulnerable: childhood, adolescence, and old age. Children are more vulnerable because they depend on others for care, while adolescents engage in risk-taking behaviors such as unprotected sexual intercourse and the use of drugs and alcohol. The elderly are more at risk because of their decreased physical ability, and their risk can be compounded with the decline in financial resources and social support that may occur at this stage of life.

Rogers also argued that both women and men could be considered vulnerable populations depending on the purpose of the classification. Women could be considered vulnerable because of their poorer self-reported health status, while men could be considered vulnerable because of their higher mortality rates and overall shorter life expectancy. For women, vulnerability is primarily derived from the stresses of childbearing, child rearing, and caregiving, reflected in a greater incidence of depression and injury from domestic conflict. Women still often have fewer financial resources at their disposal because they earn less income on average than males do.

Minority race/ethnicity is considered vulnerable in this model because these groups have higher rates of poverty, morbidity (for example, both diabetes and hypertension are more problematic for African Americans than whites), and mortality. Educational attainment is considered a marker for vulnerability because those with higher education tend to have better health, which may be due (as we discuss in Chapter Two) to better access to medical care, a greater tendency to practice prevention, or more subtle aspects of social class. One of the most interesting components of the model is that major life changes, such as a diagnosis with a major illness, the death of loved ones, the end of a close relationship, and other major transitions (such as unemployment) impair health and functioning, making these transitions vulnerable periods.

Individual Social Resources Model

Another essential model of vulnerability has been proposed by Aday (1994). It suggests that individual risks stem from lacking certain intrinsic social and personal resources that are essential to a person's well-being. According to this model, social status, social capital (or social support), and human capital (the productive potential of an individual) influence vulnerability.

Social status is associated with biological characteristics such as age, gender, and race/ethnicity, that can bring with them socially defined opportunities and rewards, such as prestige and power. African Americans, by this definition, could be viewed as a vulnerable group; they experience more barriers to obtaining material (such as income) and nonmaterial resources (such as political power) that contribute to health and social advancement. Those with a combination of characteristics that are associated with poorer social status (for example, African American and elderly) would be considered to have a higher level of vulnerability.

Social capital is defined as the quantity and quality of interpersonal ties a person has. These social ties reflect social resources that can be relied on and can be instrumental in supporting psychological, physical, and social well-being. Aday provides an example of a single mother whose social capital (or social ties with friends) may be particularly helpful in offering child care so that she can direct energies toward personal advancements such as school or work. Examples of those with less social capital are those who live alone, female-headed families, the unmarried, those who do not belong to any organizations or groups, or those who have a limited network of family or friends. Having strong ties serves as a buffer against vulnerability.

Human capital refers to the skills and capabilities of an individual that enables the person to advance and make productive contributions within society. Without human capital, individuals may experience barriers to social advancement such as exclusion from the labor force, employment in service sector jobs, or not being admitted to higher education. Higher social advancement is associated with better health (as discussed in Chapter Two); without these opportunities these populations may be considered vulnerable. Since this is a **modifiable risk,** high-quality public education or vocational training are potential ways to improve human capital.

Individual Health Behaviors Model

Many theories have been suggested for why the individual characteristics that Rogers and Aday identified as vulnerable are associated with poor health status. The next model we discuss explains this relationship through differences in individual health-promoting and **health-risk behaviors.** It is generally argued that vulnerable populations engage in fewer health-promoting activities, such as regular physical activity, healthful eating, and wearing seat belts, and in more risky activities, such as smoking, excessive alcohol consumption, and substance abuse (Power and Matthews, 1997; Lantz, House, et al., 1998; Power, Matthews, et al., 1998). These behaviors have clear and direct influences on specific health conditions (for example, smoking and lung cancer, physical activity and obesity, and alcohol consumption and car accidents) and may contribute to disparities in health among vulnerable groups (Lantz, House, et al., 1998).

Proponents of the health behavior model suggest that vulnerable populations are more likely to engage in fewer health-promoting and more health-risk behaviors due to psychosocial factors that create stress for individuals and lead to unhealthy behaviors. These factors include poorer social relationships and **social support;** reduced senses of life control and personal self-esteem; and racism, classism, or other stressors related to having less social power and resources (Lantz, House, et al., 1998). These psychosocial stressors then create mental and physical barriers to the adoption of health-promoting behaviors (depressed individuals are less likely to exercise, for example) and lead individuals to adopt risky health behaviors as coping mechanisms, such as drinking alcohol and smoking tobacco to reduce stress. Chronic mental stress can also have direct physiological effects and reduce the likelihood that a person will be motivated to obtain medical care.

Several key publications have been released supporting this health behavior model. The influence of health-promoting and health-risk behaviors on health status and mortality was first recognized among the major industrialized countries by the minister of health of Canada (Lalonde, 1974). Written by Marc Lalonde, the report suggested that lifestyle factors, or rather, "habits of indolence, the abuse of alcohol, tobacco and drugs, and eating patterns that put pleasing of the senses above the needs of the human body" (p. 5), are major contributors to health. In the United States, the first installment of the *Healthy People* reports in 1979 (U.S. Department of Health and Human Services, 1979) and a 1982 Institute of Medicine report titled *Health and Behavior* (Hamburg, Elliott, et al., 1982) summarized for U.S. audiences the evidence of the association between certain behaviors and illness. Nevertheless, the literature cautions that health behaviors explain only a modest portion of health disparities.

Individual Socioeconomic Status Model

Another explanation for why individual vulnerability characteristics are associated with poor health status is the influence of individual **socioeconomic status** (SES). In general, SES is defined by income, education, and occupation, but the same concept is often referred to as social class in other countries. In the United Kingdom, where *social class* is a common term, there is a standard measure of SES (the Registrar General's measure of occupation) using an individual's father's occupation to categorize one's social class (Hart, Smith, et al., 1998; Power and Matthews, 1997). Assessed in this way, social class is a less mutable individual characteristic, because no matter how much occupational promotion or financial wealth a person achieves, his or her social class remains entirely determined by the previous generation. Despite differences in measurement, SES remains perhaps the most commonly encountered explanation for any linkage between vulnerable populations and poor health care access and health status.

There is extensive evidence of the relationship between poor health and individual SES. Studies have demonstrated a clear inverse relationship between levels of income, education, and mortality (Lantz, House, et al., 1998). The most prominent evidence comes from the Whitehall studies of British civil servants in London that demonstrated a nearly linear relationship between **social class** (defined by occupation) and mortality from most major causes of death. Mortality was the lowest among administrators and higher for each successively lower social class, resulting in three-fold differences in mortality for the highest and lowest social classes. Interestingly, behavioral risk factors for mortality, such as smoking prevalence, in these social class groups explained fewer than half of the differences in mortality, suggesting some clear limits to the ability of the model in explaining the influences of vulnerability (Pincus, Esther, et al., 1998).

In addition to the health behavior model, two major mechanisms have been proposed for the relationship between individual SES and poor health. First, low-SES individuals have fewer financial resources to maintain and promote personal health adequately. For example, low-income groups experience greater difficulty paying for basic health and social needs, including nutritious food, safe and adequate housing, reliable transportation, and child care services, that have been shown to promote health and child development. Second, low-SES groups also have less financial access to health care services. Although health insurance programs exist for poor individuals, there are still many financial barriers, particularly for the near-poor (those living slightly above the federal poverty line), to accessing needed health services. The role of SES, in short, influences not only the ability to protect and promote health but also the ability to receive treatment when health problems occur.

Community Social Resources Model

The next set of models advances the concept of vulnerability beyond just individual risk factors and explores more of the community-level determinants of vulnerability. These models are particularly important because they emphasize that vulnerability is not simply a matter of individual bad luck or lack of personal will or resilience. Rather, they propose that community or social factors contribute to vulnerability and also highlight the responsibility that society has in addressing the consequences of vulnerability for health.

The first of these models, proposed by Flaskerud and Winslow (1998), suggests that community resources, defined broadly, strongly influence the health of a community and therefore contribute to the vulnerability of populations within the community. Although these social resources are similar to those proposed by Aday, this model is distinct in examining both community-level and individual-level social resources. Vulnerability is therefore defined at the population level as social groups that experience limited resources and consequently have a higher risk for morbidity and premature mortality.

Flaskerud and Winslow use a very broad definition of resource availability, taking into account both socioeconomic and environmental circumstances. By socioeconomic resources, the authors refer to social status, social capital, and human capital factors, but measured at the community level—for example, unemployment and poverty levels, the availability of high-quality schools, and community organizations such as churches that create social connectedness. In particular, poverty levels have been the most persistent predictors of morbidity and mortality in the United States (Wright, Andres, et al., 1996). Social status is an important socioeconomic resource to consider in that the lack of power associated with lower social status leaves those populations out of the decision making at the community level in the distribution of resources.

The authors also discuss environmental circumstances that would create vulnerability for poor health, including poor access to health care and poor quality of care. Violence and crime are considered environmental circumstances that would influence health, but the authors raise this issue only in regard to hindering access to health care and social services. Violence and crime in a community are likely to have much more direct impacts on health, including through safety and feelings of insecurity that may influence mental health. The authors finally highlight that poor health status of a population (the defining characteristic of vulnerability) may itself contribute to the poor resources in a population (for example, chronic illness may create difficulties with employment and social connectedness), creating a cycle of vulnerability. The authors suggest, however, that this influence of morbidity alone on community resources seems to be relatively small.

Community Environmental Exposures Model

Other explanations for the influence of communities in creating vulnerability include the potential role of health-impairing environmental exposures. For example, it is hypothesized that lower-SES communities have higher levels of harmful environmental exposures, such as living in substandard housing with remnants of lead paint (which contributes to lead poisoning in children), or living in inner-city or other crowded living areas that have much greater exposure to air pollution. Such living situations (for example, unventilated shelters) also promulgate the transmission of tuberculosis and increase the likelihood of exposure to violent crime. Workplace safety also varies by community, depending on the primary industry in the area. Rural areas, for example, primarily revolve around agriculture and meat-packing, which have high rates of manual labor injury.

One study provides a particularly cogent picture of the influences of environmental risk exposures on individual health over time. The study was designed to collect data longitudinally on a cohort of people from birth to thirty-three years of age (Power and Matthews, 1997). Accumulation of environmental risk factors during these years was measured by childhood respiratory illness and atmospheric pollution levels. Individual risk factors such as SES and smoking status were also taken into account, and both environmental and individual risk factors were clearly related to adult respiratory morbidity. The study demonstrated a strong occupational gradient for the prevalence of these respiratory symptoms and several other measures, including health status, psychological distress, and job strain.

Community Medically Underserved Model

Community resources, as the community-focused models suggest, also include the availability of medical care. The lack of available medical care services in a community (referred to as medical underservice) has been commonly proposed as an explanatory factor for why certain populations have poorer health status. While it is generally recognized that medical care contributes only a small portion to the overall health status of a population, this model suggests that rural populations, for example, have poor health status, or at least remain in poorer health once they become ill, because few health care providers are available in these areas.

One guideline for examining medical underservice has been proposed by Wright, Andres, et al. (1996). Four components are used to define why certain populations might be medically underserved. The first stems from the health care provider perspective and refers to the limited physical availability of health care resources. For example, there are not enough health care workers, including doctors and nurses, to meet the demand for care. Second, there may be financial barriers to obtaining health services, such as patients who lack insurance or are underinsured, meaning that their insurance does not fully cover their costs. Third, there may be nonfinancial barriers such as the lack of transportation, language difficulties, or insufficient provider cultural sensitivity that leads to medical underservice in a community.

Wright, Andres, et al. (1996) discuss some of the current inadequacies in how **medically underserved areas** (MUAs) are defined. The current definition of an MUA incorporates some specific criteria based on the physician-to-population ratio, infant mortality rates, poverty rates, and proportion of the population that is elderly. The four criteria constitute MUAs, which then receive government funding and are highlighted in encouraging providers to serve in these areas.

Wright, Andres, et al. (1996) argue that these current definitions allow some populations who are medically underserved to be missed. Individuals may live in areas with high provider-to-patient ratios, but this does not mean these providers are willing to accept low-income patients or those covered by Medicaid, which reimburses physicians at rates much lower than private insurance. In addition, women and children may be considered vulnerable populations but are not accounted for by the current criteria, and infant mortality rates are a relatively rare outcome and could be augmented by using low-birth-weight rates (which can cause substantial health and developmental problems for children and is much more common than infant mortality). Such changes to the criteria for MUAs may provide a more realistic picture of medical underservice and may lead to greater action to address the health needs of vulnerable populations.

Individual and Community Interaction Model

Aday (1993) has developed perhaps the most comprehensive vulnerability model to date that combines many previous models and incorporates both the individual- and community-level risk factors that determine vulnerability for poor physical, psychological, and social health (see Figure 1.1). Individual-level resources include social status, social capital, human capital, and health needs. Community-level resources include community cohesion (or ties between people) neighborhood characteristics (such as unemployment rates, availability of parks and recreation opportunities, and community violence), and community health needs. Based on these individual and community risk factors, Aday identifies nine specific subpopulations as those who are the most vulnerable: the physically vulnerable (high-risk mothers and infants, chronically ill and disabled, and persons living with HIV/AIDS), the psychologically vulnerable (mentally ill and disabled, alcohol or substance abusers, and the suicide or homicide prone), and the socially vulnerable (abusing families, the homeless, and immigrants and refugees). These specific groups are considered vulnerable and are focal points for intervention.

In considering interventions, Aday suggests that vulnerability is presumably influenced by ethical norms and values at both the individual level (for example, individual rights, independence, and autonomy) and the community level (for example, belief in the common good, a sense of reciprocity, and interdependence). Vulnerability is also influenced by both social and health policies (for example, welfare assistance, community regulations, public health programs, and health insurance coverage). Thus, interventions should take into account these factors when trying to prevent vulnerability or modify the consequences of vulnerability.

The Vulnerability Model: A New Conceptual Framework

Each of the models discussed reflects an evolution in defining, researching, and developing approaches to reducing or eliminating the health effects of vulnerability. Some of the more progressive models have recognized the overlap between

FIGURE 1.1. ADAY'S FRAMEWORK FOR STUDYING VULNERABLE POPULATIONS

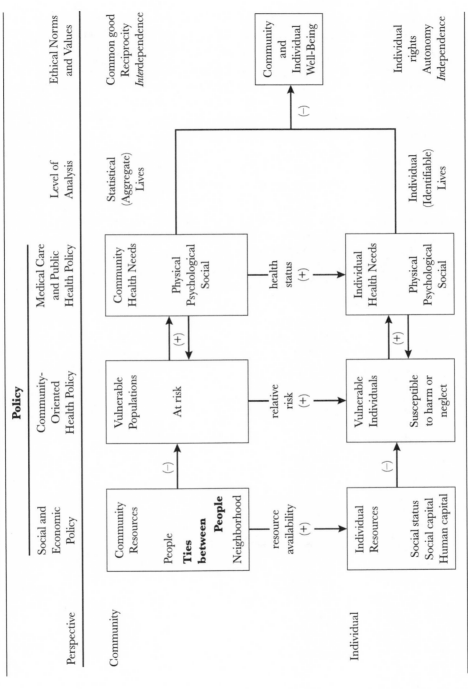

Note: A plus sign indicates a direct relationship (the likelihood of outcomes increases as the predictor increases). A minus sign indicates an inverse relationship (the likelihood of outcomes decreases as the predictor increases).

Source: Aday (2001, p. 3).

individual and community-level determinants of vulnerability, and others include the availability of medical care services as a predictor of vulnerability. The next evolutionary step, which we propose, requires a model that synthesizes previous work and recognizes the convergence of individual, social, community, and access-to-care risks that lead to vulnerability. We now turn to a discussion of this new model that we propose for both studying and assisting vulnerable populations (Figure 1.2).

In this book, vulnerability denotes susceptibility to poor health or illness. Poor health can be manifested physically, mentally, developmentally (as with language delays in children), or socially (as with poor job performance). Since poor health along one dimension can be compounded by poor health along others, the health needs are considerably greater for those with multiple health problems than for those with single health problems.

Vulnerability for poor health is determined by a convergence of predisposing, enabling, and need characteristics at both the individual and ecological levels. In laying out the now-well-known access-to-care framework (Aday, 1993), Aday and Andersen (1981) have defined predisposing characteristics as those that describe the propensity of individuals to use services, which include basic demo-

FIGURE 1.2. A GENERAL FRAMEWORK TO STUDY VULNERABLE POPULATIONS

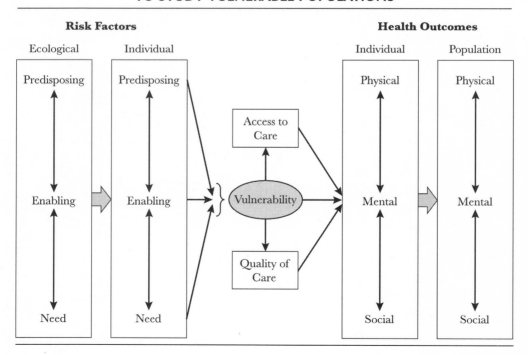

graphic characteristics, such as age, sex, and family size; social structure variables, such as race/ethnicity, education, employment, and occupation; and health beliefs, such as beliefs about health and the value of health care. Enabling characteristics are the means that individuals have available to them for the use of services, including resources specific to individuals and families (examples are income and insurance coverage) and attributes of the community or region in which an individual lives (for example, the availability of health care services). Need factors are specific illness or health needs that are the principal driving forces for receipt of health care.

These predisposing, enabling, and need characteristics converge and interact, and they work to influence health care access, health care quality, and health status. Translated into the terms of our vulnerability model, health needs directly imply vulnerability, predisposing characteristics indicate the propensity for vulnerability, and enabling characteristics reflect the resources available to overcome the consequences of vulnerability. Therefore, individuals are most vulnerable if they have a combination of health needs, predisposing risk factors, and enabling risk factors. For example, individuals who have asthma (a need factor), are Latino (a predisposing factor), and lack health insurance (an enabling factor) would be considered more vulnerable than individuals who have asthma alone.

In our model, we emphasize the importance of vulnerability determinants at community or ecological levels. This implies that vulnerability does not represent any personal deficiency of the populations defined as vulnerable, but rather that they experience the interaction of many risks over which individuals have little or no control (Aday, 1999). It also implies an important role for society in addressing the health and health care needs of vulnerable populations.

Distinctive Characteristics

The vulnerability model has a number of distinctive characteristics. First, it is a comprehensive model, including both individual and ecological (contextual) attributes of risk. A person's vulnerability status is determined not only by his or her individual characteristics, but also by the environment in which this person lives and the interactions among individual and environmental characteristics. Inclusion of ecological factors suggests that many attributes of vulnerability are beyond individuals' control, and their reduction requires government and societal efforts. Compared to models that focus on individual characteristics, a multilevel model (including both individual and ecological elements) not only more accurately reflects realities but also avoids the tendency of "blaming the victims."

Second, this is a general model focusing on attributes of vulnerability for the total population rather than a specific model focusing on vulnerable traits of subpopulations. Although we recognize individual differences in exposure to risks, we also think there are common, cross-cutting traits affecting all vulnerable populations. Due to current public funding options, a categorical approach to finding ways of assisting vulnerable subpopulation groups will likely continue. We believe such an approach is piecemeal, inefficient, duplicative, and uncoordinated. It tackles symptoms rather than causes and is unlikely to improve the situations of vulnerable populations fundamentally. Our general model calls for a global and integrated approach that focuses on the most critical and common vulnerability traits in the community. Such a practice is more efficient and likely to bring more tangible improvement in the situations that vulnerable populations in the community face.

Third, a major distinction of our model is the emphasis on the convergence of risk factors. The effects of experiencing multiple vulnerable traits may lead to cumulative vulnerability that is additive or even multiplicative. Individuals showing multiple vulnerability traits may have especially poor health status. Examining vulnerability as a multidimensional construct can also demonstrate gradient relationships between vulnerability status and outcomes of interest and thus improve our understanding of the patterns and factors related to the outcomes of interest. The findings are likely to be more precise and can provide better guidance to policymakers. For example, if we are able to demonstrate a gradient relationship between vulnerability status and health care access, quality, and health outcomes, our understanding of the patterns and factors in being vulnerable in the United States is enhanced, and policymakers can thus use limited resources to target those groups that are most vulnerable.

Components of the Model

Based on the overview presented above, we provide a graphical representation of our model of vulnerability (see Figure 1.2) and describe components of this model. Vulnerability, which is at the center of the figure, is most closely affected by individuals' predisposing, enabling, and need attributes (in the second left column) and also influences these same risk factors at an ecological or community level. It is important to note that in our model, the predisposing, enabling, and need attributes are more than just risk factors for poor access; they also reflect risks for poor quality of health care and poor health status. These risk factors then combine, interact, and work together to create a level of vulnerability for each individual that is associated with negative health care access, quality of care, and health outcomes (right columns) at individual or population levels.

Individual Risk Factors. Individual predisposing attributes in our model, reflecting risk factors for poor access to care, quality of care, and health status, include demographic factors, belief systems, and social structural variables that are associated with social position, access to financial and nonfinancial resources, and health behaviors that influence both health and health care access (Exhibit 1.1). These factors are also often foci for discrimination; patients may be discriminated against, intentionally or even unintentionally, by health care providers due to race/ethnicity, gender, sexual preference, or other factors. Individuals generally have relatively little control over most predisposing attributes.

Individual enabling attributes include SES, financial and nonfinancial social resources, and factors such as health insurance coverage associated with the use

EXHIBIT 1.1. MEASURES OF PREDISPOSING, ENABLING, AND NEED ATTRIBUTES OF VULNERABILITY AT THE INDIVIDUAL LEVEL

Predisposing factors

- Demographic characteristics associated with variations in health status, for example, age or gender.
- Inherited or cultivated belief system associated with health behaviors, for example, attitude, conviction, culture, or health belief.
- Social structural variables associated with social position, status, and access to resources, such as race/ethnicity or gender.

Enabling factors

- Socioeconomic status associated with social position, status, access to resources, and variations in health status, such as income, education, employment status, and occupation.
- Individual assets (human capital) that contribute to one's ability to be economically self-sufficient, such as inheritance, wealth, or skills.
- Mediating factors associated with using health care services, such as health insurance, access to health care, or quality of health care. Health care is broadly defined as services rendered at the individual level conducive to individual health including preventive, medical (primary, secondary, tertiary), and human services.

Health need

- Self-perceived or professionally evaluated health status, such as self-perceived physical and mental health status, diagnoses for diseases, and illness.
- Quality-of-life indicators, such as activity of daily living performance, instrumental activity of daily living performance, social limitations, cognitive limitation, and limitation in work, housework, or school.
- Certain subpopulation groups known to be at higher health risks, such as physical health (high-risk mothers and infants, chronically ill and disabled individuals, persons with AIDS), mental health (mentally ill and disabled, alcohol or substance abusers, suicide or homicide prone), and social well-being (abusing families, homeless people, immigrants and refugees).

of health care services. Perhaps the most commonly cited enabling risk factors are being low income or lacking health insurance coverage. While low income has some direct influences on health status (described more fully in Chapter Two) that having health insurance does not, both risks create substantial barriers to obtaining needed health care.

Low educational level and language barriers are also commonly cited as important risk factors for poor health care access, quality, and health status. Education has a direct impact on health (for example, less educated individuals are more likely to smoke), but both low education and difficulty speaking English produce substantial barriers to appropriate health care, which include difficulty speaking with health care providers, communicating treatment preferences, reading health materials and prescription drug instructions, and following through on recommended treatments. Overall, enabling risk factors are generally more modifiable than predisposing factors; for example, educational opportunities can be expanded through programs such as affirmative action.

Individual need attributes include self-perceived or professionally evaluated health status and quality-of-life indicators. Certain subpopulations are defined by their health; these include infants born with low birth weight, chronically ill or disabled individuals, persons with HIV/AIDS, those who are mentally ill and disabled, alcohol or substance abusers, and those who have been abused (Aday, 1999, 2001) and have greater health care needs that contribute to vulnerability. For example, persons who are chronically ill or who have other functional disabilities, such as the frail elderly or children with disabilities, may have particular difficulty obtaining needed health services due to special challenges created by their physical illness or mental condition; examples are extensive reliance on caregivers for accessing health care or difficulty communicating health needs. Such individuals may be in need of highly specialized providers or even teams of providers, and access to these specialists is not always facilitated or well coordinated by insurance plans.

In our model, the bidirectional arrows linking predisposing, enabling, and need attributes at both the individual and ecological levels indicate that these risk factors influence one another. For example, racial/ethnic minorities (a predisposing attribute) are disproportionately represented in the low-SES groups (an enabling attribute). Having health insurance (an enabling attribute) is less available to low-income groups (an enabling attribute) and is essential for ensuring access to health care, particularly for subpopulations with chronic illnesses (a need attribute). Poorer health status (a need attribute) reduces the ability to maintain stable employment and earn income (an enabling attribute), and incomes are generally reduced for older individuals (a predisposing attribute) who are retired and may receive income only through the **Social Security** system.

Predisposing, enabling, and need attributes in our model each independently influence vulnerability status, as reflected by the three separate arrows. In addition, these three attributes converge and interact and jointly determine one's vulnerability status, as indicated by the larger bracket encompassing the three attributes. Indeed, the major difference between this framework and other models is the emphasis on the convergence of risks. Operationalizing vulnerability as a combination of disparate attributes is preferred to studying individual factors separately, since a population group that is considered more vulnerable rarely experiences only one particular risk and is more likely to have multiple risks.

Ecological Risk Factors. Since individuals live in communities, they are clearly influenced by the environment around them. Our model indicates that individual attributes of risk are influenced by ecological attributes of risk (first left column in Figure 1.2) and that they combine to influence vulnerability. As with individual risks, there exist predisposing, enabling, and need risk factors at ecological levels (see Exhibit 1.2).

Ecological predisposing attributes include neighborhood demographic composition; the physical environment; political, legal, and economic systems; and cultural and social norms and beliefs. Geographical areas composed of larger populations of older individuals or inner-city areas with a larger number of teenage mothers create greater vulnerability since they require a higher intensity of medical care, financial, and social resources. For example, the low-birth-weight rate is higher among teenage mothers, and low-birth-weight babies require much more intensive care, monitoring, and social assistance than other infants, which draws resources from other medical or social services for the community. Similarly, areas that are characterized by dilapidated housing or substandard public low-cost apartments have substantial health risks, such as lead poisoning from lead-based paint, and they may offer inadequate safety protections; there may be nonfunctioning smoke detectors and dark and unmonitored halls, for example. Social and political systems that tolerate high levels of health disparities (such as the United States) are also considered predisposing risks.

Ecological enabling attributes include socioeconomic position and social class in relation to others, workplace environments, social resources, and health care delivery system factors. For example, rural communities tend to have fewer economic opportunities besides agriculture, and therefore tend to have higher rates of unemployment or employment in lower-wage sectors. Poor areas similarly tend to have fewer high-quality educational systems, since local taxes account for a substantial proportion of school system budgets and revenues generated through taxes are lower in low-income areas. These community SES barriers also contribute to medical underservice, in part determining where health care providers will work

EXHIBIT 1.2. MEASURES OF PREDISPOSING, ENABLING, AND NEED ATTRIBUTES OF VULNERABILITY AT THE ECOLOGICAL LEVEL

Predisposing factors

- Residence or geographical location, for example, MSA versus non-MSA, rural versus urban
- Neighborhood composition, for example, racial/ethnic integration or segregation
- Physical environment, for example, pollution, population density, climate, urban violence
- Political, legal, and economic system, for example, industrialization, market domination
- Cultural and social norms and beliefs, for example, religions, notion of justice, level of tolerance

Enabling factors

- Socioeconomic status and social class, for example, median household income, percentage of population with high school or college education, unemployment rate, quality of housing
- Disparities and inequalities, for example, social inequality, income inequality, wealth inequality
- Workplace environment, for example, occupational safety, health promotion practice, workplace stress, health benefits
- Social assets (social capital) and social cohesion, for example, characteristics of individuals' social network that provide emotional and instrumental support, such as family structure, friendship ties, neighborhood connections, and religious organizations, and attributes of the community or region in which individuals live
- Health care delivery system, for example, availability and accessibility of preventive, medical, public health, and human services care

Need factors

- Population health behaviors, for example, smoking, exercise, diet, alcohol consumption, drug abuse, seat belt use
- Population health status trend, for example, trends in mortality and morbidity rates for leading causes of death, life expectancy, infant mortality, low birth weight
- Population mental health and social well-being trend, for example, mental illness, suicide, quality of life
- Health disparities/inequalities, for example, race/ethnic disparities in health, SES disparities in health

(shortages are due to quality of living conditions and the lack of incentives for health care professionals to practice in these areas), and limiting health insurance coverage opportunities, since large companies that offer such coverage are generally not attracted to these areas.

Ecological need attributes include community health-risk factors such as pollution levels, health-promoting community behaviors such as health fairs and recreational opportunities, and trends in health status and health disparities. For example, rural areas and inner-city urban areas experience much higher population rates of asthma due to the presence of dust and pollution in the air, which aggravates the lungs of potential asthmatics and increases the severity of conditions among those with asthma. Communities plagued with crime and violence create unsafe living conditions for community members, increase the risk of personal injury from violence (more so for teenagers), and may sabotage community feelings of solidarity and degrade mental health.

Like individual attributes, ecological attributes also influence one another. For example, compared with other industrialized nations, the United States (a predisposing attribute) tolerates a higher level of disparities in income, education, and access to health care (all enabling attributes), despite the fact that these SES and health care access disparities are causally linked to poor population health (a need attribute). Another example is that inadequate employment opportunities (an enabling attribute) may contribute to population health behaviors such as alcohol abuse (a need attribute) that are tolerated by a community based on cultural norms (a predisposing attribute) despite their contributing to neighborhood insecurity and levels of violence (a need attribute). Relationships such as these are demonstrated in the model with the bidirectional arrows, and their independent and combined relationships with individual risk factors and, ultimately, vulnerability are visible.

The Consequences of Vulnerability. Vulnerability has direct influences on health care access, health care quality, and health status measured at the individual and population levels. The right side of our model in Figure 1.2 depicts aspects of health care access, quality, and health outcomes that vulnerability may impact (see Exhibit 1.3). Whereas the ultimate effect of vulnerability is related to declining health status, initial consequences may be observed in reduced access to health care and lower quality of care among those who are able to obtain access. Access can be measured by insurance coverage, having a usual source of care, and the use of preventive, acute, rehabilitative, and specialized care. Quality of care may be measured in many ways, including assessments of accessibility of providers or facilities, the quality of the interpersonal relationship with providers, the comprehensiveness of services, coordination of care among health providers, family-centered care and community centeredness of care, and satisfaction with care.

EXHIBIT 1.3. MEASURES OF HEALTH CARE ACCESS, QUALITY OF HEALTH CARE, AND HEALTH OUTCOMES

Access to Health Care

- Insurance coverage, for example, whether insured and type of insurance
- Usual source of care, for example, whether having primary care doctor as a usual source of care
- Preventive care, for example, regular health examination, up-to-date immunization, dental care, well-child visit
- Acute care, for example, number of primary care visits
- Specialist care, for example, those with special health needs receiving at least one subspecialty care per year, and number of specialist visits
- Emergency care, for example, number of emergency room visits
- Hospitalization, for example, number of hospitalizations

Quality of Health Care

The following can be measured by asking survey questions from the Johns Hopkins Primary Care Assessment Tool:

- First-contact and accessibility:

  When the office is open and you get sick, would someone from there see you that same day?

  When the office is closed on Saturday or Sunday and you get sick, would someone from there see you the same day?

  When the office is closed and you get sick during the night, would someone from there see or talk with you that night?

  When the office is closed, is there a phone number you can call when you get sick?

- Continuity

  When you go to the regular source of care, do you see the same doctor or nurse each time?

  If you have a question, can you call and talk to the doctor who knows you best?

  Do you think your doctor understands what you say or ask?

  Does your doctor know what problems are most important to you?

  Does your doctor know your complete medical history?

  Does your doctor know about all the medications you are taking?

  Does your doctor know you very well as a person?

  Would you change your doctor if it was easy to do?

  Would your doctor let you look at your medical record if you wanted to?

  When you go to your doctor, is your record always available?

  Does your doctor call or send you the results of your lab tests?

  If the doctor who knows you best is not available and you have to see someone else, would your doctor get the information about that visit?

  Would you recommend your doctor to a friend or relative?

  Would you recommend your doctor to someone who does not speak English well?

EXHIBIT 1.3. MEASURES OF HEALTH CARE ACCESS, QUALITY OF HEALTH CARE, AND HEALTH OUTCOMES *(continued)*

- Coordination

  Does your doctor have to get approval from someone else to refer to a specialist?

  Did your doctor know about these visits to the specialist or special service?

  Did your doctor discuss with you different places you could have gone to get help with that problem?

  Did someone at the doctor's office help you make the appointment for that visit?

  After going to a specialist or special service, did your doctor talk with you about what happened at the visit?

  Does your doctor know what the results of that visit were?

  Does your doctor seem interested in the quality of care you get from that specialist or special care?

- Comprehensiveness

  Can you get the following services from your regular source of care: (a) meeting with someone to talk about nutrition, (b) immunizations or "shots," (c) checking to see if your family is eligible for any social service programs or benefits such as WIC Services (supplemental milk and food program), (d) family planning or birth control, (e) substance or drug abuse counseling or treatment, (f) counseling for behavior or mental health problems, (g) tests for lead poisoning, (h) sewing up a cut that needs stitches, and (i) counseling and testing for HIV/AIDS?

  Have you got the following services from your regular source of care: (a) ways to keep you healthy, such as nutritional foods, or getting enough sleep? (b) ways to keep you safe? (c) home safety, like using smoke detectors and storing medicines safely? (d) ways to handle problems with your child's behavior? and (e) changes in growth and behavior that you can expect at certain ages?

- Family/community orientation

  Would anyone at the doctor's office ever make home visits?

  Does your doctor know about all of the important health problems of your neighborhood?

  How does your regular source of care get opinions and ideas from people that will help them provide better health care? Do they . . . (a) do surveys of their patients to find out their experiences with the doctor and the doctor's office? (b) do surveys in the community to find out about health problems? (c) ask family members to be on the Board of Directors or advisory committee?

Health Outcomes

Physical

- Symptoms. Measures of symptoms reflect acute and chronic problems involving one or more of the body's functional systems. Examples are a toothache, a sore throat with fever, and swollen ankles when you wake up.
- Mortality. Mortality-based measures, such as total death rate, condition-specific death rates, infant mortality, maternal mortality, life expectancy at birth, and

(continued)

EXHIBIT 1.3. MEASURES OF HEALTH CARE ACCESS, QUALITY OF HEALTH CARE, AND HEALTH OUTCOMES *(continued)*

remaining years of life at various ages are probably the most often used indirect indicators of health.

- Morbidity. The most traditional direct measures of morbidity are those that measure the incidence or prevalence of specific diseases. Examples are whether or how many times individuals are sick within a given time, the occurrence of certain diseases, and the conditions of illness.

- Disability. Disability related to illness and injury consists of event-type and person-type indicators. Examples of event-type indicators are restricted activity days, including bed days, work loss days, school loss days, and other "cutdown" days, used to measure the impact of both acute and chronic illness. Person-type indicators are usually used to reflect the long-term impact of chronic conditions, such as measures of limitation of mobility and limitation of functional activity. Examples of mobility limitation are confinement to bed, confinement to the house, and needing the help of another person or special aid in getting around either inside or outside the house. Activities of daily living (ADL) is often used to measure functional activity limitation of the elderly and the chronically ill. A set of measures somewhat related to ADL indicators are measures of functional capacity, including items such as the ability to walk a quarter mile, walk up or down a flight of stairs, stand or sit for long periods, use fingers to grasp or handle, and lift or carry a moderately heavy or heavy object. These are called instrumental activities of daily living (IADL), which require a finer level of motor coordination than is necessary for the relatively gross activities covered in ADL scales. IADL scales are used to measure less severe functional impairments and to distinguish between more subtle levels of functioning. The content of IADL scales stresses an individual's functioning within his or her particular environment. A person who is unable to

Health status and health outcome measures represent a critical end point for assessing the influences of vulnerability. The World Health Organization (WHO) has defined *health* as a "state of complete physical, mental, and social well-being and not merely the absence of disease or infirmity" (World Health Organization, 1948; Hanlon and Pickett, 1984). This definition recognizes that health is influenced by a combination of biological, social, individual, community, and economic factors. In addition to its intrinsic value, health is a means for personal and collective advancement. It is not only an indicator of an individual's well-being, but a sign of success achieved by a society and its institutions of government in promoting well-being and human development.

While good or positive health is a major component of broad conceptual definitions of health, most commonly used indicators are actually measures of poor health (Wilson and Drury, 1984; Bergner, 1985; Dever, 1984; U.S. Department of Health and Human Services, 1991; Rice, 1991; McGinnis and Foege, 1993). The major reason is that measurements of health status have been defined historically in terms of health problems, such as disease, disability, and death.

EXHIBIT 1.3. MEASURES OF HEALTH CARE ACCESS, QUALITY OF HEALTH CARE, AND HEALTH OUTCOMES *(continued)*

perform numerous IADL activities (usually more than five) for an extended period of time and is not acutely ill is designated as disabled.

Mental

- Self-assessed psychological state, such as self-reports of the frequency and intensity of psychological distress, anxiety, depression, and psychological well-being.
- General health perceptions, such as whether the person describes his or her health in general as excellent, very good, good, fair, or poor.

Social

- Social contacts refer to the number of social activities one performs within a specified time period, such as visits with friends and relatives and participation in social events such as conferences and workshops.
- Social resources or ties represent personal evaluations of the adequacy of interpersonal relationships, such as linkages with people who will listen to personal problems and provide tangible support and needed companionship.

Health outcome: Population

- Physical: Rates of mortality, morbidity, preventable hospitalizations, disability and functional status, leading causes of death, life expectancy, infant mortality, low birth weight, percentage of families satisfied with health care and cost, and percentage of primary care physicians satisfied with providing care, for example.
- Mental: Suicide rates and mental illness, for example.
- Social: Health disparities, quality of life, and labor force participation, for example.

Health status can be measured along physical, mental, or social dimensions for individuals, and similarly for populations. Individual physical health reflects symptoms, mortality, morbidity, and disability. Individual mental health reflects psychological states and health perceptions. Individual social health reflects social ties and resources. Although mental and social dimensions of health are less frequently measured, at least nationally, they are becoming widely recognized as important features of health status. Newer health status measures are capturing more of these domains.

Health problems affect the length and quality of life. Longevity can be expressed in terms of life expectancy, mortality rates, number of deaths from specific causes, and other similar indicators. Quality-of-life measures encompass such factors as personal well-being, the ability to function independently, family circumstances, income, housing security, and job satisfaction. Economic consequences of ill health are reflected by the "burden of illness," which refers to both the direct and indirect economic costs associated with health care utilization and any functional restrictions imposed by illness.

Measuring Vulnerability in Research

In research, vulnerability may be studied by using distinct population groups defined by one or more vulnerable attributes. Examples of vulnerable groups defined by one risk attribute are racial/ethnic minority (predisposing characteristic), uninsured (enabling characteristic), and chronically ill (need characteristic). Examples of vulnerable groups defined by two risk attributes include uninsured racial/ethnic minorities (predisposing and enabling), children with chronic illness (predisposing and need), and low-income persons with AIDS (enabling and need). Examples of vulnerable groups defined by the convergence of predisposing, enabling, and need attributes of risk include children in low-income families with poor health or uninsured minorities in poor health.

Sample sizes permitting, it is possible to include more than one risk attribute within predisposing, enabling, or need factors. For example, one can study minority children in low-income, uninsured families (two predisposing and one enabling attributes). Conceptualization of vulnerable subpopulations should be guided by the study purpose and availability of sufficient sample sizes and accurate and reliable measures for both the vulnerable groups and the groups with which they are compared. Ultimately, however, the operationalization of vulnerability should always be based on the presumption that the interaction between multiple individual and ecological factors contributes to a higher level of vulnerability and a greater risk of poor health.

Focus on Three Key Risk Factors

Although there are many predisposing, enabling, and need attributes of vulnerability, this book primarily focuses on three key risk factors—race/ethnicity, SES, and health insurance coverage—because they are three of the most powerful predictors of poor health care access and health, and therefore vulnerability. These three factors are closely intertwined but exert independent effects on health. They are also indirectly associated with, or contribute to, other vulnerability traits.

Race/ethnicity has long been a major basis of social stratification in the United States (Power and Matthews, 1997). While race and ethnicity are closely associated with SES and health insurance indicators, SES is not entirely equivalent across racial/ethnic groups. For example, even within categories of SES, racial/ethnic minorities often have higher rates of morbidity and mortality than whites. The failure of SES to account for racial variations in health status completely emphasizes the need to give attention to the unique factors linking race and ethnicity with health. One of these is discrimination, which incorporates ideologies of superiority, negative attitudes and beliefs toward racial/ethnic minorities, and differential treatment of members of these groups by both individuals and societal institutions (Williams and Collins, 1995). Because race/ethnicity and socioeconomic position in the United States are so closely intertwined, it is difficult to address socioeconomic or health insurance disparities without examining racial/ethnic disparities.

The relationship between SES and health care access and quality of care, and health is quite well known. Variations in income and wealth, educational attainment, and occupational position as markers of socioeconomic inequality have long been associated with variations in health status and mortality (Moss, 2000; Kaplan, Pamuk, et al., 1996; Amick, Levine, et al., 1995). Persons with high income, education, or occupational status live longer and have lower rates of diseases than those with lower SES. SES is also closely linked with health insurance status (due to health coverage provided primarily through employers and to income-based eligibility for safety net insurance programs like Medicaid), but both have independent effects on health.

In the United States, health insurance coverage has long been regarded as a marker for access. Recently, the IOM concluded that health insurance is also predictive of health outcomes. The IOM's Committee on the Consequences of Uninsurance (2002) concluded that providing health insurance to uninsured adults would result in improved health, including longer life expectancy. Increased health insurance coverage would especially contribute to improving the health of those in the poorest health and those who are most disadvantaged in terms of poor access to care and thus would likely reduce health disparities among racial and ethnic groups.

Given the well-established disparities in race/ethnicity, SES, and health insurance in access to health care, quality of care, and health status, timely and accurate knowledge of these three aspects of diverse vulnerable population groups is of critical importance in developing and assessing targeted interventions to reduce these disparities. Focusing on racial and ethnic, SES, and health insurance disparities is also consistent with current and future national health policies. *Healthy People 2010* (U.S. Department of Health and Human Services, 2000) focuses national attention on racial/ethnic and SES disparities in health and health care and, in a bold step forward from *Healthy People 2000*, called for the elimination of disparities in health and health care access.

The vast availability of health data according to race and ethnicity, SES, and health insurance coverage also makes it easier to demonstrate the vulnerability status associated with these factors. National protocols have institutionalized the collection and reporting of health data according to these factors. For example, the U.S. Office of Management and Budget (1978) requires that federal agencies report health statistics for four race groups (American Indian/Alaskan Native, Asian and Pacific Islander, black, and white) and one ethnic category (Hispanic origin). Regarding SES, in 1998, the U.S. Department of Health and

Human Services (1998) issued its first annual report of *Health, United States, 1998,* which included a special chart book on SES and health, and later editions have continued to report health data using these characteristics of SES. Finally, almost all major national health surveys have included health insurance coverage data in addition to SES and race/ethnicity.

Summary

Over the years, studies on vulnerable populations have used different paradigms or models in examining the characteristics that make populations vulnerable. These include individual demographic, behavioral, and socioeconomic characteristics; health care system characteristics; community characteristics; and the interaction of individual, system, and community characteristics. Each of the models reflects an evolution in defining, researching, and developing approaches to reducing or eliminating the health effects of vulnerability. Some have recognized the overlap between individual and community-level determinants of vulnerability, and others include the availability of medical care services as a predictor of vulnerability.

We have defined vulnerability as a multidimensional construct reflecting convergence of predisposing, enabling, and need attributes of risk at both individual and ecological levels. This broad definition of vulnerability presumes that vulnerable populations experience risks in clusters and that those susceptible to multiple risk factors, such as being of racial/ethnic minority background and living in poverty, are likely to be more vulnerable than those susceptible to a single risk, such as high-income minorities. Although there are many predisposing, enabling, and need attributes of vulnerability, this book primarily focuses on race and ethnicity, SES, and health insurance coverage because they are three of the most powerful predictors of poor health and, thus, vulnerability. These three factors are closely intertwined but exert independent effects on health. They are also indirectly associated with, or contribute to, other vulnerability traits.

In the next chapter, we delve further into the mechanisms of vulnerability and the pathways through which these influence health care access, quality, and health status disparities.

Review Questions

1. What is vulnerability? How can this concept be applied to the field of health and health care?
2. Identify three possible risk factors that could be used to characterize vulnerable populations. Why might these risk factors be associated with vulnerability?

3. What are the five main reasons to focus our national attention on vulnerable populations? Briefly describe the rationale for each reason.

Essay Questions

1. Why should the concept of vulnerability focus not just on independent risk factors but also on profiles of multiple risks? How might this understanding change daily business in the pursuit of good health for everyone in the United States, including how politicians, health care administrators, local health programs, and health care providers operate or practice?
2. How is the concept of equity a guiding principle in focusing national efforts on vulnerable populations? What does equity mean in terms of health and health care access? How does the concept of health care as a right illustrate this concept of equity? Given that health and health care equity for vulnerable populations will likely require extensive political intervention and large national financial costs, should this rationale of equity be prioritized over other factors, such as economics and politics? If so, why?

CHAPTER TWO

THE COMMUNITY DETERMINANTS AND MECHANISMS OF VULNERABILITY

In the previous chapter, we outlined our general model of vulnerability, which highlights the importance of understanding the overlap and interplay of multiple risk factors in leading to poor health status and creating barriers to health care access. Before presenting the evidence of the impact of individual and multiple risk factors on health and health care access, one needs to have sufficient knowledge about why vulnerability factors exist and how certain risk factors can lead to inadequate health care access and poor health outcomes. Understanding the determinants and mechanisms of the main risk factors highlighted in this book (race/ethnicity, SES, and insurance coverage) will help guide the interpretation of the detailed data presented in Chapters Three and Four.

Such an understanding will also provide a basic foundation to assess the effectiveness of programs that aim to prevent the occurrence of these risk factors through primary prevention or to disrupt or negate the effects of vulnerability through secondary prevention. Developing more effective solutions will require this understanding of determinants and mechanisms, so that interventions and policies can be developed to interrupt these mechanisms and pathways at critical junctures.

This chapter describes how vulnerability characteristics are produced and how they are allowed to persist in the United States. Vulnerability is a relative term that implies a particular susceptibility to adverse health and health care events beyond those normally experienced. How a population obtains the characteristics or risk factors that make it vulnerable must be viewed in relation to the community in which they occur because many of these risks are based on interactions among members of the community and may be affected by social policies. In this chapter, we examine each characteristic of vulnerability, discuss trends in its occurrence, its determinants, and the potential mechanisms of its relationship with adverse health outcomes and health care experiences.

Race and Ethnicity

Racial and ethnic differences are common determinants of disparity and conflict. Apartheid in South Africa, ethnic cleansing in Croatia, and tribal wars in Rwanda, for example, suggest a global preoccupation with racial and ethnic identity. In many countries around the world, access to medical care breaks down across racial and ethnic lines (World Health Organization, 2001). Often, vulnerable populations within a country are made up of minorities who are underserved in many ways, with health care delivery being only one of them.

Historical Development of the Importance of Race and Ethnicity

Although the preoccupation with race and ethnicity is not unique to the American culture, the United States has its own distinctive racial history that has contributed to current racial issues and diverse racial identities. Historically, race in the United States has played a significant role as a determinant of individual rights, opportunities, and social privilege. Laws and institutions catering to the interests of America's privileged class protected these rights and reinforced the significance of race. As a result, deficits in nearly every aspect of modern social life—education, employment, income, and health, for example—have accumulated for minorities throughout most of American history.

Starting in the 1950s, the national milieu began to improve for minorities as the civil rights movement ushered in proactive policies to reduce discrimination and level the playing field between whites and minorities. The Civil Rights Act of 1964 passed equal employment opportunity, a law requiring federal contractors to provide minorities and women with a proportion of jobs equivalent to their representation in the labor force or population. In the 1970s, American universities sought to increase the diversity of their student bodies with **affirmative action.** The 1978 ruling by the Supreme Court in *University of California Regents v. Bakke* supported this effort by permitting race to be used as an admission criterion under certain circumstances. The intended result was to counter the earlier effects of discrimination in excluding minorities from higher education. A controversial issue, affirmative action policies and their efficacy are the center of much debate even today.

The civil rights movement awarded value to minority status and provided minorities with the chance to compete against nonminorities for the same educational and professional opportunities; however, racial and ethnic identity continues to be associated with substantial vulnerabilities. In a report to the United Nations in 2000, the U.S. State Department noted a significant reduction in overt and institutionalized discrimination but acknowledged a strong "legacy of segregation, ignorance, stereotyping, discrimination and disparities in opportunity and achievement" for minorities (Lobe, 2000, p. 3). Racial and ethnic identity will likely continue to fragment the nation as long as race influences individual access to fundamental rights and privileges.

Defining Race/Ethnicity

Most policymakers, practitioners, and researchers are quick to use *race/ethnicity* in most discussions of disparities. But what does this term really mean? And why has it become an almost daily point of discussion in the media and created such division in society and politics, given that we know so little about its meaning? At its simplest, race and ethnicity reflect skin color and, in some instances, cultural heritage or language. In nearly all of medical care and health care policy, it has been simple enough to classify individuals as black, white, Asian, or Hispanic. Even without attention to the many possible inaccuracies in measuring race/ethnicity, such as self-reported race/ethnicity versus how others would identify a person's background, why should we challenge these simple classifications?

Race/ethnicity, when measured as skin color or physical appearance, is rarely the cause of disparities in health and health care (LaVeist, 1994). Although there is evidence that the lightness or darkness of skin color may indeed be a risk factor for a few health outcomes, including incidence of skin cancer (Klag, Whelton, et al., 1991; Dwyer, Prota, et al., 2000; Fuller, 2000, 2003; Dwyer, Blizzard, et al., 2002), there is generally little support for the direct correlation of skin color and most health outcomes or health care experiences. For example, if we find that blacks are less likely to receive high-quality primary care (say, they receive fewer preventive services, have less continuity of care with an ongoing provider, and are less likely to find their patient-provider relationships satisfactory), can this be attributed to the color of skin alone? The answer is most definitely not. Skin color does not transport a person to the doctor, choose and pay for what preventive services are delivered, or obtain the health insurance to maintain a continuous pairing with a specific provider. These differences in quality are much more likely to be explained by other factors, such as health insurance coverage or other factors that are related to race/ethnicity.

It has been proposed that race/ethnicity frequently serves as a **proxy measure** for other factors that are more appropriate explanatory factors than skin color alone. Race/ethnicity can be a reflection of biological factors; socioeconomic status; cultural practices, beliefs, or acculturation; political factors; or discrimination (King and Williams, 1995). Race/ethnicity may also serve as a proxy measure of discrimination. In the case of health outcomes, race/ethnicity may serve as a proxy for biological factors (blacks are more prone to sickle cell anemia, for example), cultural behaviors or practices regarding health, or access to material goods and services that support health. In the case of health care experiences, race and ethnicity may serve as a proxy for socioeconomic factors (enabling the purchase of services), language factors (creating barriers to accessing services), or discrimination based on skin color. This is not to say that race/ethnicity may not reflect other unmeasured or unknown factors, as is found in some research studies, but in any interpretation of the research literature, one should seek to understand the mechanisms linking race and ethnicity with health and health care outcomes. LaVeist (1994) argues that where possible, measures of the actual mechanisms should be used instead of race/ethnicity so that more accurate interventions and health policies can be made. But in many cases, adequate measures such as cultural factors and measures of discrimination have not been developed or implemented, so we are left with race/ethnicity measures serving as relatively inaccurate proxies (LaVeist, 1994).

One final aspect of race/ethnicity to consider is how politics may influence the definition. While we have come to understand the complexity of race/ethnicity in modern research and now acknowledge combinations of racial/ethnic groups (such as black/Asian pairings) in national statistics as mixed-race groups, this highlights the political nature of how race and ethnicity is constructed. Within the past decade, the U.S. Census has attempted to capture some of this complexity in the self-reporting of race/ethnicity. Similar changes have been made in other countries, including Japan and Brazil (LaVeist, 1994). Due to these changes in coding, substantial changes in the reported prevalence of racial/ethnic groups have occurred or are pending. Since race/ethnicity is frequently used to determine affirmative action policies in universities, decide funding allotments for health care workforce and other training programs, or allocate money to some underserved areas and is used in a range of national and local programs, these changes are made with political scrutiny and not without political consequences. Changes in simple terms such as *minority* will have to be redefined in the coming years to reflect these changes in racial/ethnic group prevalence due to measurement.

And these changes will potentially influence the dynamics of health and social policies, how they are constructed, and how and to whom they are targeted. In short, although a solution has proven evasive, it is important to be aware of these issues in discussions of disparities for vulnerable populations.

National Trends in Race/Ethnicity and Diversity

Minority racial and ethnic background has increasingly become an important consideration in the U.S. health care system. Recent creation of large national initiatives to reduce these racial and ethnic disparities in health and health care has reaffirmed the nation's commitment to the elimination of one of its most enduring problems. In fact, the surgeon general, a unifying voice of the nation's public health goals, has prioritized the elimination of racial and ethnic disparities at the top of the nation's health agenda (Satcher, 2000).

Even apart from the socioeconomic status factors that it is closely associated with, minority race and ethnicity have been shown to independently predict poorer health status, access to care, and quality of care. Race/ethnicity is a relatively immutable personal trait that, when conceptualized as skin color alone, is unlikely to be the cause of adverse events. Minority race and ethnicity, however, usually serves as a proxy for other factors such as SES, language ability, or cultural behaviors that are correlated with health status and health care experiences (LaVeist, 1994; Schulman, Rubenstein, et al., 1995). Understanding historical trends and patterns related to the growth and distribution of minority populations is therefore essential.

Traditional use of the term *minority* is slowly becoming inapplicable in the United States. During the decade between 1990 and 2000, the minority population (consisting of black, Hispanic, Asian and Pacific Islander, and American Indian or Alaskan Native) grew by nearly 31 percent, making the United States one of the most ethnically diverse countries in the world. As of the year 2000, minority groups represented about 29.7 percent of the population compared with 24.3 percent of the population at the start of the decade (U.S. Census Bureau, 2001b).

Not every racial and ethnic group was equally represented in this growth. Hispanics and Asians grew faster in number than other minorities, and this was due primarily to the increasing momentum of immigration among these groups. Hispanics, who accounted for 9 percent of the total population in 1990, grew by over 10 million, to account for 11.9 percent of the population in 2000. The number of Asians grew at a slower rate during this period, increasing by about 2 million, from about 2.8 percent to 3.5 percent of the population. Blacks and Native Americans accounted for approximately the same proportion of the total population (12.2

percent and 0.7 percent, respectively) during this decade. In the most recent census, 2.5 percent of the population reported associating with two or more racial groups (U.S. Census Bureau, 2001c).

The growth of racial and ethnic diversity varies by geographic region. **Diversity,** measured by the percentage of times that two randomly selected people in a specific area would be of different racial and ethnic backgrounds, is currently reported to be 49 percent (U.S. Census Bureau, 2001b). In general, racial diversity is greatest in the western and southern states, with rates of diversity occurring well above 60 percent in certain areas of California and Texas. The rate of change in diversity, however, is greatest in the Northwest, the Midwest (Oklahoma, Kansas, and Nebraska), and the Southeast, particularly Florida (see Figures 2.1 and 2.2). These geographical changes in diversity are important because health care resources also vary by geography and may influence racial differences in health and health care experiences.

Theoretical Pathways of Racial and Ethnic Vulnerability

We present a summary conceptual model in Figure 2.3 that builds on the original work of Stevens and Shi (2003), Aday and Andersen (1981), and King and Williams (1995) to describe several potential pathways linking race and ethnicity with health and health care. The pathways begin with family characteristics that include socioeconomic status, cultural factors, discrimination, and health need. The model then traces the pathways through the health care delivery system and identifies provider and system factors that may contribute to disparities in care. Several pathways are likely to operate simultaneously, leading to adverse health and health care outcomes (Stevens and Shi, 2003).

Socioeconomic Status. One theory behind racial and ethnic differences in health care experiences is that they are attributable to differences in socioeconomic status that include family income, parent education or occupation, and insurance status and type. African Americans, Hispanics, and certain other racial/ethnic groups are more likely than whites to have lower family income and lower education levels (DeNavas-Walt, Cleveland, et al., 2001). They are also less likely to have insurance coverage and, when insured, are more likely to be covered by public payers such as Medicaid and the **State Children's Health Insurance Program** (SCHIP; Mills and Bhandari, 2003). These SES factors often combine to affect health care utilization, the presence and type of a regular source of care, and health status. Race/ethnicity is so closely intertwined with SES factors that it is often difficult to separate SES effects from the effects of other racial/ethnic pathways.

FIGURE 2.1. DIVERSITY BY U.S. COUNTY

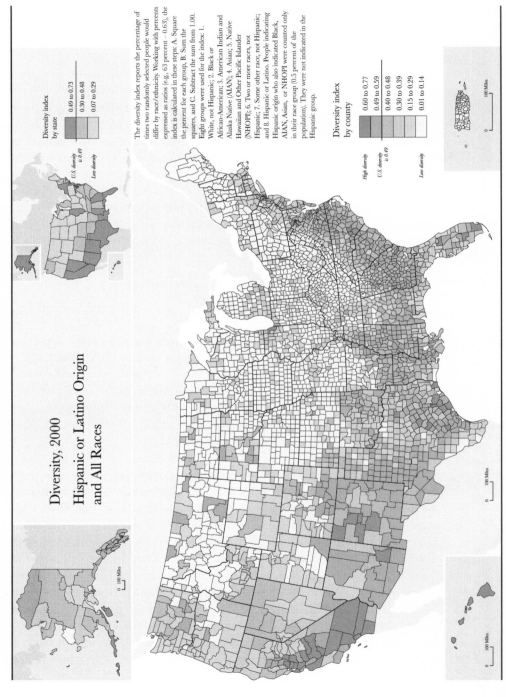

Diversity, 2000

Hispanic or Latino Origin
and All Races

The diversity index reports the percentage of times two randomly selected people would differ by race/ethnicity. Working with percents expressed as ratios (e.g. 63 percent = 0.63), the index is calculated in these steps: A. Square the percent for each group, B. Sum the squares, and C. Subtract the sum from 1.00. Eight groups were used for the index: 1. White, not Hispanic; 2. Black or African-American; 3. American Indian and Alaska Native (AIAN); 4. Asian; 5. Native Hawaiian and Other Pacific Islander (NHOPI); 6. Two or more races, not Hispanic; 7. Some other race, not Hispanic; and 8. Hispanic or Latino. People indicating Hispanic origin who also indicated Black, AIAN, Asian, or NHOPI were counted only in their race group (0.5 percent of the population). They were not indicated in the Hispanic group.

Diversity index
by state

High diversity

0.49 to 0.73
0.30 to 0.48
0.07 to 0.29

U.S. diversity
≈ 0.49

Low diversity

Diversity index
by county

High diversity

0.60 to 0.77
0.49 to 0.59
0.40 to 0.48
0.30 to 0.39
0.15 to 0.29
0.01 to 0.14

U.S. diversity
≈ 0.49

Low diversity

0   100 Miles

Source: U.S. Census Bureau (2001a).

FIGURE 2.2. CHANGES IN DIVERSITY BY U.S. COUNTY

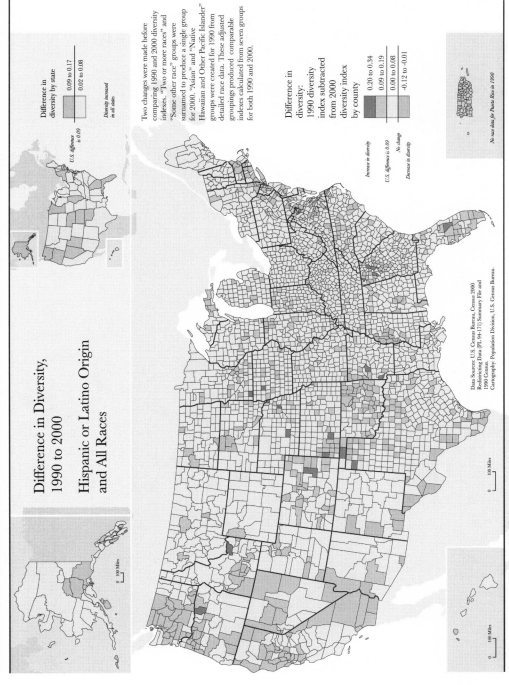

Difference in Diversity, 1990 to 2000

Hispanic or Latino Origin and All Races

Difference in diversity by state

0.09 to 0.17

0.02 to 0.08

Diversity increased in all states

U.S. difference is 0.09

Two changes were made before comparing 1990 and 2000 diversity indexes. "Two or more races" and "Some other race" groups were surnamed to produce a single group for 2000. "Asian" and "Native Hawaiian and Other Pacific Islander" groups were created for 1990 from detailed race data. These adjusted groupings produced comparable indexes calculated from seven groups for both 1990 and 2000.

Difference in diversity: 1990 diversity index subtracted from 2000 diversity index by county

0.20 to 0.34

0.09 to 0.19

0.00 to 0.08

-0.12 to -0.01

Increase in diversity

U.S. difference is 0.09

No change

Decrease in diversity

No race data for Puerto Rico in 1990

Data Sources: U.S. Census Bureau, Census 2000 Redistricting Data (PL 94-171) Summary File and 1990 Census. Cartography: Population Division, U.S. Census Bureau.

0   100 Miles

0   100 Miles

0   100 Miles

Source: U.S. Census Bureau (2001a).

FIGURE 2.3. CONCEPTUAL MODEL LINKING RACE AND ETHNICITY WITH HEALTH CARE EXPERIENCES

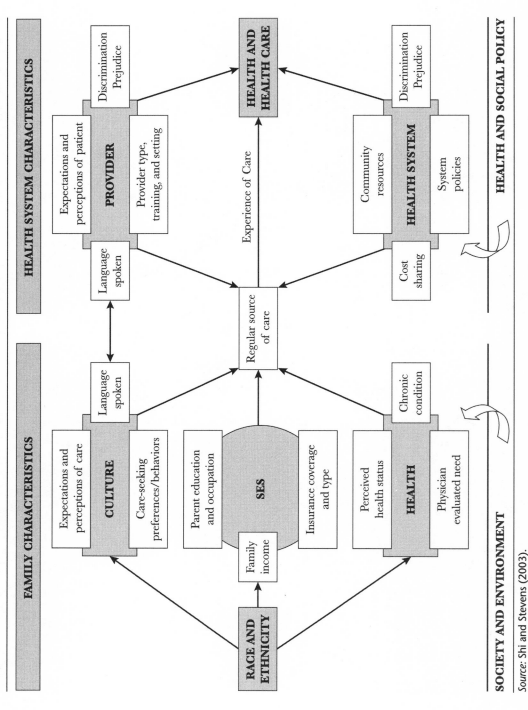

Source: Shi and Stevens (2003).

Cultural Factors. Perhaps offering the most potential for future research into racial disparities are family cultural factors, including language ability, family preferences or beliefs leading to various health behaviors and health-care-seeking practices, and differences in perceptions and expectations for health care. Language, in particular, is a well-known barrier to accessing health care (Aday, Fleming, et al., 1984; Ferguson and Candib, 2002) and may also be an important barrier to effective **continuity of care** and developing a strong patient-provider relationship. Language concordance between patient and provider may be a more accurate explanatory variable (rather than patient language alone), but it is often absent from health care research.

Culturally based, care-seeking practices may also be associated with disparities in health and health care experiences. Controlling for SES, racial and ethnic minorities seek and obtain primary care more frequently from emergency rooms and non-office-based sources of care. These settings are not generally designed to deliver the continuity of care necessary for achieving high-quality primary care (Halfon, Inkelas, et al., 1995). Moreover, cultural values and beliefs may influence the decision to seek health care and whether to adhere to medical advice (Flores, Abreau, et al., 1998; Flores and Vega, 1998). *Respeto* in Hispanic culture, for example, refers to the particularly high valuation of, and authority given to, physicians (American Medical Association, 1994). This may lead Hispanic patients to interact and collaborate with physicians differently than other patients do.

Racial and ethnic differences in family expectations or preferences for care are not well identified and catalogued, but may uniquely affect parent ratings of experiences with care. Without documentation and recognition of these cultural differences, however, it is difficult to know whether disparities in ratings of care reflect actual variations in provider behaviors. Nonetheless, perceptions of care are invaluable because negative perceptions may lead to more frequent switching of providers and health plans (Safran, Montgomery, et al., 2001), thus resulting in more fragmented delivery of health care.

Discrimination. Discrimination provides another potential pathway linking race and ethnicity to health. Recent studies have shown that experiences of discrimination are often negatively associated with health. These experiences, most commonly reported by minorities, and the resulting effects on minority health and receipt of health care are another piece of the puzzle of racial disparities.

Defined as the differential action toward an individual or group based on race, discrimination is a manifestation of prejudice, the assumption of individual or group abilities, motives, and intentions according to race (Jones, 2000). Discrimination at the institutional level directly affects the health of minorities, who are treated differently once they enter the health care system. For example, in a study comparing bypass procedures given to a group with similar levels of severe illness and expected postoperative benefit, whites in the group received the surgery more often than black patients (Peterson, Shaw, et al., 1997). Other studies have found comparable results even when adjusting for SES and health insurance (AMA Council on Ethical and Judicial Affairs, 1990; McBean and Gornick, 1994). In some cases, differences in minority patient preferences and refusals have contributed to corresponding differences in health outcomes; however, a study by Hannan, van Ryn, et al. (1999) considered patient preferences and patient refusals as a cause for racial differences in the receipt of bypass surgeries and found that neither played a significant role in the differential treatment of minorities.

Perceived discrimination and self-reported racism is also negatively associated with health. Recent research has shown a relationship between perceived discrimination and poor mental health, including conditions of psychological distress, major depression, and generalized anxiety (Jackson, Brown, et al., 1996; Kessler, Mickelson, et al., 1999; Brown, Williams, et al., 2000; Karlsen and Nazroo, 2002a, 2002b). Studies have found that hypertension and poor self-rated health are associated with perceived discrimination (Dressler, 1990; Williams, Yu, et al., 1997; Ren, Amick, et al., 1999; Schulz, Israel, et al., 2000; Finch, Hummer, et al., 2001; Guyll, Matthews, et al., 2001; Karlsen and Nazroo, 2002a, 2002b). It is important to note that individual coping skills, however, can modify, for better or worse, negative effects of discrimination on mental and physical health (James, LaCroix, et al., 1984; Krieger, 1990; Krieger and Sidney, 1996; LaVeist, Sellers, et al., 2001).

Experiences of self-reported discrimination have been linked to destructive behavior patterns such as problem drinking and cigarette smoking, as well as low levels of compliance with medical recommendations (Cohen, Kessler, et al., 1995; Landrine and Klonoff, 1996, 2000; Yen, Ragland, et al. 1999a, 1999b). Considering discrimination to be a form of stress, and in some cases a form of chronic stress, helps illustrate one likely pathway ultimately connecting race/ethnicity with health. Current literature on stress suggests a process beginning with stress-induced anxiety or depression that either affects physical health directly or results in negative health behavior, which in most cases will eventually worsen physical health.

Evidence suggesting that discrimination contributes to racial disparities in health is increasing. The research continues to be challenged by limits in methodology and the difficulty of standardizing a subjective variable such as perceived discrimination. Additional investigation is necessary to learn more about the impact of discrimination on minority health and how great a role it plays in racial disparities.

Health Needs. Health care needs drive the seeking of health care services. Health needs derive from both acute and chronic illnesses, as well as from recommendations for preventive care visits. Illness includes both clinically evaluated health problems and patient perceptions of health risks and needs. Racial and ethnic minorities generally have poorer health status than whites (Montgomery, Kiely, et al., 1996; Weigers, Weinick, et al., 1998; National Center for Health Statistics, 2003). Thus, minorities have greater health needs that present both opportunities and challenges for the delivery of high-quality care. Even before entering the health care system, individuals are influenced and distinguished by family characteristics that will govern their health care experience and outcome.

Provider Factors. Individuals enter the primary health care system when they seek care from a provider or clinic of providers. Patients may identify the provider or clinic as a regular source of care, indicating they have prior experience with the source of care and will seek care in the future from this source. Alternatively, patients may obtain care from a variety of sources or in team care settings such that there is no single regular provider of care that is relied on. The presence or absence and type of regular source of care are determined by SES, cultural factors, and health needs (among other health system factors), and it may influence both perceptions and actual delivery of care.

Once a person has entered the health care system, several provider factors may influence the delivery and experience of health care (Halfon, Inkelas, et al., 1995). Provider specialty, training, and setting of care may reveal differences in experience or preferences for delivering health care. Pediatricians may, for example, spend more time delivering preventive health services to minority children, while family practitioners may develop better knowledge of a minority family and then use that information when caring for the children. Differences by race/ethnicity in the types of providers who are seen may contribute to some disparities.

In addition, providers have preferences and expectations for the delivery of care to their patients. Research suggests, in fact, that physician perceptions and beliefs about patients are affected by race, ethnicity, and socioeconomic status (van Ryn and Burke, 2000; van Ryn, 2002; van Ryn and Fu, 2003). These perceptions may affect physician treatment decisions, feelings of affiliation with patients, and beliefs about risk behaviors that influence the type and degree of care delivered. Perhaps for this reason, racial and ethnic concordance between provider and patient has been associated in some cases with better patient perceptions of partnership and satisfaction with the patient-provider relationship (Cooper-Patrick, Gallo, et al., 1999; Saha, Komaromy, et al., 1999; Malat, 2001; Cooper and Roter, 2002; LaVeist and Nuru-Jeter, 2002; LaVeist, Nuru-Jeter, et al., 2003; Saha, Arbelaez, et al., 2003). These measurably improved interactions may lead families to seek care from racially concordant providers (Gray and Stoddard, 1997; Saha, Taggart, et al., 2000). In the only study among children, no disparities in primary care quality were found according to patient-provider racial/ethnic concordance, due perhaps to the attenuation in pediatric care of provider biases or patient expectations that may contribute to disparities (Stevens, Shi, et al., 2003).

Health System Factors. Apart from provider characteristics, health care system factors such as community resources, health plan cost-sharing requirements, and other various health plan policies may influence the experiences of minorities in health care. The availability of health resources in the community may affect the ability of individuals to access care and may determine the setting in which care is delivered. Cost sharing has been shown to affect utilization of health services, and it may have a further impact on perceptions of the care received (Leibowitz, Manning, et al. 1985; Valdez, Brook, et al. 1985; Anderson, Brook, et al. 1991). For example, patients in public health insurance programs that do not require copayments or deductibles may hypothetically feel less enfranchised to voice criticism of their health care simply because they are not directly paying for it.

Health care plan policies may be even more important in influencing the delivery of primary care to families. For example, managed care policies such as gatekeeping and networks that limit patient choice of providers may strengthen relationships by linking patients with a specific provider. Alternately, restrictions in patient care may place an unnecessary burden on minority patients by reducing flexibility in finding race- or language-concordant providers. Either way, the effects of managed care are likely to be particularly pronounced for vulnerable populations and children (Szilagyi, Rodewald, et al., 1993; Hughes, Newacheck, et al., 1995; Hughes and Luft, 1998; Simpson and Fraser, 1999; Miller and Luft, 1994, 1997, 2002).

Finally, health and social policies play an important role in mediating racial and ethnic minorities' experiences with health care. Health care policy shapes, for example, the nature and provision of **safety net insurance** coverage, regulates organizations such as managed care, and subsidizes the education and training of health providers, particularly those of minority background. Many of the factors in this model are amenable to policy intervention, and thus policy may play an overarching role in reducing racial and ethnic disparities in health care.

Front-Line Experience: Nurses Reaching Beyond School Borders

Jane Lyon, Liz Mercer, and Lorraine Lemus, respectively the director of health services and nursing staff at an urban school district in southern California, provide an account of how school nurses in one school district have reached far beyond the borders of the school grounds to help children and families struggling with multiple risk factors to interact with a sometimes daunting system of medical care.

Juan was diagnosed with leukemia during kindergarten. (The child's name and identifying information have been altered.) Despite the difficulty of chemotherapy, he returned to school for grades 1 and 2 and was living a relatively normal child's life. During the summer after third grade, he went to his school health office complaining of a sore throat, and by the next week he was back in the hospital with a reoccurrence of leukemia. The hospital that could take Juan was more than forty miles away from his home and the school district. The drive from our community to the hospital regularly takes one to two hours due to traffic.

Because of our ongoing relationship with Juan's family—Juan has three sisters who also attend our school district—we visited Juan in the hospital to see how he and his family were faring. Juan's mom and dad were at his bedside, and his grandmother was in the hospital courtyard with his three young sisters. Although Juan's dad was very complimentary about his son's care, we became uncomfortable with the care Juan received at the hospital. Despite being at risk of infection due to the chemotherapy, he was inappropriately placed in an adult intensive care unit with a patient coughing in the next bed, and not a single person washed his or her hands before interacting with Juan.

Because Juan's family did not speak English and we knew they did not feel comfortable enough to inquire about why he was not being better protected from infection, we felt it was important to intervene ourselves to help his family obtain a better situation. We asked Juan's parents if they would be more comfortable with Juan staying in a hospital closer to home. Both agreed that this would be a much better situation; staying with him at a far-away hospital was causing some difficulties with their employers because they were spending so much time away from work.

We made telephone calls to local hospitals closer to Juan's home but had no luck with transferring him to another facility because his Medicaid insurance was accepted only in certain locations and these locations were already overwhelmed with patients. We had almost reached the end of our resources when a lifesaving event occurred: in response to an article that we and Juan's family placed in the local newspaper about his difficult health situation, a parent at our school came forward as chief of oncology at a local hospital and offered her services to help this child. Juan's family required our assistance in communicating and negotiating the transfer with this doctor; they were also somewhat reluctant to request a transfer because they did not want to hurt the original doctor's feelings. However, this rally of support from their community encouraged and empowered them to be advocates for their son's health care.

Juan was in the hospital for one year and received a bone marrow transplant from one of his sisters. Despite these difficult times and procedures involving multiple family members, Juan's mother amazes us to this day with the level of self-confidence she has developed in dealing with Juan's health problems and in advocating for her family. Given just a little encouragement and support from our nursing staff and the community, she has learned to boldly face the many obstacles of language, culture, and emotional and physical exhaustion to continue to fight for her family and Juan's health.

When she believes things are not in Juan's best interest, she speaks up in Spanish until she can get an interpreter. She will ask over and over for services that she knows Juan needs. During this process, Juan's mother has built a strong network of advocates who are always willing to fight for her son. We believe that one of the most important things that a school nurse can do for the vulnerable students in a community is to teach and empower parents to advocate strongly for their families. Juan's mother has learned to ask for help when she needs it and knows that she can call on her resources when she needs assistance.

Juan is back in school part time. Even with his health difficulties, Juan and his sisters always come on time to school with their homework completed. They are clean and well cared for, and his sisters wear their hair in ribbons and bows. With his condition, Juan still requires toilet changing and feeding supplies at school, and thanks to our efforts and the friendly reminders from Juan's mother, we have never run low on supplies. Given the barriers that Juan's family faces—being low income, maintaining Medicaid insurance coverage, not speaking English, raising four young children, and dealing with a complex medical condition—we do not know how Juan's family can get everything done. When we visit their modest home to check on Juan's progress, it is clean and neat, and there always is food simmering on the stove. It is a heartwarming sight considering how much time this family has spent with Juan in the hospital.

As school nurses, we are grateful for the opportunity to work with such loving, hard-working parents who are devoted to their children and, when needed, have been willing to explore and rely on the recommendations of school nurses with confidence and determination.

Socioeconomic Status

An unfortunate truism in the United States, and in nearly every other developed country in the world, is that individuals with the greatest financial resources have the best health. They also have the greatest ability to access health services and obtain the highest-quality care. The apparent explanation is that income translates into purchasing power for health care services. In fact, based on national spending, one would think that purchasing medical care is the only determinant of a population's health. However, research has revealed much more substantial and complex effects of income on health than just purchasing power. On closer review, income appears to be just part of a larger concept of social position, generally referred to as socioeconomic status (SES) that most commonly incorporates measures of income, education, and occupation, to provide a broader picture of a person's status in a community or society.

Historical Development of the Importance of Socioeconomic Status

Before examining the relationship between SES and health, it is important to take a step back and consider what determines an individual's socioeconomic status. Because SES has a significant impact on health, it is essential to understand what factors influence it and how modifying these factors could improve population health well before public health efforts or medical care are required. Environment, and place of residence in particular, influence all three measures of an individual's SES: income, education, and occupation. Changes made at the environmental level may ultimately improve community health through SES pathways.

First, in the United States, residence dictates which public school students can attend. Because public school funding depends on the local tax base, a community's financial resources partially determine the quality of a neighborhood's public school. In areas of concentrated poverty where financial resources are limited, public schools have lower average test scores, more restricted curricula, fewer qualified teachers, less access to more broadly experienced academic advisers, less interaction with potential colleges and employers, higher levels of teen pregnancy, and higher dropout rates than public schools in middle-class areas.

Minorities are the most common residents in areas of high poverty concentration and disproportionately suffer the consequences of low-quality educational opportunities compared to whites (Orfield and Eaton, 1996; Willms, 1999). Differences in educational opportunities contribute to racial/ethnic disparities in educational attainment, competency levels among graduates, and preparation for enrollment in college or employment, all factors that shape an individual's ability to seek higher education, stable employment, and steady income (Williams and Collins, 2001; Acevedo-Garcia, Lochner, et al., 2003).

Second, residence further dictates employment opportunities by determining access to convenient and well-paying entry-level job opportunities. Since the 1950s, low-skilled, higher-paying jobs have been migrating out of poor, urban communities to suburban areas (Kasarda, 1989; Wilson, 1996). Minorities living in urban areas are the most affected by this migration, or "spatial mismatch," and among minorities, blacks are the most disadvantaged by their geographical distance. In fact, sociologists argue that spatial mismatch is a significant factor contributing to the consistently low employment rates of blacks and potentially poor health status (Raphael and Stoll, 2002; Schulz, Williams, et al., 2002).

Discrimination based on negative racial stereotypes may also be a factor in low employment rates and fewer opportunities for minorities. Corporations seeking to expand, relocate, or build new facilities have used geographical racial composition in deciding where to place these facilities. The location of black communities, in particular, has been a significant negative factor in some of these decisions (Wilson, 1987, 1996; Cole and Deskins, 1988; Kirschenman and Neckerman, 1991; Neckerman and Kirschenman, 1991). Thus, it follows that white residential areas have more convenient and well-paying job opportunities than black residential areas (Raphael and Stoll, 2002).

The effect that residential segregation has on employment opportunities further demonstrates the role that discrimination plays in creating poor labor markets for blacks. Cities such as Detroit, New York, and Chicago, which have high levels of residential segregation, have greater spatial mismatches between blacks and job locations. Conversely, blacks living in cities with less residential segregation such as Portland, Oregon, and Charlotte, North Carolina, have better access to jobs. This relationship persists even as cities change over time. Cities that became less segregated from 1990 to 2000 showed a concurrent improvement in spatial mismatch between blacks and job opportunities (Raphael and Stoll, 2002). Corporate and geographical discrimination contributing to segregation leaves inner-city communities isolated and further impoverished by high unemployment.

Communities with high unemployment can entangle themselves in a cycle of poverty as fewer employment and job-networking opportunities limit an economic escape and fewer consistently employed adults are able to act as role models for young adults in the next generation (Wilson, 1987). Furthermore, living in areas of concentrated poverty over an extended period of time can weaken a strong work ethic, devalue academic achievement, and reduce the social stigmas of incarceration, low educational attainment, and economic failure (Shihadeh and Flynn, 1996). Moreover, such devaluations and lower achievement may discourage future companies from moving into the economically deprived area, extending the cycle.

Factors leading to limited educational and employment opportunities in poor communities are made worse by political neglect. Social services have the potential to buffer disadvantaged communities from the stress and circumstances of poverty. Politicians, however, are more likely to cut funding for services in poor areas because these communities are less politically organized and less empowered to successfully protest the funding cuts compared to more economically and socially advantaged communities (Wilson, 1987; Wallace, 1990, 1991). Even for conscientious politicians, providing essential social services in areas of concentrated poverty is challenging. As individuals who are able to afford better neighborhoods move from urban to suburban areas, the urban tax base shrinks, making it difficult to continue to fund social services (Bullard, 1994; Wilson, 1996).

Environmental factors, including racial and ethnic segregation and political neglect, influence the education options, employment opportunities, and income of individuals residing in a community. Not only do these factors determine where individuals will rank along the SES gradient, they also govern mobility up and down the social classes.

National Trends in Income and Poverty and Their Distribution

The importance of SES to health has been recognized in Europe since the early 1900s, when mortality statistics were first reported according to occupation. The United States, however, has been slower to adopt this practice. In 1976, the U.S. Department of Health and Human Services released its inaugural report of the nation's health, revealing substantial differences in mortality, morbidity, and access to care according to SES. Numerous studies since the 1976 report have concluded that lower-SES populations have increased incidence of chronic disease and depression, as well as increased reports of disability. What characteristics define this vulnerable population? Who has low SES in the United States?

Household income has changed substantially in the past thirty years. In 1970, the median adjusted household income in the United States was about $34,600. By 2000, the annual household income had reached $42,100, the highest median income recorded in the nation's history. Per capita income grew similarly during this period, increasing from $12,300 in 1970 to $22,200 in 2000. Changes in annual income, however, have not been consistent across all demographic groups (Proctor and Dalaker, 2003).

Some of the most striking differences in income are across racial/ethnic groups. Since 1970, Asians and whites have consistently had higher annual incomes than blacks and Hispanics. In 2000, the median household income of Asians and whites reached $55,500 and $45,900, respectively, but Hispanic and black households reached new historic highs in household income of $33,500 and $30,500 respectively. The new highs reflect seven years of significantly greater percentage gains in income for black (32.5 percent), Hispanic (24.3 percent), and Asian (23.1 percent) households compared to whites (14.2 percent). (See Figure 2.4.)

These racial differences in household income look somewhat different when one considers per capita income. Although Asians had the highest median household income in 2000, income for each household member was lower for Asians ($22,700) compared to whites ($25,000). Asian and Pacific Islander households are typically composed of more members than white households (3.1 versus 2.5 members). Similarly, blacks and Hispanics had lower per capita income than whites ($15,000 and $12,200, respectively).

Another important way to examine household income is through the concept of poverty. The federal government annually determines a level of income that will qualify individuals for government assistance programs. This poverty threshold is adjusted for age, family size, and number of children. For example, in

FIGURE 2.4. MONETARY INCOME BY RACE AND ETHNICITY

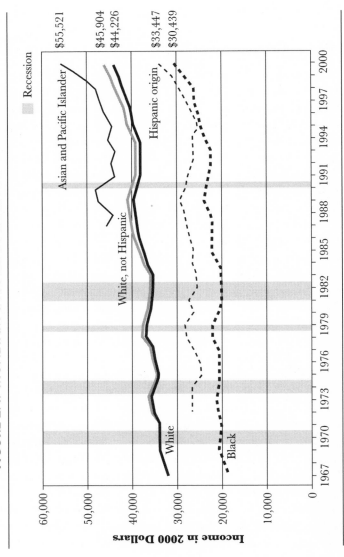

■ Recession

Asian and Pacific Islander — $55,521

White, not Hispanic — $45,904

White — $44,226

Hispanic origin — $33,447

Black — $30,439

Income in 2000 Dollars

60,000

50,000

40,000

30,000

20,000

10,000

0

1967 1970 1973 1976 1979 1982 1985 1988 1991 1994 1997 2000

aHispanics may be of any race. Data are not available prior to 1972.

Source: DeNavas-Walt, C., R. Cleveland, et al. (2001).

2000, the poverty threshold for a two-parent household with one child was about $11,900. Families making less than this amount are considered poor and therefore qualified to participate in several governmental health and social welfare programs developed to provide assistance in obtaining adequate food, income, and health care.

Trends in poverty generally mirror the changes in income (Figure 2.5). In 2002, 12.1 percent of the population was living in poverty, up from 11.3 percent in 2000, which was then statistically similar to the lowest recorded rate of poverty in history (11.1 percent), set in 1979. Even the seemingly small change in the poverty rate from 2001 (11.7 percent) to 2002 reflects an increase of about 1.7 million people living in poverty, bringing the total to 34.6 million people. Substantial variation in the rates of poverty between 1960 and 2002 shows that is closely tied to the changes in the national economy (Proctor and Dalaker, 2003).

As with income, some of the most striking differences in poverty rates are across racial and ethnic groups. Blacks and Hispanics have traditionally experienced the highest rates of poverty. In 2002, 24.1 percent of blacks and 21.8 percent of Hispanics were living in poverty, close to the lowest recorded rates in history (in 2000) but still much higher than the 8.0 percent rate for whites (see Figure 2.6). However, the disparity in poverty rates between blacks and whites has decreased substantially. In 1959, for example, over 50 percent of blacks were poor compared to 18 percent of whites, a difference of 32 percent. This gap has narrowed significantly since that time, such that the size of the disparity in poverty rates between blacks and whites was 23.2 percent in 1993 and 16.1 percent in 2000. Similarly, the difference between Hispanics and whites decreased from 20.2 percent in 1993 to 13.8 percent in 2002 (Proctor and Dalaker, 2003).

Finally, there are several interesting smaller trends in both income and poverty according to region and household type. Since the 1970s, the South has consistently had a lower median household income compared to other regions of the country ($38,400 versus about $45,000). In 2002, people in the South and West were more likely to be in poverty (13.8 percent and 12.4 percent, respectively) than those in the Midwest and Northeast (10.3 percent and 10.9 percent, respectively). Single-parent households headed by women have generally had lower incomes and higher rates of poverty than other household types. But in recent years, there has been a general trend of increasing household income for these families, and in 2000 their rate of poverty (although still very large) had decreased to 24.7 percent, its lowest level in history. By 2002, this rate had climbed to 26.5 percent (Proctor and Dalaker, 2003).

Children are an important consideration because they are more likely than adults to live in families with incomes below poverty. In 2002, 16.7 percent of children lived in poverty, with 9.4 percent of white children living in poverty compared to 11.7 percent of Asians, 28.6 percent of Hispanics, and 32.3 percent of

FIGURE 2.5. POVERTY (NUMBERS AND RATES) FROM 1959 TO 2001

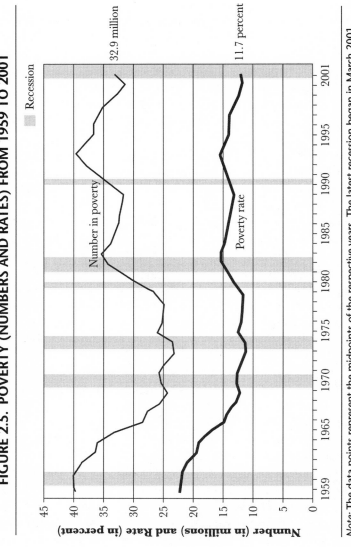

Note: The data points represent the midpoints of the respective years. The latest recession began in March 2001.

Source: Proctor and Dalaker (2002).

FIGURE 2.6. U.S. POVERTY RATES BY RACE AND ETHNICITY, 1959–2001

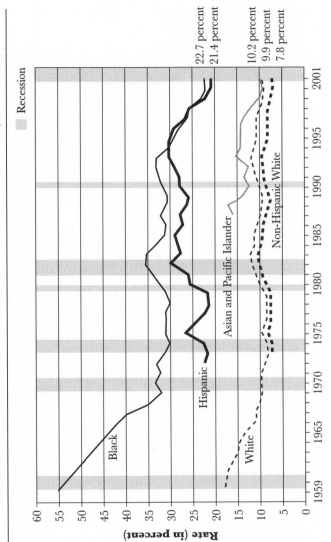

Recession ▨

Note: The data points represent the midpoints of the respective years. The latest recession begin in March 2001. Data for blacks are not available from 1960 to 1965. Data for the other races and Hispanic origin are shown from the first year available. Hispanics may be of any race.

Source: Proctor and Dalaker (2002).

black children. This means that in 2002, more than one of every four Hispanic children and nearly one in every three black children lived in poverty (Proctor and Dalaker, 2003).

Trends in Income Inequality. Both absolute income and the distribution of income in a population are important considerations in determining the health and health care experiences of a population. The U.S. Census Bureau has traditionally used two measures of income distribution to describe the income inequality in the population. The first measure is the **Gini index,** which uses a single statistic (ranging from 0 to 1) to summarize the degree of income dispersion across a population. A score of 0 indicates perfect equality, where everyone receives an equal share of income, and a score of 1 indicates complete inequality, where all of the income is received by a single person.

The second measure of income distribution uses shares of income to describe the level of income inequality in a population. This approach ranks households according to income and divides them into groups of equal population size such as quartiles or quintiles. The aggregate income of the group is then described as a proportion of the total income, such that each quartile or quintile holds a certain percentage of all the income. The more income that a single group holds, the greater the level of income inequality is.

According to both of these measures, income inequality in the United States has increased significantly in the past thirty years. In 1970, the top quintile of households held 43.3 percent of all income, and the top 5 percent of households held 16.6 percent. In 2002, the amount of total income held by the top quintile increased to 49.6 percent and the top 5 percent held about 22 percent. According to the Gini index, the degree of income inequality increased between 1970 and 2002 from 0.394 to 0.462. It is important to note that regardless of the measure used, income inequality increased most substantially between 1970 and 1993, but has risen slowly since then (DeNavas-Walt, Cleveland, et al., 2003).

When defining income inequality as the percentage of total household income received by the poorest 50 percent of households in each state, there are significant differences found among the states. Based on 1990 census data, Louisiana and Mississippi had the highest levels of income inequality. Alabama, Kentucky, and New York also had distinctively high levels. States with the lowest income inequality were New Hampshire, Utah, and Vermont. One theory suggests that income inequality is associated with racial/ethnic diversity and that it is more characteristic of states that originally had a vertically designed, plantation-based economy instead of a horizontally structured, freeholder economy (Hertzman, Power, et al., 2001). Consistent with the results found using the Gini index and shares of income measurements, household income data also showed an increase in income inequality for all states except Alaska between 1980 and 1990 (Kaplan, Pamuk, et al., 1996; Lynch, Kaplan, et al., 1998).

When comparing the inequality rates for the United States to Organization for Economic Cooperation and Development (OECD) countries, the United States has much greater income inequality than most other developed countries. Of the twenty countries ranked highest in human development in the 2002 *Human Development Report* published by the United Nations, the United States had the greatest inequality (a Gini Index coefficient of 0.41). The United Kingdom had the second greatest inequality (.368), followed by Ireland with a Gini coefficient of 0.36. Denmark and Japan had the lowest levels of inequality, with Gini coefficients of 0.25 for both (United Nations Development Program, 2002).

Global distribution of wealth is even more dramatically disproportionate. According to the same United Nations report, the richest 5 percent of the world population has income 114 times higher than that of the poorest 5 percent. The United States earns much of this global wealth. The income for the wealthiest 25 million Americans is equivalent to the aggregate income of the 2 billion poorest people in the world, suggesting significant income inequality among the world's nations. Since the mid-1980s, income inequality measures of differences across countries has risen 20 percent, to just under 0.54. Global income inequality was relatively constant between 1960 and the early 1980s, with an average Gini coefficient of 0.460. After the 1980s, the greater level of inequality in the world has been attributed to recessions among Latin American countries and weaker economies in Eastern Europe and the former Soviet Union in the 1990s.

Trends in Education. Income and education are strongly correlated, such that more highly educated individuals generally earn higher wages. Trends in education, however, vary somewhat from trends in income. The most common measure of education is whether a person has completed high school, and statistics on this measure have changed dramatically over the years. In 1940, only 24.5 percent of the population age twenty-five and over had completed high school. By 1970, high school completion had nearly doubled to 55.2 percent. Since then, even greater increases have occurred, and by 2000 high school completion had increased to 84.2 percent.

Similarly, college completion has accelerated dramatically in the past sixty years. In 1940, only 4.6 percent of the population age twenty-five and over had completed college. By 1970, college completion had more than doubled, to 11.0 percent. Like high school completion, even greater increases occurred in college completion in the thirty years after 1970, more than doubling again by 2002 to 26.7 percent. Years of educational attainment have increased in a slightly less dramatic manner, rising from 8.6 years of education in 1940 to about 12.8 by 2000. This change in years of education suggests there is a growing majority of individuals seeking at least some college education (Stoop, 2004).

Educational attainment is not equally distributed across all demographic groups. In particular, there have been dramatic differences in education across racial/ethnic groups. In 2002, 84.8 percent of whites and 87.4 percent of Asian Americans completed high school or higher, but only 78.7 percent of blacks and 57.0 percent of Hispanics had done so (Kaufman, Alt, et al., 2001). Even greater disparities exist in college education, with rates of completion ranging from 47.2 percent for Asian Americans and 27.2 percent for whites, to 17.0 percent for blacks and 11.1 percent for Hispanics (U.S. Census Bureau, 2001a).

Similar disparities in educational attainment also exist according to gender. Men age twenty-five and over complete college at a rate 3.4 percent higher than the rate for women (28.5 percent versus 25.1 percent), but this disparity is closing with each passing year. Women have now slightly outpaced men in high school graduation rates (84.4 percent versus 83.8 percent), which is the first statistically significant difference in high school completion rates since the 1980s, when men graduated from high schools at higher rates than women. Even more evidence of this progress for women is seen among younger ages, where women ages twenty-five to twenty-nine now complete college at a rate higher than men of the same ages (89.4 percent versus 86.7 percent) (Kaufman, Alt, et al., 2001).

There are also substantial differences in education according to region. In the most general terms, southern states have consistently had lower high school and college completion rates than other regions. States in the Midwest and Northeast have commonly had completion rates well above the national average. Historically, there have been few changes in these regional patterns (see Figures 2.7 and 2.8).

To compare how well the United States ranks globally in education is difficult because of diverse educational systems and variations in census data collected in different countries. Using adult functional literacy rates as a proxy for education, it is interesting to note that 10 to 20 percent of people in most OECD countries are functionally illiterate. Norway and Sweden have the lowest illiteracy rates among the OECD nations, with rates of 8 to 9 percent. In contrast, Ireland, the United Kingdom, and the United States have illiteracy rates greater than 20 percent (United Nations Development Program, 2002).

Trends in Occupation. Occupation is closely tied to income and education. In general, higher education is associated with the ability to obtain higher-level

FIGURE 2.7. HIGH SCHOOL COMPLETION RATES BY STATE, ADULTS TWENTY-FIVE YEARS AND OVER, 2002

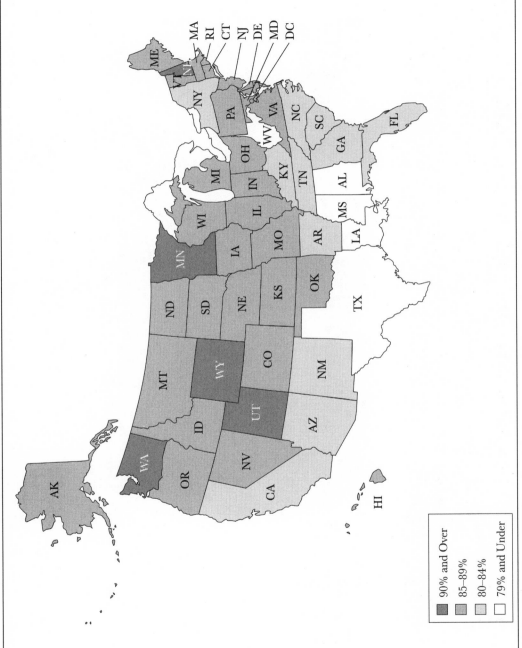

Legend:
- 90% and Over
- 85–89%
- 80–84%
- 79% and Under

Source: U.S. Census Bureau (2003).

FIGURE 2.8. COLLEGE COMPLETION RATES BY STATE, ADULTS TWENTY-FIVE YEARS AND OVER, 2002

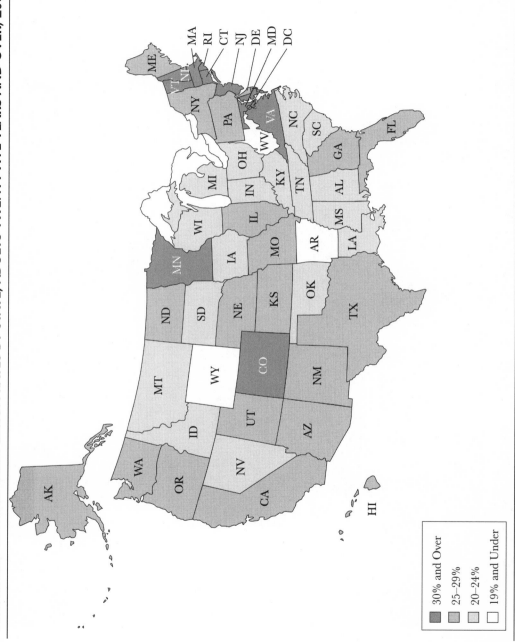

Legend:
- 30% and Over
- 25–29%
- 20–24%
- 19% and Under

Source: U.S. Census Bureau (2003).

occupations with higher salaries and greater benefits. Understanding the trends in employment and occupation is particularly important because occupation plays a role in determining aspects of personal lifestyles and because it is a primary source of health insurance coverage for many Americans.

The unemployment rate in the United States has fluctuated significantly over the years, frequently in response to variations in national economic growth. In 2002, about 5.8 percent of the workforce reported being unemployed, and the average length of unemployment was just about thirteen weeks. This reflects an increase of about 1.8 percent compared to 2000, when the unemployment rate was just 4.0 percent, the lowest rate of unemployment in national history. In the past forty years, the rate of unemployment reached a high of 9.7 percent in 1982, and the longest duration of employment reached a high of about 16.5 weeks in 1995 (U.S. Department of Labor, Bureau of Labor Statistics, 2002).

Relative to other OECD countries, the United States has a lower average unemployment rate. Only 5.8 percent of the U.S. population experienced unemployment in 2002, lower than the OECD average of 6.9 percent. Luxembourg and Austria had the lowest unemployment rates in 2002, with 2.4 percent and 4.1 percent, respectively. The OECD countries with the highest unemployment were the Slovak Republic (19.4 percent) and Spain (11.4 percent) (United Nations Development Program, 2002).

As with income and education, there are differences in unemployment rates across racial/ethnic groups. In general, minorities have higher rates of unemployment than whites, and these disparities have remained relatively consistent over the years. In 2002, the rate of unemployment was 10.2 percent for blacks, 7.4 percent for Hispanics, and only 5.1 percent for whites, all showing increases from their lowest points in 2000. Though substantial differences remained in 2000, these rates reflect a trend of a narrowing gap between minorities and whites in unemployment. Figure 2.9 shows the changes in employment for these groups between 1970 and 2002.

There are also some differences in employment rates across genders. Among labor force participants, men have had slightly lower unemployment rates than women. In 2000, for example, the unemployment rate for males was 3.9 percent compared to 4.1 percent for females. Perhaps more interesting are the gender differences in labor force participation. In the 1970s, the participation rate for males was 79.7 percent but only 43.3 percent for females. By 2000, there were major changes in female participation. The difference between males and females narrowed to only 14.5 percent, with the rate for females reaching 61.1 percent. Marital status also makes a difference in the participation rates of men and women in the labor force. In 2000, the rate for single women was 69.0 percent, and the rate for married women was 61.3 percent. The figures were reversed

FIGURE 2.9. UNEMPLOYMENT RATES BY RACIAL AND ETHNIC GROUP, 1980–2002

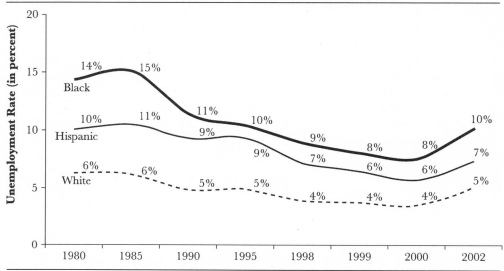

Source: U.S. Department of Labor, Bureau of Labor Statistics (2002).

for men, with single men having a lower rate (73.5 percent) than that for married men (77.3 percent) (U.S. Department of Labor, Bureau of Labor Statistics, 2002).

Unemployment rates are lowest in managerial or professional occupations (1.7 percent) compared to service occupations (5.3 percent) and blue-collar positions (6.3 percent). Technical and administrative support positions, along with production, craft, and repair positions, all have rates of unemployment of 3.6 percent. Not only do individuals in service and blue-collar occupations experience greater rates of unemployment, but the incomes for these individuals (often based on the minimum wage) are shrinking. Adjusting for inflation, the minimum wage has decreased steadily over the past thirty years, dropping from $7.10 per hour in 1970 and $6.48 in 1980 to only $5.15 per hour in 2000. Finally, these jobs are also less likely to offer basic employee benefits. Employer-sponsored health insurance coverage, for example, is available in 79 percent of professional and managerial positions, but only in 74 percent of full-time service and blue-collar positions.

Theoretical Pathways of Socioeconomic Status

Levels of income, education, and occupation together characterize an individual's relative position along the socioeconomic gradient. But by what means does this position or status affect health outcomes and health care experiences?

We present a model (Figure 2.10) that synthesizes the work of Evans, Barer, et al. (1994), Seeman and Crimmins (2001), Starfield and Shi (1999), and researchers from the MacArthur Network on SES and Health (Adler and Ostrove, 1999), to describe potential pathways linking socioeconomic status with disparities in health and health care. In its simplest form, SES is related to health and health care in two ways that have been previously labeled **material deprivation** and lack of **social participation** (Marmot, 2002).

Material deprivation includes access to material goods that are required for good health, including clean water and good sanitation, adequate nutrition and housing, reliable transportation, and a safe and comfortable environment. Social participation includes having time for leisure activity and group participation, having friends or family around for entertainment and support, receiving chances for professional achievement, and ultimately having sufficient opportunities and life control to lead a fulfilling and satisfying life. Without access to material goods and supportive social participation, health may falter, and greater barriers may be experienced in obtaining needed health care services. In the following section, we take a closer look at the pathways linking material deprivation and social participation to population health.

Material Deprivation. Material deprivation is the lack of material resources that enable the protection or promotion of health. These resources also enable a person to obtain adequate health care when faced with ill health. Steady income is fundamental to obtaining clean water and adequate housing, proper nutrition, electricity for warmth, and a safe environment. These factors are most clearly associated with health in developing countries, but they also play an important role in areas of developed countries, such as many rural and inner-city areas of the United States, that experience poverty and deprivation resembling that of developing countries.

In addition to affording basic life necessities, absolute personal income allows the purchase of health insurance coverage and specific health care services. Education and occupation also play an important role in obtaining health insurance coverage and health care. Most people in the United States receive their health insurance coverage through their employer, though recent research has revealed a decline in the percentage of employers offering this benefit, particularly in lower-paying, nonprofessional positions. However, the U.S. government provides safety net health insurance coverage to many low-income individuals; a growing proportion of individuals who do not qualify for safety net coverage and also earn insufficient income to purchase health insurance may experience some of the greatest difficulties in obtaining care.

A unique consideration with regard to SES and health is the likely presence of an income threshold above which simple material deprivation may no longer

FIGURE 2.10. CONCEPTUAL MODEL LINKING SOCIOECONOMIC STATUS WITH HEALTH

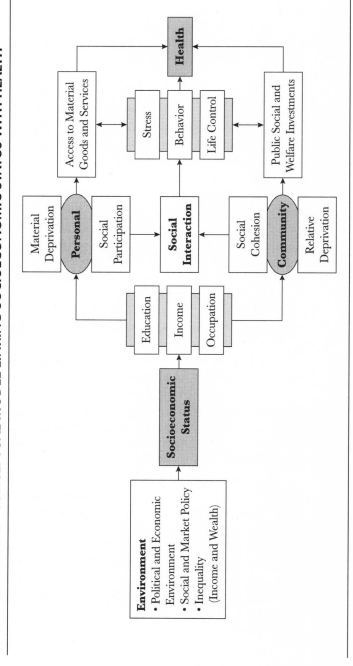

play a primary role in determining health. Above this proposed threshold, people are universally able to afford basic material necessities, and any higher income is less likely to affect or improve health through the purchase of material goods. Interestingly, however, there still exists a stark SES gradient in health above this income threshold, suggesting the presence of SES effects other than material deprivation.

Social Participation. There is substantial debate regarding the correlation of SES and health above the proposed income threshold. Social participation provides a possible explanation for the SES gradient above the income threshold, with greater income being associated with greater social participation. At the individual level, there is substantial evidence of the effects of social participation on health across all levels of income. Social participation includes having time for leisure and group participation, support of family and friends, chances for professional achievement, and sufficient opportunities and control to lead a fulfilling and satisfying life.

Specifically, there are three main mechanisms through which social participation may be correlated with health: the effects of stress and coping, health-related behaviors, and life control. Other mechanisms have been proposed, including reciprocal influences of health on SES, such that being in poor health limits the ability to earn income. There is some evidence of this direction of causality, but this is likely limited to only the most disabling long-term conditions (Adler and Ostrove, 1999).

Social participation links SES to health by providing a protective effect against the deleterious health effects of chronic stress associated with lower incomes. It has been demonstrated that stressful life events or high levels of stress that persist over time result in physical and psychological strains, enhancing vulnerability to infectious diseases, heart disease, cancer, HIV, and depression (Baum, Garofalo, et al., 1999; Kaplan and Manuck, 1999). There is also substantial evidence to suggest that these strains can be reduced or even reversed when effective coping mechanisms are present (Taylor, Repetti, et al., 1997; Taylor and Seeman, 1999). Coping mechanisms can be individual coping behaviors or skills, or they can be buffers such as social support from family and friends. Therefore, the lack of social participation that may be associated with lower income may also weaken the ability of low-SES individuals to cope with stress, placing health at even greater risk.

The second mechanism by which social participation links SES with health is the presence of socioeconomic differences in deleterious health-related behaviors. Extensive research has documented an SES gradient in health risk behaviors, such that individuals of lower SES are more likely to smoke, drink excessively, and participate in less physical activity than individuals of higher SES (Colhoun, Ben-Shlomo, et al., 1997; Marmot, 1998; Winkleby, Cubbin, et al., 1999; Seeman and Crimmins, 2001). Why these differences exist is not entirely clear, but one likely hypothesis is that risk behavior is a negative coping response to the chronic stress that is more common in lower-SES groups (Gallo and Matthews, 1999, 2003). If this hypothesis is true, there may be a particularly important role for social participation in protecting against the adoption of health risk behaviors. In fact, social support is associated with lower rates of smoking and drinking, better nutrition, and higher rates of health prevention behavior and seeking of preventive care (Franks, Campbell, et al., 1992; Yarcheski, Mahon, et al., 2001, 2003; Ross and Mirowsky, 2002; Geckova, van Dijk, et al., 2003).

The third mechanism linking SES with health is the presence of socioeconomic differences in feelings of personal control over life circumstances. Research has shown that populations with low SES are more likely to lack a sense of control over their life, particularly with regard to the daily work environment. Studies have shown that SES differences exist in employment security, opportunities for occupational advancement, control over work, and the variety and pace of work (Marmot and Theorell, 1988; Steptoe and Appels, 1989; Marmot, Smith, et al., 1991; Taylor and Seeman, 1999; Levi, Bartley, et al., 2000; Steenland, Fine, et al., 2000). Moreover, there is a large body of empirical literature showing that these aspects of control in the work environment are related to cardiovascular disease and other measures of health (Syme, 1989; Karasek, 1990; Seeman and Lewis, 1995; Marmot, Bosma, et al., 1997; Lundberg, 1999). In addition, there is evidence that a lack of social support at work, when coupled with high demands and low control, substantially increases health risks (Johnson and Hall, 1995). It is plausible that these feelings of control affect health through additional stress or health-related behavior mechanisms, making it difficult to delineate the separate effects of each.

Community and Relative Deprivation. So far, we have considered the pathways between individual SES and health that operate through either the ability to purchase goods and services (material deprivation) or through the interrelated elements of social participation (such as stress, health behaviors, and control). Interestingly, a growing body of literature suggests that individual determinants of health have their community-level counterparts and that these may play an even larger role in determining the health of a population.

The first mechanism by which community-level socioeconomic inequalities may be associated with health is through community-based material deprivation (sometimes termed *relative deprivation*). With community-based deprivation, the socioeconomic characteristics of the community play an important role in determining health above and beyond the effects of personal income. A handful of studies have demonstrated this relationship between disadvantaged communities and poorer health outcomes, even after controlling for individual-level demographic and socioeconomic factors (Diez-Roux, Nieto, et al., 1997; LeClere, Rogers, et al., 1998; Smith, Hart, et al., 1998; Diez-Roux, Merkin, et al., 2001; Lee and Cubbin, 2002).

Exploring the potential pathways between community deprivation and health, studies have shown that both adults and youth living in disadvantaged communities have poorer dietary habits, less physical activity, higher rates of smoking, and greater exposure to environmental risks compared to those living in more advantaged communities (Diez-Roux, Nieto, et al., 1997, 1999; Smith, Hart, et al., 1998; Yen and Kaplan, 1998; Evans and Kantrowitz, 2002; Lee and Cubbin, 2002). Although these intermediary factors provide an explanation for the relationship between community disadvantage and health, they fail to offer an explanation for why these higher-risk factors occur in disadvantaged communities.

No one would dispute that absolute poverty is bad for health. But a relatively new and major change in thinking about the health effects of socioeconomic status is revealed in evidence showing that mortality rates in a population are strongly related to the degree of inequality (typically income) in a population (Ben-Shlomo, White, et al., 1996; Kaplan, Pamuk, et al., 1996; Wilkinson, 1996; Lynch, Kaplan, et al., 1998; Lynch, Smith, et al. 2000). Such findings have been reported in the United States, the United Kingdom, Canada, and a dozen or more European and Latin American developed and developing countries. Repeated corroboration that inequitable distribution of resources in a population is associated with poorer health has prompted research into the mechanisms underlying this relationship.

Social Cohesion. One frequently proposed explanation of the relationship between inequality and health is the intermediary role of **social cohesion** (Kawachi and Kennedy, 1997; Kawachi, 1999). Social cohesion is the community-level equivalent of social participation, and is used to characterize social relationships on a larger scale. Social cohesion (also often referred to as *social capital*) reflects concrete elements of the social fabric—such as the forming of associations, church groups, and political organizations—and also less tangible aspects of social interaction—such as interpersonal trust and community norms—that shape individual identities, norms, beliefs, and practices (Coleman, 1990; Collins, 1994; Kawachi and Kennedy, 1997; Kawachi, 1999; Macinko and Starfield, 2001; Lochner, Kawachi, et al., 2003; Subramanian, Lochner, et al., 2003).

There is abundant literature suggesting that as social status differences in society and community deprivation increase, the quality of social relations deteriorates. Circumstantial evidence was derived from analyses of a number of countries (including Japan and the Kerala state in India) that were found to be unusually egalitarian, socially cohesive, and healthy (Wilkinson, 1996). Additional studies have confirmed this pattern, showing that areas with greater inequality and deprivation are less socially cohesive: they have lower trust, less participation in community and civic groups, greater hostility, and more violent crime (Hseih and Pugh, 1993; Putnam, Leonardi, et al., 1993; Williams, Feaganes, et al., 1995; Kawachi and Kennedy, 1997; Kennedy, Kawachi, et al. 1998). Moreover, income inequality has been related to mortality from homicides and alcohol-related causes, both of which are health outcomes that have strong social roots, which suggests that social mechanisms are involved (Wilkinson, 1997).

The evidence linking social cohesion to health outcomes is still somewhat sparse, reflecting the relatively recent application of this concept to the field of population health. It is now well established that socially isolated individuals are at an increased risk of mortality, reduced survival after major illness, and poor mental health (House, Robbins, et al., 1982; House, Landis, et al., 1988; Berkman, 1995). Two studies, however, have strongly linked social cohesion at the community level to health outcomes (Kawachi and Kennedy, 1997; Kawachi, 1999), and it is plausible that social cohesion affects health through the same mechanisms through which social participation operates at the individual level, such as anxiety and stress, health-related behaviors, and life control (Wilkinson, 1999).

There have been several key criticisms of the community deprivation and income inequality determinants of health theories. One of these recognizes the close association between wide income disparities in SES and lower public investments in social welfare, education, and health care (Kaplan, Pamuk, et al., 1996; Ross, Wolfson, et al., 2000). Thus, disparities in health and health care are more attributable to the public health and welfare safety nets in place to assist those of lower SES than to any psychosocial mechanisms of inequality. While not refuting the effects of income inequality, additional critiques have pointed to the importance of including race, the political context, and class relations in analyses of social inequalities in health (Muntaner, Lynch, et al., 1999; Williams, 1999; Navarro and Shi, 2001).

Health Care System. Although the literature indicates some skepticism as to the overall contribution of medical care to the improvement of population health worldwide (McKeown, 1976), there is evidence that access to certain types of medical care may be more beneficial than others in reducing a country's overall burden of disease (Starfield, 1994, 1998). In particular, **primary care,** defined as "that level of a health service system that provides entry into the system . . . provides person-focused care over time, provides care for all but very uncommon or unusual conditions, and coordinates or integrates care provided elsewhere or by others" (Starfield, 1998, p. 19), has been shown to have an important impact on health outcomes for some of the most common medical problems. Furthermore, several studies have demonstrated that the level of primary care orientation (as opposed to physician specialists) has a statistically significant effect on improving life chances, particularly among the disadvantaged (Shi, 1992, 1994, 1995).

Moreover, studies have found that greater access to primary health care can mediate some of the effect of the SES differentials (Shi, Starfield, et al., 1999; Shi and Starfield, 2001; Shi, Macinko, et al., 2003). Shi, Macinko, et al. (2003), in an ecological study in the United States, found that income inequality and primary care (measured by primary care physicians per ten thousand population) exerted a strong and statistically significant influence on state-level mortality and life expectancy. Path analysis suggested that primary care might overcome some of the adverse health impacts of income inequality on population health.

In a multilevel model including individual, community, and state-level variables, Shi and Starfield (2000) present stronger evidence for the ability of primary care to partially attenuate the adverse health effects of income inequalities. In multivariate analyses, income inequality and primary care were significantly associated with self-rated health (odds ratio [OR] = 1.33 and 1.02, respectively; $p <$ 0.01). Primary care significantly attenuated the effects of income inequality on self-reported health status. Adding individual-level SES variables somewhat reduced the magnitude of the association between income inequality, primary care, and self-reported health. The study found that while controlling for all covariates, an increase of one primary care physician per ten thousand population was associated with a 2 percent increase in the odds of reporting excellent or good health.

Although the authors do not propose any specific mechanisms, there may be several possible explanations for the observed relationship between income inequality, primary care, and health. One mechanism is that access to a regular source of primary care may improve prevention and early detection of diseases such as complications of hypertension (Shea, Misra, et al., 1992). It may be that the preventive aspects of primary care reverse some of the negative health effects of inequalities because these effects may work through long-term stressors that are likely to develop into chronic ailments. Furthermore, because primary care implies person-oriented, longitudinal, and first-contact care, it is expected that in the best of circumstances, individuals living in areas with high levels of primary care providers may develop an important social tie with their primary care provider. And fourth, primary care may function as a sensitive measure of social transfer that allows individuals to compensate for their relative income deprivation with an essential social service.

Health Insurance

The United States is the only developed nation that does *not* guarantee its citizens access to health care through a system of **universal health coverage.** In 2000, the World Health Organization released a report ranking countries on the quality of their health systems (see Exhibit 2.1). The report placed the United States in the thirty-seventh spot for health system performance and seventy-second for health outcome performance (out of 191), primarily because of its failure to ensure access to care for the uninsured and because of the relatively low life expectancy and high infant mortality despite the fact that the United States spends more than all the other nations on health care (World Health Organization, 2000). Although there is substantial controversy surrounding the validity of the methodology of the report (Navarro, 2000; Almeida, Braveman, et al., 2001; Braveman, Starfield, et al. 2001), few have contested the placement of the United States far below most other developed countries that provide universal health insurance coverage.

Historical Development of the Importance of Health Insurance Coverage

Policymakers have not ignored the irony of spending more than any other industrialized nation on health care without providing universal coverage. There have been numerous attempts by various presidents to establish universal coverage. Administrations under Presidents Truman, Kennedy, Nixon, and most recently Clinton have all tried and failed (Bodenheimer, 2003). There are two likely reasons that a universal coverage system has not been established in the United States. First, a majority of the American public and the politicians who represent them have not decided that health care access is a fundamental right of U.S. residents. The belief in health care as a given personal "right" that is the foundation for universal coverage in other countries is not well enough established in the United States (Brown and Sparer, 2003; Rekindling Reform Steering Committee, 2003). Moreover, inherent in American culture is the belief that large, government-run programs are inefficient (Tooker, 2003).

However, despite the doubts of some American voters and policymakers, the tragedy of almost 45 million people consistently without health insurance continues to motivate the nation toward improving affordable access to health care. Another barrier to establishing universal coverage is determining the best way to extend service to the uninsured. Policymakers are currently mired down by the complex array of solutions including public programs, such as the extension of Medicaid and SCHIP and funding for community health centers, and private programs including employer mandates and tax credit plans (Bodenheimer, 2003).

EXHIBIT 2.1. WORLD HEALTH ORGANIZATION RANKINGS OF INTERNATIONAL HEALTH SYSTEMS

	Performance on Health Level (DALE)					Overall Performance			
Rank	Uncertainty Interval	Member State	Index	Uncertainty Interval	Rank	Uncertainty Interval	Member State	Index	Uncertainty Interval
1	1 – 5	Oman	0.992	0.975 – 1.000	1	1 – 5	France	0.994	0.982 – 1.000
2	1 – 4	Malta	0.989	0.968 – 1.000	2	1 – 5	Italy	0.991	0.978 – 1.000
3	2 – 7	Italy	0.976	0.957 – 0.994	3	1 – 6	San-Marino	0.988	0.973 – 1.000
4	2 – 7	France	0.974	0.953 – 0.994	4	2 – 7	Andorra	0.982	0.966 – 0.997
5	2 – 7	San-Marino	0.971	0.949 – 0.998	5	3 – 7	Malta	0.978	0.965 – 0.993
6	3 – 8	Spain	0.968	0.948 – 0.989	6	2 – 11	Singapore	0.973	0.947 – 0.998
7	4 – 9	Andorra	0.964	0.942 – 0.980	7	4 – 8	Spain	0.972	0.959 – 0.985
8	3 – 12	Jamaica	0.956	0.928 – 0.986	8	4 – 14	Oman	0.961	0.938 – 0.985
9	7 – 11	Japan	0.945	0.926 – 0.963	9	7 – 12	Austria	0.959	0.946 – 0.972
10	8 – 15	Saudi Arabia	0.936	0.915 – 0.959	10	8 – 11	Japan	0.957	0.948 – 0.965
11	9 – 13	Greece	0.936	0.920 – 0.951	11	8 – 12	Norway	0.955	0.947 – 0.964
12	9 – 16	Monaco	0.930	0.908 – 0.948	12	10 – 15	Portugal	0.945	0.931 – 0.958
13	10 – 15	Portugal	0.929	0.911 – 0.945	13	10 – 16	Monaco	0.943	0.929 – 0.957
14	10 – 15	Singapore	0.929	0.909 – 0.942	14	13 – 19	Greece	0.933	0.921 – 0.945
15	13 – 17	Austria	0.914	0.896 – 0.931	15	12 – 20	Iceland	0.932	0.917 – 0.948
16	13 – 23	United Arab Emirates	0.907	0.883 – 0.932	16	14 – 21	Luxembourg	0.928	0.914 – 0.942
17	14 – 22	Morocco	0.906	0.886 – 0.925	17	14 – 21	Netherlands	0.928	0.914 – 0.942
18	16 – 23	Norway	0.897	0.878 – 0.914	18	16 – 21	United Kingdom	0.925	0.913 – 0.937
19	17 – 24	Netherlands	0.893	0.875 – 0.911	19	14 – 22	Ireland	0.924	0.909 – 0.939
20	15 – 31	Solomon Islands	0.892	0.863 – 0.920	20	17 – 24	Switzerland	0.916	0.903 – 0.930
21	18 – 26	Sweden	0.890	0.870 – 0.907	21	18 – 24	Belgium	0.915	0.903 – 0.926
22	19 – 28	Cyprus	0.885	0.865 – 0.898	22	14 – 29	Colombia	0.910	0.881 – 0.939
23	19 – 30	Chile	0.884	0.864 – 0.903	23	20 – 26	Sweden	0.908	0.893 – 0.921
24	21 – 28	United Kingdom	0.883	0.866 – 0.900	24	16 – 30	Cyprus	0.906	0.879 – 0.932
25	18 – 32	Costa Rica	0.882	0.859 – 0.898	25	22 – 27	Germany	0.902	0.890 – 0.914
26	21 – 31	Switzerland	0.879	0.860 – 0.891	26	22 – 32	Saudi Arabia	0.894	0.872 – 0.916
27	21 – 31	Iceland	0.879	0.861 – 0.897	27	23 – 33	United Arab Emirates	0.886	0.861 – 0.911
28	23 – 30	Belgium	0.878	0.860 – 0.894	28	26 – 32	Israel	0.884	0.870 – 0.897
29	23 – 33	Venezuela, Bolivarian Republic of	0.873	0.853 – 0.891	29	18 – 39	Morocco	0.882	0.834 – 0.925
30	23 – 37	Bahrain	0.867	0.843 – 0.890	30	27 – 32	Canada	0.881	0.868 – 0.894

Source: World Health Organization (2000).

National Trends in Public and Private Health Insurance Coverage

Before the 1960s, the U.S. government was mostly uninterested in assisting its citizens with the ability to access health care. In 1965, however, a monumental change occurred. As part of President Lyndon Johnson's Great Society, the federal government enacted two major health insurance programs that would help the poor (**Medicaid**) and the elderly (**Medicare**) obtain care. These **entitlement programs** have expanded over the years into major federal and state efforts, so much so that they have consistently occupied the top spots in the federal budget. In 1997, the federal government took the next major incremental step toward universal coverage by enacting a program to provide health insurance coverage for children who are from low-income families but were not categorically poor. After discussing demographic trends in insurance coverage, we review these programs separately. The promotion of community health centers for the uninsured and medically underserved will be discussed in Chapter Five.

In 2002, an estimated 15.2 percent of the population (43.6 million people) under age sixty-five was without health insurance coverage during the entire year, up from 14.6 percent of the population in 2001, reflecting an increase of about 2.4 million people from the previous year (Mills and Bhandari, 2003). The percentage of the population with no coverage has varied somewhat over the past fifteen years and responded primarily to changes in the economy (since most citizens receive their health insurance coverage through their employer) and to expansions of public coverage through national programs. In 1987, 12.9 percent of the population was uninsured, but this increased steadily to a peak of 16.3 percent uninsured in 1998. Since then, there have been steady improvements in the economy, and as new public insurance programs like SCHIP began their full implementation, the result has been a decrease in the number of uninsured.

The problem of lacking insurance coverage has evolved into an issue primarily among the working poor. These individuals are generally employed in low-paying jobs that do not offer health insurance coverage or enable individuals to purchase insurance, but also produce earnings too high to qualify the individual for government assistance in programs like Medicaid. So while the United States has insured the poorest individuals, there are still many families living on meager wages for which health coverage remains out of reach. Figure 2.11 shows the dramatic picture of uninsured rates among those who are employed.

Because health insurance coverage is closely tied to education, occupation, and income, there are substantial demographic disparities in insurance coverage and type (Figure 2.12). For example, Hispanics were the most likely racial/ethnic group to be uninsured (33.2 percent). Blacks and Asians had similar rates of being uninsured (19.0 percent and 18.2 percent, respectively), which were much higher than the rate for whites (10.0 percent) (Mills and Bhandari, 2003). Coverage rates

FIGURE 2.11. UNINSURED RATES AMONG THE WORKING POOR

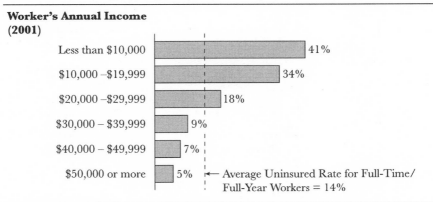

Worker's Annual Income (2001)

Source: Kaiser Commission on Medicaid and the Uninsured (2003, p. 19).

also vary across geographical areas and reflect some of the distribution of racial/ethnic groups and income levels in various states (see Figure 2.13).

Despite the presence of Medicaid and SCHIP safety net insurance programs, 30.7 percent of the poor (10.1 million) were still uninsured in 2002 (Mills and Bhandari, 2003). Among the near-poor (those with family income greater than the poverty level but less than 125 percent of poverty), 27.9 percent (or 3.5 million people) were uninsured, highlighting the need to fill important gaps in insurance coverage. Finally, in the general population, young adults eighteen to twenty-four years old were more likely than other age groups to be uninsured (28.1 percent). This is attributable to the transitional period between when insurance coverage through a parent generally ends and individual employment and insurance coverage begins.

Medicaid. Medicaid is a combined federal and state initiative to provide health insurance for the poor. Authority over the Medicaid program is somewhat complex, with the federal government paying 50 to 80 percent of the costs of the program, depending on the state and its per capita income. Following broad national guidelines, the states are allowed to establish the eligibility for the program, the range of covered services, and the rate of payment to providers for those services. Medicaid was initially tied to state welfare programs (to simplify administration of the program), but this was undone recently so that being poor no longer automatically makes a person eligible for Medicaid. In fact, most people become

FIGURE 2.12. INDIVIDUALS WITHOUT HEALTH INSURANCE COVERAGE, 2001

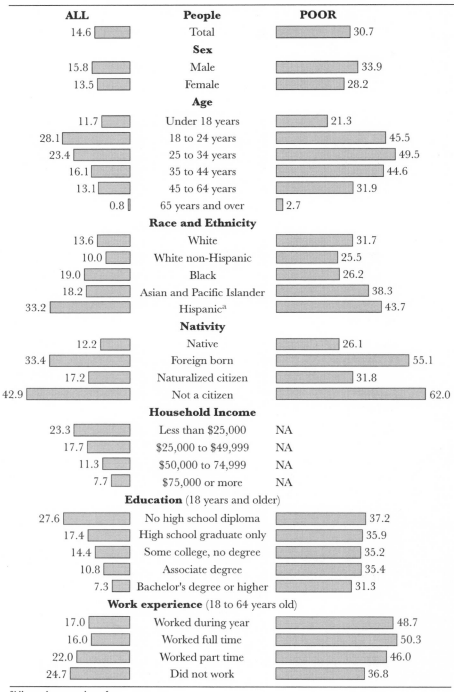

ALL	People	POOR
	Total	
14.6	Total	30.7
	Sex	
15.8	Male	33.9
13.5	Female	28.2
	Age	
11.7	Under 18 years	21.3
28.1	18 to 24 years	45.5
23.4	25 to 34 years	49.5
16.1	35 to 44 years	44.6
13.1	45 to 64 years	31.9
0.8	65 years and over	2.7
	Race and Ethnicity	
13.6	White	31.7
10.0	White non-Hispanic	25.5
19.0	Black	26.2
18.2	Asian and Pacific Islander	38.3
33.2	Hispanic[a]	43.7
	Nativity	
12.2	Native	26.1
33.4	Foreign born	55.1
17.2	Naturalized citizen	31.8
42.9	Not a citizen	62.0
	Household Income	
23.3	Less than $25,000	NA
17.7	$25,000 to $49,999	NA
11.3	$50,000 to 74,999	NA
7.7	$75,000 or more	NA
	Education (18 years and older)	
27.6	No high school diploma	37.2
17.4	High school graduate only	35.9
14.4	Some college, no degree	35.2
10.8	Associate degree	35.4
7.3	Bachelor's degree or higher	31.3
	Work experience (18 to 64 years old)	
17.0	Worked during year	48.7
16.0	Worked full time	50.3
22.0	Worked part time	46.0
24.7	Did not work	36.8

[a]Hispanics may be of any race.

Source: Mills and Bhandari (2003).

FIGURE 2.13. UNINSURED RATES AMONG THE NONELDERLY BY STATE, 2001–2002

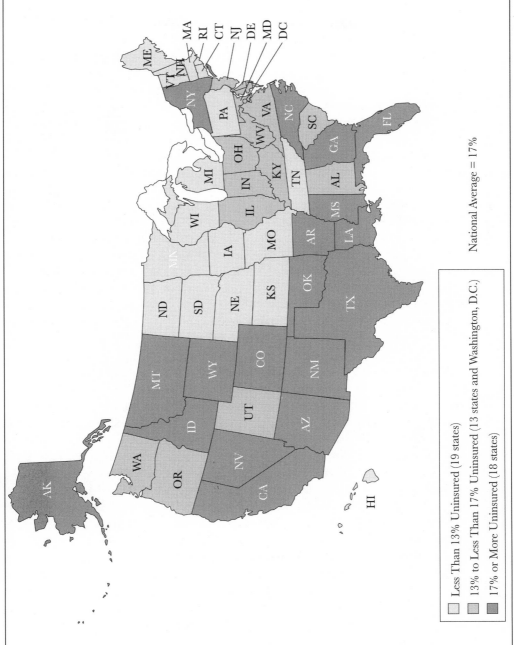

National Average = 17%

☐ Less Than 13% Uninsured (19 states)
☐ 13% to Less Than 17% Uninsured (13 states and Washington, D.C.)
☐ 17% or More Uninsured (18 states)

Source: Kaiser Commission on Medicaid and the Uninsured (2003).

eligible for the program by meeting a specific criterion: advanced age, blindness, disability, or membership in a single-parent family with dependent children. Within this rubric, states may set very different eligibility criteria (Iglehart, 1999; Rosenbaum, 2002). Because Medicaid is partially funded by state governments, eligibility and other factors are dependent on the state's economic success, as well as the percentage of federal matching funds to help expand Medicaid services and enrollment (Kronebusch, 2001).

In 2002, approximately 11.6 percent of Americans received health insurance coverage through the Medicaid program, up from 11.2 percent in 2000 (Mills and Bhandari, 2003). Among poor individuals, nearly 40.5 percent (13.3 million people) were covered by Medicaid. Overall, there has been little variation in the proportion of people covered by Medicaid in the past fifteen years. For example, the greatest variation in coverage rates was between 1987 (8.4 percent covered) and 1993 (12.2 percent covered). There are differences in Medicaid enrollment according to race and ethnicity. Blacks (23.1 percent) and Hispanics (20.2 percent) were more likely than whites (7.7 percent) and Asians (10.4 percent) to be covered by Medicaid. Children are more likely than adults to be covered by Medicaid (23.9 percent), although this too varies by race/ethnicity. In 2002, more than one of every three black and Hispanic children (41.2 percent and 37.3 percent, respectively) was covered by Medicaid compared to only 15.5 percent of white and 18.1 percent of Asian and Pacific Islander children.

Medicare. By the time Medicare was enacted in 1965, the legislative contributors envisioned the combined programs of Medicaid and Medicare as only a preliminary step toward achieving the inevitable goal of universal health insurance coverage. Although this goal has never materialized, Medicare alone has become the nation's single largest payer for medical care services, covering about 40 million beneficiaries. Most of these recipients are over sixty-five years of age, but the architects of the program included eligibility for two smaller categorical groups: those who are permanently disabled and those with end-stage renal disease.

Medicare is financed through a form of social insurance that requires employers and employees to contribute to a fund that finances the coverage for those who are currently enrolled in the program. Medicare offers two major benefit categories: Part A, which covers hospital and limited long-term care costs, and Part B, which covers physician services and most other ambulatory care services. Those who are eligible for Medicare are automatically enrolled in Part A and are offered the opportunity to purchase Part B through monthly premiums (Iglehart, 1999). While the U.S. Congress in 2004 passed a prescription drug bill to pay for prescription services under Medicare, this bill remains extremely controversial and may be subject to additional amendments and substantial changes.

Because Medicare is universally available after age sixty-five, there are few differences in coverage rates across racial or socioeconomic groups. There are, however, challenges to maintaining the solvency of the program (Boccuti and Moon, 2003). Since its creation, spending in this program has increased by a factor of ten (to nearly $2.2 billion in 2000), and the eligible population has increased by about 14 million beneficiaries. Predicted continuing growth of the elderly population, coupled with increasing rates of chronic illness among the elderly, is expected to place considerable strain on the Medicare program. In 1997, Congress opened the program more substantially to managed care plans in order to contain costs, but due to low reimbursement rates and substantial administrative burden, participation was weak, and many managed care organizations (MCOs) have abandoned the program (Iglehart, 1999; Henry J. Kaiser Family Foundation, 2001).

State Children's Health Insurance Program. Despite the large safety net role of Medicaid, children were continuing to account for a large proportion of the uninsured in the early 1990s. Recognizing this and building on the work of several states, including Massachusetts, that had successfully and inexpensively expanded coverage to children (McDonough, Hager, et al., 1997), the federal government passed the State Children's Health Insurance Program as part of the Balanced Budget Act of 1997. The program provides about $40 billion for states to expand coverage to children in low-income families. Within broad federal guidelines, SCHIP allowed states the choice of expanding coverage through the Medicaid program, through a new child health insurance program developed by the state, or a combination of both (Rosenbaum, Johnson, et al., 1998). As of 2001, seventeen states had chosen to expand Medicaid coverage, sixteen created a new child health program, and eighteen chose to implement a combination. By 2002, coverage was available for children in families whose income was 200 percent of the federal poverty level or higher in thirty-nine states.

In 2001, SCHIP was providing comprehensive insurance coverage to 4.6 million previously uninsured children. This number represents an increase of about 38 percent from the number of children covered in 2000 (3.3 million), and nearly double the number of children originally predicted to have been covered. By 2001, four states had obtained permission to use some SCHIP funds to insure parents of eligible children, in order to spur enrollment and improve the retention of children in the program. The four states—Minnesota, New Jersey, Rhode Island, and Wisconsin—additionally enrolled over 230,000 adults as part of the SCHIP funds in 2001. Because many states had not spent their allocated funds, there has been some congressional discussion about reducing SCHIP funding in the coming years (Park and Greenstein, 2002).

Theoretical Pathways of Health Insurance Coverage

We present a model (Figure 2.14) that synthesizes a growing body of literature on the role of health insurance coverage in supporting health and determining experiences in the health care system. With the exception of individuals living in close proximity to free health care clinics or community health centers, the uninsured are particularly vulnerable to financial barriers in accessing health care. Once a person is insured, there are three mechanisms by which insurance may be related to health and health care experiences: (1) health plan policies may affect care-seeking and cost-sharing behaviors of beneficiaries, (2) providers' incentives and reimbursement strategies may influence provider behavior, and (3) perceptions of health insurance plans may create feelings of stigma and affect the use of services and reports of quality.

Health Plan Policies. Since 1950, insurance companies have developed a variety of plans and strategies that implement a range of care-seeking and cost-sharing policies that are intended to improve care and reduce costs simultaneously. Plans range from **fee-for-service** (FFS) coverage (which pays for each service rendered), to a variety of prepaid health plans (which generally pay a specified monthly amount to a selected provider to care for all of a patient's health care needs). The most common prepaid plans are **health maintenance organizations** (HMOs), point of service (POS) plans, and preferred provider organizations (PPOs). These prepaid plans, referred to categorically as managed care, often combine into a single organization owned by the insurance company that contracts with the providers and manages the health care facilities. **Managed care organizations** (MCOs) have been on the rise since the late 1970s and currently cover about 90 percent of the population. Among these MCO enrollees, 26 percent are enrolled in an HMO, 52 percent are in PPOs, and 18 percent are in POS plans (Rabin, 2002).

Many MCOs and some FFS plans have adopted a range of care-seeking policies that may affect access to and quality of health care. The most common policies include **gatekeeping,** where a beneficiary is required to seek primary care and obtain referrals for specialty care only from a preselected provider. Another common policy is to require that beneficiaries seek care only within a network of health plan providers. While such policies are intended to improve the quality and efficiency of health care by improving coordination between providers and eliminating duplication of effort, some concern has been raised about unnecessarily limiting or restricting access to particular primary care and specialty care services.

Despite a vast literature on the effects of managed care, the evidence is mixed on how health plan policies affect access to care and quality. Compared with FFS plans, MCO plans with gatekeeping and network restrictions generally have more

FIGURE 2.14. CONCEPTUAL MODEL LINKING HEALTH INSURANCE COVERAGE WITH HEALTH CARE EXPERIENCES

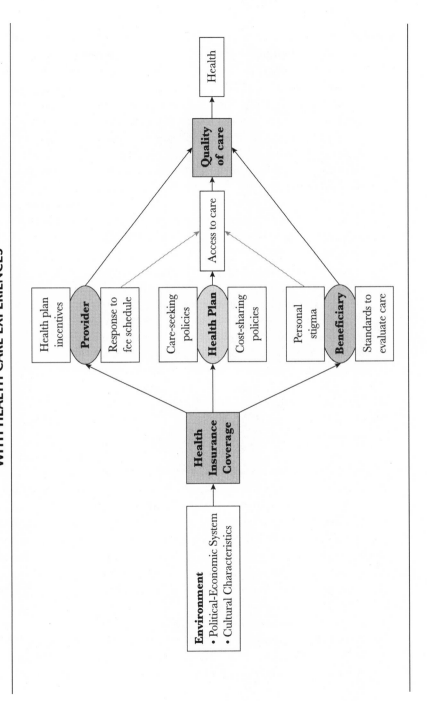

physician office visits per beneficiary, less use of expensive procedures and tests, and greater provision of preventive services, but also poorer patient-provider relationships and lower patient satisfaction (Szilagyi, Rodewald, et al., 1993; Miller and Luft, 1994, 1997, 2002; Safran, Tarlov, et al., 1994; Starfield, Cassady, et al., 1998; Szilagyi, 1998; Safran, Rogers, et al., 2000; Stevens and Shi, 2002b). Although a handful of studies have shown that these care-seeking policies reduce the use of specialty care by restricting direct access to these providers, the debate is far from over (Halm, Causino, et al., 1997; Forrest, Glade, et al., 1999; Ferris, Perrin, et al., 2001; Ferris, Chang, et al., 2002). Moreover, because most states have used managed care to serve an extensive proportion of their Medicaid populations, there is considerable concern about whether MCOs make care sufficiently accessible to these vulnerable populations (Hughes, Newacheck, et al., 1995; Deal and Shiono, 1998; Fox, Limb, et al., 2000; Phillips, Mayer, et al., 2000; Draper, Hurley, et al., 2004).

Health plans generally require that beneficiaries share some portion of the costs of care, through premiums, deductibles, or copayments, or a combination of these. Although contributions are usually fairly small, they serve the purpose of making consumers sensitive to the costs of care and have been shown to reduce use of services significantly. Though this may reduce some costs for health insurance plans, cost sharing has been shown to reduce use of needed services in addition to unnecessary care (Leibowitz, Manning, et al., 1985; Valdez, Brook, et al., 1985; Anderson, Brook, et al., 1991). In response, Medicaid has a regulation that does not allow any patient cost sharing, state SCHIP programs have very low cost sharing (if any at all), and many MCOs and FFS plans have eliminated service costs for the receipt of preventive care.

Health Plan Influences on Providers. Not only do health plans place restrictions on care seeking and cost sharing for beneficiaries, but some managed care plans and their variants place similar restrictions on providers. Though not exactly restrictions, there are a handful of incentives and reimbursement mechanisms that may influence the behaviors of providers in both positive and negative ways. Some MCOs offer providers financial bonuses for limiting the number of referrals or for seeing more patients to reduce costs or increase revenue. Other plans offer education or systems of peer review that are intended to improve the quality of care. Studies have indeed found that incentives to increase productivity or limit referrals may compromise patient care (Barr, 1995; Mechanic and Schlesinger, 1996; Grumbach, Osmond, et al., 1998; Williams, Zaslavsky, et al., 1999). The main criticism of this approach is that most physicians are not able to remember the incentives attached to each patient. But this finding has at least been debunked by research showing that the presence of any health plan incentive increases the perception of pressure to alter services for patients (Hadley, Mitchell, et al., 1999; Mitchell, Hadley, et al., 2000).

The most common incentive that MCOs use to influence the behavior of primary care physicians is reimbursement through **capitation,** that is, paying a physician a specified monthly amount to provide all the necessary care for a particular patient. Approximately 60 percent of HMOs reimburse primary care physicians using this mechanism (Dalzell, 2002). From the perspective of the health plan, shifting the financial risk of care to providers helps predict and stabilize the MCOs expenditures. For the provider, this helps stabilize income (albeit capitation rates are generally low) but also places the provider in an awkward position of needing to provide all necessary care for a patient or losing personal income. The more care the provider refers, the less income he or she takes home. From the perspective of the patient, knowledge of this provider role may reduce patient trust in the physician and inhibit development of the patient-provider relationship.

Reimbursement is also a factor for physicians providing services to Medicaid beneficiaries. From 1997 to 2001, the proportion of physicians serving Medicaid patients decreased by about 2 percent (Perloff, Kletke, et al., 1987, 1995; Norton and Zuckerman, 2000; Cunningham, 2002). Physician surveys show that the primary reason for decreasing Medicaid service is low reimbursement rates. When Medicaid payment rates lag too far behind private insurance or Medicare payments, physicians stop accepting new Medicaid patients. It is interesting to note that physicians in areas of high market saturation are more willing to maintain all or less limited Medicaid services (Tooker, 2003).

Health Plan Influences on Beneficiaries.

Health Plan Influences on Beneficiaries. Although Medicaid and SCHIP provide health insurance coverage to many low-income families, some advocacy groups have recognized the possible presence of stigma created by the long-standing correlation between Medicaid and welfare programs. Not much research has been conducted on this issue, but it is plausible to recognize that beneficiaries of such programs for low-income families may have some reservations about seeking care for fear of unfair judgment about their socioeconomic position.

In the same regard, it has been proposed that beneficiaries of public programs may be less likely to voice concerns about their experiences in medical care. Researchers have argued that because these beneficiaries are paying very little for their coverage, they may not feel they have a right to evaluate the care they receive negatively. Again, this has not been well researched, but does suggest some caution when interpreting ratings of health care quality or satisfaction with care among beneficiaries in public programs.

Multiple Risk Factors

Vulnerability characteristics or risk factors, while having independent influences on both health status and health care access and quality, tend to be very closely associated. Although most of this chapter has been devoted to describing these individual risk factors and how they affect a range of health care access, quality, and health status outcomes, it is not trivial to discuss how the risk factors we have studied tie together, overlap, and often recycle themselves across decades in populations and families.

One very simplified model demonstrates the linkage between minority race/ethnicity, low SES, and health insurance coverage (see Figure 2.15). This model incorporates some additional risk factors as stepping-stones or bridges between the three main risks, highlighting an important point: that there is a range of other risk factors for poor health care access and health status that could be appropriately addressed in this book. Although this book attempts to be as comprehensive as possible with regard to the range of risk factors, addressing more than a handful of risks in the context of this review is not feasible to allow sufficient detail and focus.

The generic model can be interpreted as follows: because of a long history of social segregation and exclusion from educational resources, African Americans and Hispanics remain less likely than other racial/ethnic groups to obtain higher education. Without higher education, employment opportunities for these individuals are frequently limited to low-wage or service sector jobs. These jobs rarely pay sufficiently well to support a family and also frequently do not provide health insurance coverage. Although insurance is available for private purchase, individuals working in low-wage jobs are less able to spend their already sparse dollars on insurance to protect against incurring future possible health care costs.

This interconnection of risk factors can be carried through even further, such that lacking health insurance coverage creates major barriers to obtaining high-quality medical care and reduces the chances that needed preventive and acute health care services will be obtained. For adults, this likely means more sick days from work, and for children this means more sick days from school, and ultimately a greater likelihood that both major and minor health problems will go undetected or untreated. For adults, this means that problems such as hypertension, depression, and diabetes go untreated, and for children this means that some learning problems may go undiagnosed and a host of other social barriers to achieving at school may remain unaddressed.

These interactions and pathways between risk factors create the potential for a sort of vicious cycle where vulnerable adults and children have much greater

FIGURE 2.15. SIMPLIFIED INTERCONNECTIONS BETWEEN RISK FACTORS AND THE CYCLING OF VULNERABILITY

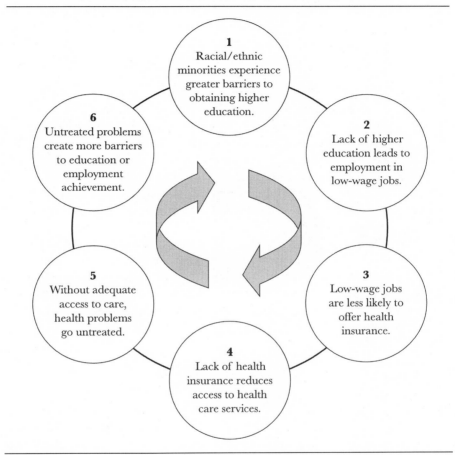

1
Racial/ethnic minorities experience greater barriers to obtaining higher education.

2
Lack of higher education leads to employment in low-wage jobs.

3
Low-wage jobs are less likely to offer health insurance.

4
Lack of health insurance reduces access to health care services.

5
Without adequate access to care, health problems go untreated.

6
Untreated problems create more barriers to education or employment achievement.

difficulty obtaining higher education, obtaining jobs that can provide sufficient income to support a family and offer health insurance, and obtain needed health care services. While this one model is oversimplified and it assumes a continuous and uninterrupted flow from each of the risk factors to another, it describes a general process by which risks may co-occur, interact, and recycle across generations.

Many other risk factors could easily be used to constitute vulnerability. A list of a range of predisposing, need, and enabling risk factors might include genetics (which influences the biological likelihood of developing health conditions), marital status and social support (which have been shown to predict adult mortality), and primary language and cultural beliefs about medical care (which affect how health care needs are reported and may create barriers to obtaining and using health services). Additional risk factors include depression, which not only creates a need for health services among adults but influences child development and also reduces the chances that a person will effectively seek health care for self or family.

Many health system factors may also constitute vulnerability. Geographical inaccessibility (a rural or inner-city setting) of health services may limit the availability of medical providers from whom to seek care, health insurance type (managed care versus fee for service) may influence how and what services are obtained, and both cost sharing and provider type could potentially influence the technical quality of care. Community factors such as community SES and community social cohesion may influence health status through factors such as stress and the availability of basic health and social resources, such as recreational parks and community safety.

Granted, this list is just the beginning of enumerating potential vulnerability factors. This book details many of the most commonly cited risk factors in the process of discussing the mechanisms and pathways of race/ethnicity, SES, and health insurance. Some of these additional risk factors are also discussed in Chapter Four, where we present data from other studies on the influences of multiple risk factors.

Summary

This chapter described how vulnerability characteristics (race/ethnicity, socioeconomic status, and health insurance coverage) are produced and how they are allowed to persist in the United States. It then discussed the mechanisms or pathways by which these vulnerability characteristics are associated with negative health and health care experiences. The models we have presented summarize the relationships between the vulnerability characteristics and either health or health care experiences, but the mechanisms are similar for both outcomes.

In the pathways of racial and ethnic vulnerability, we present a summary conceptual model that describes several potential pathways linking race and ethnicity with health and health care. The pathways begin with family characteristics that include SES, cultural factors, discrimination, and health need. The model then traces the pathways through the health care delivery system and identifies provider and system factors that may contribute to disparities in care. Several pathways are likely to operate simultaneously, leading to adverse health and health care outcomes.

In the pathways of SES, levels of income, education, and occupation together characterize an individual's relative position along the socioeconomic gradient. SES is related to health and health care in two ways: material deprivation and lack of social participation. In the pathways of health insurance coverage, we present a model of the role of health insurance coverage in supporting health and determining experiences in the health care system. Uninsured individuals are particularly vulnerable to financial barriers in accessing health care.

By understanding these mechanisms and pathways, one can begin to understand why disparities persist and how they influence health and health care within the United States. In the next chapter, we present current evidence of the individual contributions of risk factors to health care access, quality of care, and health status. Interpreting these findings with a broader grasp of how these disparities are created will improve the ability to design more effective ways to enhance equity in health and health care.

Review Questions

1. Define *race* and *ethnicity.* Identify three factors for which race/ethnicity is often used as a proxy measure. Why is skin color rarely the main reason that race/ethnicity is associated with health status or health care access and quality?

2. What is socioeconomic status, and how is it usually measured? Briefly describe two possible individual-level pathways through which SES is related to health care access (that is, getting health care when one needs it).

3. Define *Medicaid* and *SCHIP.* What are the main criteria that determine eligibility for these programs, and how large a proportion of the population is covered by these programs? Does this proportion vary by race/ethnicity?

Essay Questions

1. Describe how vulnerability is created through social (as opposed to personal) forces. Identify these social forces for risk factors such as race/ethnicity, SES, and health insurance coverage. What are the strengths and weaknesses of focusing national efforts on both social determinants and individual determinants of vulnerability? Make sure to discuss how a focus on these social determinants of vulnerability creates a societal obligation to address the consequences of vulnerability on health.

2. Vulnerability can be composed of many different risk factors. Identify three risk factors besides race/ethnicity, SES, and health insurance coverage risk for

poor health care access. Examine some of the peer-reviewed research litera-ture on these risk factors, and present a short synopsis of why and how these factors are related to access to care. Be sure to describe how strongly these fac-tors are related to health care access in comparison to race/ethnicity, SES, and health insurance.

CHAPTER THREE

DISPARITIES IN HEALTH CARE ACCESS, QUALITY, AND HEALTH STATUS

The Influence of Individual Risk Factors

In this chapter, we present findings regarding disparities according to the three main vulnerability characteristics addressed in this book: race/ethnicity, socioeconomic status, and health insurance coverage. For each characteristic, we present evidence of disparities in access to health care, quality of care, and health status. Highlighting disparities in health care access, quality, and health status across racial/ethnic, socioeconomic, and insurance groups reflects an overarching concern for equity. These vulnerable populations, in terms of health and health care, are groups for which the current system is not equitable. In recent years, there has been a growing interest in the concept of equity in health care access and utilization (Caplan, Light, et al., 1999; Glick, 1999; Peacock, Devlin, et al. 1999; Ubel, Baron, et al. 2000). Much of the literature reviewed presents findings on health, health care access, and utilization for vulnerable groups relative to nonvulnerable groups or the population as a whole. These comparisons help in understanding whether equitable distribution of optimal health, as well as timely and effective access to and use of health services, exists in the United States.

The evidence for this review comes from a variety of sources. First, a systematic review of MEDLINE was conducted to identify empirical studies addressing disparities in access to health care, quality of care, and health status across racial/ethnic, SES, and insurance groups. We have chosen to present data from nationally representative studies when they are available because they are the most useful starting points for policymakers and can often be supplemented with state or regional data. Preliminary or innovative research on disparities, however, is usually available only from smaller nonrepresentative samples. Second, we incorporated our own analyses of national surveys sponsored by the federal government (for example, the National Health Interview Survey and the Medical Expenditure Panel Survey) and private **foundations** (for example, the Community Tracking Survey and the Kaiser Family Foundation Survey of American Families). Third, many of the sources of evidence in this chapter are derived from the publication of annual national reports, *Health, United States,* by the Centers for Disease Control, National Center for Health Statistics, that synthesizes results from many of these national data sources. The studies and analyses presented do not attempt an exhaustive review of the literature. This task could fill several books. Rather, the goal of this chapter is to present the most recent and seminal research that best illustrates the pervasive influence of vulnerability.

Racial and Ethnic Disparities

Because of the recent national attention given to eliminating racial/ethnic disparities in health and health care, there has been an explosion of research documenting these disparities. The available evidence strongly and consistently suggests that racial/ethnic minorities have poorer access to health care, receive poorer quality of care, and experience greater deficits in health status and health outcomes.

Health Care Access

One of the most consistent findings across decades of research is that minorities have poorer access to health services compared to their white counterparts, even after controlling for SES, insurance coverage, and health status. A commonly used measure of access to care is whether a person has a **regular source of care** (RSC). In most research studies, an RSC is defined as a single provider or place where patients obtain, or can obtain, the majority of their health care. Having an RSC is associated with greater coordination of care, a greater likelihood of receiving **preventive care,** better treatment for chronic and acute health conditions, and fewer delays in care (Moy, Bartman, et al., 1995; Caplan and Haynes, 1996; Ettner, 1996; Mark and Paramore, 1996; Martin, Calle, et al., 1996).

Figure 3.1 shows the likelihood of having an RSC by race and ethnicity. According to 2000–2001 national data, about 16.5 percent of the total adult population does not have a regular source of health care. Minorities are less likely than

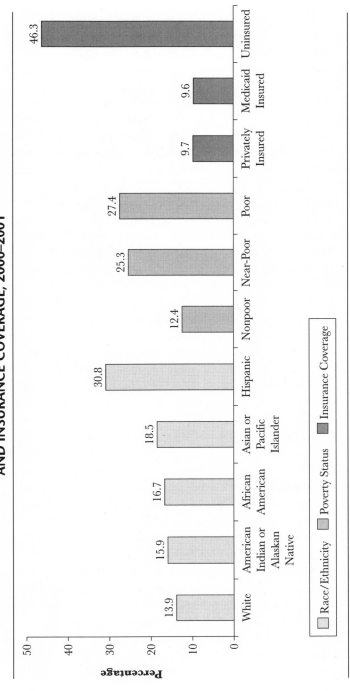

FIGURE 3.1. RESPONDENTS REPORTING NO REGULAR SOURCE OF CARE AMONG ADULTS EIGHTEEN TO SIXTY-FOUR YEARS, BY RACE/ETHNICITY, POVERTY STATUS, AND INSURANCE COVERAGE, 2000–2001

Source: National Center for Health Statistics (2003).

whites to report having an RSC. Almost one-third of Hispanic adults (30.8 percent) reported not having an RSC, followed by 18.5 percent of Asians and Pacific Islanders, 16.7 percent of African Americans, and 15.9 percent of American Indians and Alaska Natives. These rates of lacking an RSC are higher than for whites (13.9 percent).

The finding that Hispanics have a much greater likelihood of lacking an RSC than other racial/ethnic groups has been repeated in many studies. A nationally representative study that examined nearly two decades of access to care (from 1977 to 1996) demonstrated that Hispanics have had an increasingly difficult time obtaining access to care. In 1977, about one in five of the nation's Hispanic adults (19.7 percent) did not have an RSC. By 1996, this had increased to nearly one in three Hispanics (29.6 percent) without an RSC (Zuvekas and Weinick, 1999). The authors attribute the increase primarily to the deterioration of private health insurance coverage and decreases in the likelihood of having an RSC for the uninsured overall during the period under study. According to the results, 55 to 77 percent of the observed disparities for Hispanics remain even after controlling for the effects of income and health insurance coverage.

Children have similar difficulties in obtaining access to care. A study by Weinick and Krauss (2000) examined racial/ethnic differences in having an RSC for children. The study used three analytical models that controlled for different sets of variables and found that Hispanic, black, and Asian children were significantly less likely than white children to have an RSC (OR = 0.35, 0.54, and 0.85; all p < .01). Even after controlling for insurance coverage, family income, maternal education, and employment status (all factors strongly associated with adult access to care), the disparities in having an RSC remained the same for black children (OR = 0.57, p <.01) and decreased slightly, but remained significant, among Hispanic children (OR = 0.52, p < .001). Finally, after controlling for the potential influences of language on access to care, the disparities in having an RSC decreased further for Hispanic children (OR = 0.71) such that they became nonsignificant, and increased slightly for black children (OR = 0.55, p < .01). This suggests that many, but certainly not all, of the racial/ethnic disparities in having an RSC for children is attributable to factors such as health insurance coverage, family income, and language (Weinick and Krauss, 2000).

There are many reasons that individuals (adults or children) do not have a regular source of health care. In one important analysis of national data from the 1996 Medical Expenditure Panel Survey (MEPS), Weinick and Drilea (1998) examined the most common reasons for individuals to report lacking an RSC. Among all individuals who did not have an RSC, the most commonly reported reason was that the individual seldom or never got sick. Among minority racial/ethnic groups that did not have an RSC, however, Hispanics were more likely than other groups to report cost as being the main reason for not having an RSC (16.4 percent versus 7.1 percent blacks and 7.4 percent whites) (Weinick and Drilea, 1998). This provides further evidence of the importance of ensuring adequate health insurance coverage and minimal **cost sharing** to improve access to care.

Even among individuals who have an RSC, racial/ethnic minorities still report much less flexibility in their choices of where to seek medical care. Factors including language difficulty, poor geographical proximity to health care providers, and the absence of providers and clinics offering **culturally appropriate** services may be the reasons for the lower flexibility in where minority individuals can easily obtain care. Data from the 2001 Commonwealth Fund Health Care Quality Survey show that a substantial proportion (18 percent) of all adults report "very little" or "no choice" of where to seek medical care. Hispanic and Asian respondents are the most likely to report having very little or no choice (28 percent and 24 percent, respectively), compared to 22 percent of blacks and only 15 percent of whites (Collins, Hughes, et al., 2002). Lesser flexibility in where to seek medical care may lead to greater dissatisfaction and may lead individuals to delay or forgo obtaining some needed medical services.

Perhaps because of this lack of choice in where to seek care, there are differences in the types and settings of RSC reported by each racial/ethnic group. Many adults report seeking care in an emergency room or urgent care facility as their regular place for obtaining care. These sites are generally places of last resort for indigent patients and are rarely designed to deliver the most efficient and highest-quality primary care services. There remains debate even about the quality of care in hospital outpatient clinics, **community health centers,** and health department clinics, all of which are reported as an RSC more frequently by racial/ethnic minorities.

In 2001, about 76 percent of the population reported having a doctor's office as their RSC. Whites were the most likely racial/ethnic group to report a doctor's office (80 percent) and Hispanics least likely (59 percent). Hispanics reported seeking care from a community health center more frequently than any other racial/ethnic group (20 percent versus 7 percent of whites), and both Hispanics and blacks cited emergency departments as their RSC with similar frequency (about 13 percent) (Collins, Hughes, et al., 2002).

Although a person may have a regular source of care, organizational or health system barriers may prevent the timely and appropriate use of primary health care services. Forrest and Starfield (1998), in a study reviewing barriers to access and their effects on seeking primary care, found that Hispanic and black adults faced significantly more barriers to timely access compared to whites. Five barriers to primary care access were measured: (1) no after-hour care, (2) a wait time of five or more days for an appointment, (3) a wait time of thirty or more minutes in the office, (4) travel time of thirty or more minutes to the health care site, and (5) no insurance for part or all of the year. The study showed that racial/ethnic minorities faced more barriers to accessing care than whites. Whites faced an average of 0.96 access barriers per person, while Hispanic and black respondents faced an average of 1.22 and 1.14 ($p < .001$) barriers, respectively (Forrest and Starfield, 1998).

Poor access to care is also frequently documented through delayed or forgone health services. There has been a relatively recent movement to document more directly the effects of poor access to care by assessing the degree to which patients experience delays in seeking care. These **unmet health care needs** can be measured directly by asking patients if they delayed or did not seek care for any health problems that they believed required medical attention. In addition, a few studies have attempted to assess unmet health needs by examining whether patients sought care for specific health symptoms that the medical community generally agrees should receive medical attention. These studies focus predominantly on children, however, and have not found any consistent pattern of disparities for minority children (Stoddard, St. Peter, et al., 1994; Newacheck, Hughes, et al., 1996, 2000).

In 2001, almost one in every ten adults in the United States (about 9.5 percent) reported delaying medical care that they thought was needed. Delays in seeking medical care vary according to race/ethnicity, but not as expected given the previously presented evidence about disparities in access to care. Black and white adults have a similar tendency to report delayed or forgone care (9.7 percent and 9.2 percent, respectively), but Hispanics appear less likely to delay seeking care (8.4 percent) than these other groups. Although there is not yet a clear explanation for these unique findings, this may be attributable to racial/ethnic differences in how adults perceive their health needs. Hispanics may underestimate their health needs or feel disinclined to obtain services for less acute or severe conditions because of the challenges in accessing health care. Regardless of the reason, these findings have been relatively consistent during the past five years (Center for Studying Health System Change, 2001).

So far, the measures of access that we have presented reflect **potential access** to health care services. Instead of assessing the actual use of health services, the measures reflect the potential use of services and imply appropriate and adequate use of primary care services. The other type of access measure that is commonly reported reflects **realized access** to care, or rather the actual utilization of health services such as physician visits, hospitalizations, and urgent care or emergency department visits (Andersen, 1995).

Racial/ethnic disparities in the use of health services have been examined most frequently in terms of differences between blacks and whites, and the following review reflects this pattern. It should be noted that given the multiple barriers to access faced by other minority populations, it may be assumed until further research is conducted that these groups have patterns of use similar to those of blacks. In 2000, after all health care settings are taken into account and after rates are adjusted for age, blacks have similar annual rates of health care visits for ambulatory services (nonhospital inpatient services) as whites: respectively, 353 versus 380 visits per 100 persons (National Center for Health Statistics, 2003).

It is important, however, to recognize the differences in where black and white adults receive their ambulatory care. Black adults use hospital outpatient departments (54 visits per 100 persons) and emergency departments (62 visits per 100 persons) about twice as often as white peers, who made 28 visits to outpatient departments and 37 visits to emergency rooms for every 100 persons. Whites are more likely than blacks to visit physician offices (315 visits compared to 239 visits per 100 persons) (National Center for Health Statistics, 2003).

Similar patterns can be seen in emergency department use for children under eighteen years of age. Black and Hispanic children are more likely than white children to have two or more visits to the emergency department in a given year (10.4 percent and 7.0 percent, respectively, versus 6.4 percent). Reliance on these non-primary-care-focused sources of care may have serious implications for the quality of care that racial/ethnic minorities are receiving.

Racial disparities in the use of particular health services have also been demonstrated. Reviewing health care use rates among Medicare beneficiaries of different racial/ethnic groups (who are provided the same basic level of health insurance coverage and presumably the same level of access to care), illustrates this point (see Table 3.1). Data from the 1990 census and Medicare administrative data from 1993 for over 26 million beneficiaries (age sixty-five and older) were used to compute rates of various procedures (adjusted for age and gender) to determine black-white ratios of health care **utilization rates** (Gornick, Eggers, et al., 1996). Black Medicare beneficiaries have fewer ambulatory visits to physicians, are less likely to receive mammograms, and receive fewer common services such as cardiac-related procedures and hip repairs. Blacks are also more likely to be hospitalized and are more than three times as likely as whites to receive much more aggressive treatments such as amputation for complications of diabetes (ratio = 3.64) and bilateral orchiectomy (removal of the testes) to treat prostate cancer (ratio = 3.30). After controlling for the effects of income on utilization rates, differences in the black-white utilization rates were reduced but remained significant.

TABLE 3.1. DIFFERENCES BETWEEN BLACK AND WHITE MEDICARE BENEFICIARIES IN USE OF SERVICES

Health Services Received	Black-White Rate Ratio		Black-White Rate Ratio	
	Adjusted for Age and Sex	Standard Error	Adjusted for Age, Sex, and Income	Standard Error
Visits to physician	0.89	0.003	0.93	0.003
Mammography	0.66	0.001	0.75	0.001
All hospital discharges	1.14	0.001	1.15	0.001
Coronary angioplasty	0.46	0.006	0.51	0.007
Coronary-artery bypass surgery	0.40	0.006	0.43	0.007
Reduction of hip fracture	0.42	0.007	0.43	0.007
Bilateral orchiectomy	2.45	0.065	2.32	0.062
Amputation of limb	3.64	0.034	3.30	0.032

Note: There was no age adjustment for mammography, reduction of hip fracture, and bilateral orchiectomy.

Source: Gornick, Eggers, et al. (1996); 1993 Medicare administrative files and 1990 U.S. Census data.

Health Care Quality

Recognizing that assessments of disparities in access to care are likely to reveal only the very tip of the iceberg of racial disparities in health care, there has been a growing movement to monitor racial/ethnic disparities in the **quality of care** that patients receive (Smedley, Stith, et al., 2002). National surveys have been created or revised to incorporate questions on quality of care, and several have been developed specifically to allow consumers to report on their experiences in various types of health plans. There are a variety of approaches to assessing quality of care. Quality can be measured by the receipt of preventive care, hospitalization for **ambulatory care sensitive conditions** (also known as preventable hospitalization), qualitative experiences such as patient-provider interactions, and patient satisfaction with care.

Figure 3.2 shows recent estimates of racial/ethnic disparities in the receipt of preventive services. In general, racial and ethnic minorities are less likely than whites to receive preventive services, including early childhood immunizations, receipt of prenatal care, mammography for women over forty years of age, and

FIGURE 3.2. RECEIPT OF PREVENTIVE SERVICES BY RACE AND ETHNICITY, 2000–2001

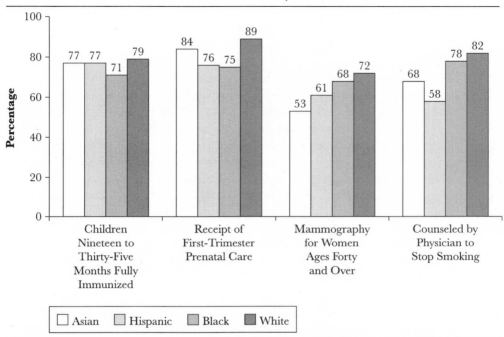

Source: National Center for Health Statistics (2003); Collins, Hughes, et al. (2002).

smoking cessation counseling for current smokers. Hispanics and Asians were least likely to receive these preventive services, with the exception that Asians were similar to whites in the likelihood of obtaining prenatal care. It is particularly interesting to note that despite nearly universal financial access to immunizations, significantly less than 80 percent of all children aged nineteen to thirty-five months were considered up-to-date with their immunization schedule.

Numerous additional studies have evaluated racial and ethnic disparities in receipt of preventive services such as immunizations, **well-child care,** health screenings, type 2 diabetes check-ups, and others. Ronsaville and Hakim (2000) used a nationally representative sample of all births that occurred in 1988 along with 1991 longitudinal follow-up data to determine factors associated with incomplete compliance with well-child guidelines. The study found that 58 percent of white, but only 35 percent of African American and 37 percent of Hispanic infants, obtained or received all recommended well-child care. After adjustment for SES, demographic factors, the number of children in the family, parent smoking, and main site of care, the strongest risks for incomplete compliance were being African American (OR 1.7; confidence interval [CI]: 1.5–1.9), Hispanic (OR 1.7; CI: 1.4–2.1), and having low family income measured as a percentage of the federal poverty level (FPL): 100–200 percent of FPL (OR 1.3; CI: 1.1–1.6) and less than 100 percent of FPL (OR 1.6; CI: 1.3–2.0) (Ronsaville and Hakim, 2000).

Similar disparities exist among patients in the Medicare population. In one study using the Health Plan Employer Data and Information Set (HEDIS) from 1998, Schneider, Zaslavsky et al. (2002) examined four quality measures: (1) breast cancer screening, (2) eye exams for diabetic patients, (3) beta blocker use for myocardial infarction, and (4) follow-up after hospitalization for mental illness. After analyzing data for more than 300,000 Medicare beneficiaries in managed care plans, the study showed significant differences in the quality of care given to white and black beneficiaries. After adjusting for individual socioeconomic factors and health plan effects, whites were significantly more likely than blacks to receive each of the services except breast cancer screening. The adjusted differences between whites and blacks were 2.5 percent (CI: 0.8–0.2 percent) for eye exams, 4.3 percent (CI: 0.3–0.8 percent) for beta blocker use, and 15.7 percent (7.98–23.1) for mental illness follow-up.

A similar pattern of racial disparity is also found in screening for cancer. Substantial gaps in breast cancer screening rates between blacks and whites have been demonstrated, even among those with insurance (Gornick, Eggers, et al., 1996; Rahman, Dignan, et al., 2003). Prostate cancer screening may be another example of preventive services that are not delivered equally to members of all racial/ethnic groups. Black, Hispanic, and Asian men have a higher risk than whites of presenting at medical visits with advanced prostate cancer, which strongly suggests that these groups have poor access to timely screening (Lillie-Blanton, Rushing, et al., 2003; Oakley-Girvan, Kolonel, et al., 2003).

In order to further understand racial/ethnic differences in preventive care, one study (Fiscella, Franks, et al., 2002) evaluated the receipt of preventive services by race/ethnicity and language for adults covered by either private insurance or Medicaid. The study found that receipt of preventive care for English-speaking Hispanic patients was not much different from that of white patients. Spanish-speaking Hispanic patients were significantly less likely than whites to have had a physician visit (relative risk [RR]=0.77; 95 percent CI: 0.72–0.83), mental health visit (RR=0.50; CI: 0.32–0.76), or influenza vaccination (RR=0.30; CI: 0.15–0.52). Adjustment for predisposing, enabling , and need factors revealed that Spanish-speaking Hispanic patients had significantly lower use than whites across all four measures. Blacks had a significantly lower relative risk of having received an influenza vaccination (RR=0.73; 95 percent CI: 0.58–0.87) and were significantly less likely than white patients to have had a visit with a mental health professional (RR=0.46; CI: 0.37–0.55). In summary, this study demonstrates that ethnic disparities in some preventive care services may be explained by differences in English-language fluency, but that other racial and ethnic disparities in care still persist despite adjustment for language and other common enabling, predisposing, and need factors (Fiscella, Franks, et al., 2002).

Another study used hospital discharge data from ten U.S. states to evaluate racial/ethnic differences in preventable hospitalization rates as an indicator of poor access to and quality of primary care (Gaskin and Hoffman, 2000). Preventable hospitalizations are hospitalizations for conditions such as asthma or diabetes that can be easily managed through high-quality primary care and should rarely require hospitalization if managed appropriately. After adjustment for individual demographics, SES, and county-level health care factors such as availability of health centers and hospital beds, the authors concluded that in 44 percent of the study's possible comparisons across states and insurance types for African Americans, Hispanics, and white patients, Hispanic children and African American adults were significantly more likely than whites to experience preventable hospitalization.

There are many studies now documenting racial and ethnic disparities in the treatment of heart disease, a leading contributor to mortality for minorities. There has long been a major gap between blacks and whites in the rate of cardiac catheterizations used to diagnose heart disease, but recently researchers have found this gap to be narrowing. In 1980, African Americans were 58 percent less likely (RR = 0.42) to undergo cardiac catheterizations than whites. By 1993, this rate had decreased to just a 9 percent lower likelihood of having this procedure (RR = 0.91) according to the National Hospital Discharge Survey. While this is some positive news, there still exist large disparities in the actual treatment of heart disease, with African Americans being 62 percent less likely than whites to receive angioplasty and 57 percent less likely to receive coronary bypass surgery (Gillum, Gillum, et al., 1997).

Exploring more subjective quality-of-care experiences requires more sophisticated measurement tools that have not been adequately tested and available until recently. Most of the instruments have been designed to assess patient-reported quality of their experiences in primary care. Subsequently, studies have begun to compare primary care quality across racial and ethnic groups. Nationally representative data for these studies come from the Consumer Assessment of Health Plans Survey (CAHPS), which incorporates detailed quality-of-care questions. In addition, a number of studies using other data sources have revealed deficits in the primary care experiences of racial and ethnic minority groups (Taira, Safran, et al., 1997, 2001; Morales, Elliott, et al. 2001; Weech-Maldonado, Morales, et al., 2001, 2003; Stevens and Shi, 2002a, 2002b, 2003).

Figure 3.3 shows the results of one study examining the primary care experiences of racial and ethnic minority adults (Taira, Safran, et al., 2001). The study revealed substantial racial and ethnic deficits in primary care quality across seven aspects of care (five are shown in the figure). The aspects of care selected for the figure are financial access, continuity of care, **preventive counseling,** interpersonal treatment, and trust in the physician. Each represents a scale score developed from between two and eight survey questions. Overall, Asian adults report the greatest deficits in primary care quality, and whites consistently report the best quality. Blacks in this study reported somewhat better interpersonal treatment despite particularly low trust in physicians. The finding of relatively low quality reported by Asians has been a common finding in many of the studies of racial/ethnic disparities in primary care.

One of the most fruitful explorations in quality of care has been examining the variations in racial/ethnic group perceptions of personal interactions in the health care system. Most of the studies evaluating primary care quality include

FIGURE 3.3. PRIMARY CARE QUALITY RATINGS BY RACE AND ETHNICITY

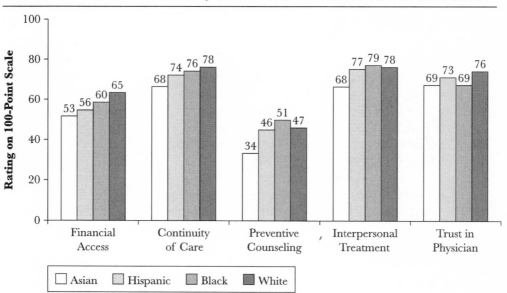

Source: Taira, Safran, et al. (2001).

a measure of patient-provider communication, interpersonal relationship, or trust in the provider. Some of these studies have shown that personal interactions in the health care system are influenced by factors such as provider race/ethnicity and health plan policies (Cooper-Patrick, Gallo, et al., 1999; Saha, Komaromy, et al., 1999; Cooper and Roter, 2002; LaVeist and Nuru-Jeter, 2002; Stevens and Shi, 2002b; LaVeist, Nuru-Jeter, et al., 2003; Saha, Arbelaez, et al., 2003; Stevens, Shi, et al., 2003) and that these disproportionately influence the reported quality experiences of minorities.

Figure 3.4 presents two unique findings regarding racial/ethnic differences in personal interactions with a provider. National data collected in the Commonwealth Fund Health Care Quality Survey (Collins, Hughes, et al., 2002) reveal that minority adults are more likely than whites to report that they were treated with disrespect because of ability to pay, English-language ability, or race/ethnicity. Hispanics, for example, report being treated with disrespect at twice the rate of whites (18 percent versus 9 percent). The figure also shows that

FIGURE 3.4. PERSONAL INTERACTIONS IN THE HEALTH CARE SYSTEM BY RACE AND ETHNICITY, 2001

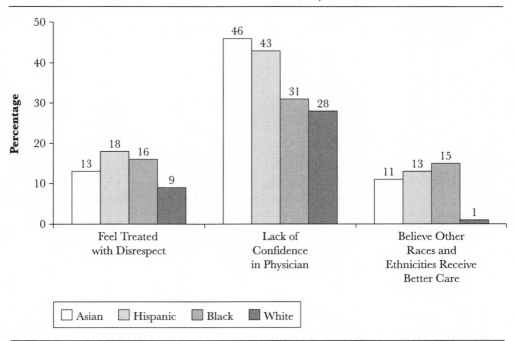

Source: Collins, Hughes, et al. (2002).

minorities have less confidence in their physicians than whites do. Asian Americans, for example, reported lacking confidence in their provider almost 50 percent of the time. Similarly, minorities are much more likely to report that they would receive better health care if they were of a different race or ethnicity. Black, Hispanic, and Asian adults all reported this feeling at a rate far greater than that for whites, which was only about 1 percent.

Patient-reported satisfaction with health care is another important component of quality. It captures the perceptions of patients in relationship to their expectations for the health care they receive. High satisfaction would suggest that patient expectations for care are met. Data from the Commonwealth Fund Health Care Quality Survey (Collins, Hughes, et al., 2001) revealed that Hispanic and Asian adults are much less likely than white adults to be "very" satisfied with the health care received in the past two years. Asian Americans were least satisfied with health care, reporting that they were very satisfied only 45 percent of the time compared to 65 percent of whites.

Changing providers is often indicative of patient satisfaction. Data from the same survey show that racial/ethnic minority adults are less likely than whites to stay with the same physician for more than five years. Asian adults are the least likely to report having the same physician for more than five years (32 percent), compared to 37 percent of Hispanics, 43 percent of blacks, and 46 percent of whites. This suggests an additional degree of evidence of Asians' higher dissatisfaction with care.

Health Status

Health status and health risk behaviors both contribute to driving the use of medical care and are important tools for assessing the effects of health care services, since they are the main purpose of health services. Many studies document that racial/ethnic minorities experience much higher incidence rates of morbidity and mortality compared to whites. Disparities in health exist between white and nonwhite Americans in terms of perceived health status as well as traditional indicators of health, such as infant mortality rates and general population mortality rates. Racial/ethnic disparities in health status are so significant and have received so much attention that the federal government has named the elimination of racial/ethnic disparities in health as one of two primary goals for the Healthy People 2010 initiative (U.S. Department of Health and Human Services, 2000).

Some of the earliest efforts in revealing racial/ethnic disparities in the United States were through the use of national statistics on health status and health risk factors. The disparities were found so prominent in early studies that now nearly all vital statistics and reports of health conditions are routinely reported according to race and ethnicity, although not all racial/ethnic subgroup populations are consistently represented in each statistic. In this section, we present key evidence illustrating racial/ethnic disparities in perceived health status, health risks, and mortality.

Figure 3.5 presents self-assessed health status by race and ethnicity. The most common way of assessing patient perceptions of health status is to use a Likert-type response scale with response options ranging from "poor" to "excellent." This method is frequently used because it has been very closely linked to future health outcomes and health care utilization among adults (McGee, Liao, et al., 1999). The figure, using data from *Health, United States 2003* (National Center for Health Statistics, 2003), shows large racial/ethnic differences in individual age-adjusted assessments of health status. For example, African Americans were the most likely to say their health status was "fair" or "poor" (15.5 percent), followed by American Indians and Alaskan Natives (14.5 percent), and Hispanics (12.7 percent). This is an important finding, showing that more than one in every ten individuals in these groups is in the two lowest reportable categories of health status. Asians and whites had lower rates of self-reported fair or poor health (8.1 percent and 7.9 percent, respectively) compared to the other racial/ethnic groups. These results are corroborated by other studies (Staveteig and Wigton, 2000) and in all earlier versions of the *Health, United States* reports (National Center for Health Statistics, 1998, 1999, 2001, 2002).

Similar racial/ethnic disparities in health status have been reported among children. One study that analyzed children from three consecutive years of the National Health Interview Survey (1989, 1990, and 1991) found that American Indian/Alaskan Native and black children were the least likely racial/ethnic groups to be rated by their parents in "excellent" or "good" health (66 percent and 68 percent, respectively). Hispanic children fared somewhat better than these groups, with 74 percent of these children reported to be in excellent or good health, but white children had the highest rate (85 percent). In the same study, after further adjustment for SES and family demographics, the odds of being in less than excellent or good health were higher for all racial/ethnic groups compared with whites: Native American (OR = 2.12; CI: 1.85–2.43), Asian/Pacific Islander (OR = 1.32; CI: 1.18–1.47), black (OR = 1.92; CI: 1.83–2.0), and Hispanic (OR = 1.23;, CI: 1.17–1.30) (Flores, Bauchner, et al., 1999). These findings have been replicated in many other studies (Montgomery, Kiely, et al., 1996; Szilagyi and Schor, 1998; Weigers, Weinick, et al., 1998; Weinick, Weigers, et al., 1998).

The poorer self-assessed health status of racial/ethnic minorities is underscored by more traditional and objective measures of health. Racial/ethnic minority groups have higher rates of infant mortality, lower birth weight, and higher

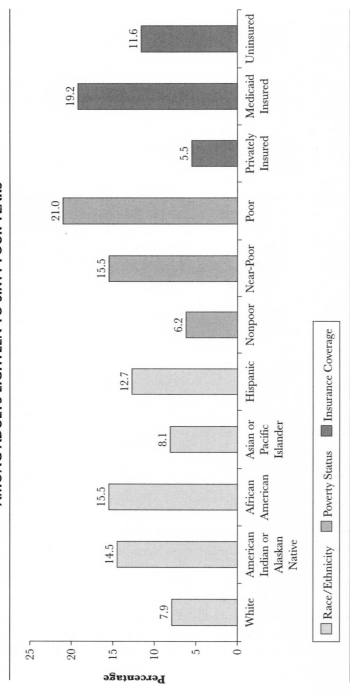

FIGURE 3.5. SELF-REPORTED FAIR OR POOR HEALTH STATUS AMONG ADULTS EIGHTEEN TO SIXTY-FOUR YEARS

Source: National Center for Health Statistics (2003).

overall and condition-specific mortality rates than whites. Between 1998 and 2000, for example, black mothers had more than twice the infant mortality rate of whites (13.9 versus 5.8 deaths per 1,000 live births), while Hispanic and Asian mothers had lower rates of infant mortality than other groups (5.7 and 5.1 deaths per 1,000 live births) (see Figure 3.6). Perhaps even more interesting is the variation in infant mortality rates within racial/ethnic subgroups in the population. For example, Puerto Rican Hispanics have a much higher rate of infant mortality than other Hispanic groups (8.1 deaths per 1,000 live births), and Cubans have a lower rate (4.3 deaths per 1,000 live births). Similarly, among Asian subgroups, Hawaiians have higher infant mortality rates (8.7 deaths per 1,000 live births), and Chinese have the lowest rates (3.5 per 1,000 live births) among all the racial/ethnic groups studied (National Center for Health Statistics, 2003).

One of the main contributors to infant mortality (death in the first year of life) is low birth weight. For the past thirty years, blacks have had higher rates of low birth weight than other racial/ethnic groups. In 2001, the rate was 13.1 percent

FIGURE 3.6. INFANT MORTALITY RATES BY RACE AND ETHNICITY, 2000

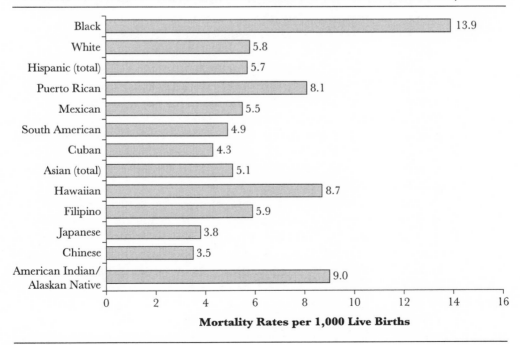

Source: National Center for Health Statistics (2003).

compared to 7.4 percent among Asian or Pacific Islanders, 7.0 percent among American Indians and Alaska Natives, 6.7 percent among whites, and 6.4 percent among Hispanics. Table 3.2 shows the stability of low-birth-weight rates across racial/ethnic groups over the past three decades. Not only do low-birth-weight rates contribute to higher infant mortality, but they also have been associated with increased risks of **developmental disabilities** such as mental retardation and cerebral palsy (Escobar, Littenberg, et al., 1991; Copper, Goldenberg, et al., 1993; Hack, Klein, et al., 1995; Avchen, Scott, et al., 2001; Holzman, Bullen, et al., 2001; Horbar, Badger, et al., 2002; Thompson, Carter, et al., 2003).

Figure 3.7 presents several other key national mortality statistics by race and ethnicity. Exploration of homicide mortality rates, mortality from breast cancer, and mortality from HIV for males reveal striking patterns of racial/ethnic disparities. For example, African Americans have mortality rates from homicide that are nearly five times that of whites, mortality rates from breast cancer that are about three times higher than Asians, and HIV mortality rates that are about eight times higher than that of whites and about thirty times higher than Asians. Asians have the lowest mortality rates for each of these causes, followed by whites (with the exception of breast cancer, for which the mortality rate is higher for white populations than among Hispanics and Asians).

These findings regarding racial/ethnic differences in mortality are particularly important because these specific causes of mortality can be prevented. Homicide mortality, for example, can be reduced with stronger gun laws, reduced availability of firearms, and violence prevention interventions. Similarly, breast cancer mortality can be reduced through mammography screens and early detection, and HIV mortality can be reduced through health education about safer sex practices, regular testing for HIV, and access to effective medications to regulate virus growth. While overall mortality rates in the United States have fallen consistently since 1930, the decreases have not been equitable for all Americans. In 2000, black individuals still had a mortality rate of 1,121 deaths per 100,000 individuals compared to just 850 deaths per 100,000 white individuals (National Center for Health Statistics, 2003).

Heart disease ranks as the top cause of death for all racial/ethnic groups. Black adults, however, suffer from the highest mortality rates from heart disease—almost 50 percent higher than white Americans. They also suffer from higher mortality rates due to cancer (specifically breast, colon, prostate, and lung cancer) and asthma than any other ethnic group (Grant, Lyttle, et al., 2000; Lillie-Blanton, Rushing, et al., 2003). Hayward and Heron, (1999) have shown that these higher rates of mortality are accompanied by reduced active life expectancy rates (the number of years of life spent in good health without disability) for racial/ethnic minority groups. This study showed that at the age of twenty, the active life

TABLE 3.2. LOW BIRTH WEIGHT BY MATERNAL RACE/ETHNICITY, 1970-2001

	1970	1975	1980	1985	1990	1991	1992	1993	1994	1995	1996	1997	2001
All races	7.93	7.38	6.84	6.75	6.97	7.12	7.08	7.22	7.28	7.32	7.39	7.51	7.62
Hispanic	—	6.12	6.16	6.06	6.15	6.10	6.24	6.25	6.29	6.28	6.42	6.42	
White	6.85	6.27	5.72	5.65	5.70	5.80	5.80	5.98	6.11	6.22	6.34	6.49	6.67
American Indian/ Alaska Native	7.97	6.41	6.44	5.86	6.11	6.15	6.22	6.42	6.45	6.61	6.49	6.75	7.08
Asian/ Pacific Islander	—	—	6.68	6.16	6.45	6.54	6.57	6.55	6.81	6.90	7.07	7.23	7.42
Black	13.90	13.19	12.69	12.65	13.25	13.55	13.31	13.34	13.24	13.13	13.01	13.01	13.14

Note: Defined as less than 2,500 grams.

Sources: National Center for Health Statistics (1999, 2003).

FIGURE 3.7. NATIONAL MORTALITY RATES BY RACE AND ETHNICITY, 2000

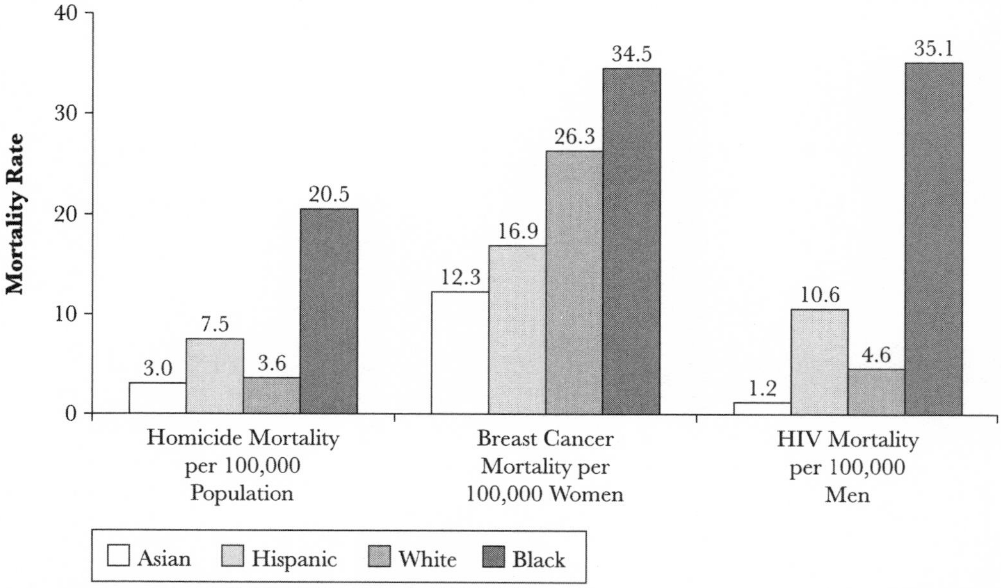

Source: National Center for Health Statistics (2003).

expectancy was about fifty-two years for Asian men, forty-five for whites, forty-two for Hispanics, thirty-nine for Native Americans, and thirty-seven for black men (Hayward and Heron, 1999).

McCord and Freeman (1990) published one of the most widely cited studies illustrating that the gains in health over time have not been felt equally by all Americans. Death certificate records from the New York City Health Department and 1980 census data were abstracted for the analysis. They examined death rates of the residents of Harlem, an inner-city neighborhood in New York City. When the 1980 census was taken, Harlem was 96 percent black, and 40.8 percent of the families living there had incomes below the federal poverty line.

The residents of Harlem had the highest mortality rates of any area in New York City. Compared to all white men in the United States in 1980, the standardized mortality ratio (SMR) for men in Harlem was almost three times higher (SMR = 2.91), resulting in 948 per 100,000 annual excess deaths for the residents of Harlem. For Harlem women, the magnitude of excess deaths was slightly lower (SMR = 2.70), but still significantly higher than for white women in the United

States. The disparities were so great that the rate of survival beyond age forty was actually lower in Harlem than in some parts of developing Bangladesh.

Taking their analyses further, the authors compared the death rates in Harlem to the remaining 342 health areas in the city of New York with a population of over 3,000 residents. They found 54 additional areas of New York with mortality rates similar to those found in Harlem. The SMR in these areas of New York was higher than 2.0, suggesting mortality rates twice that of U.S. white males. In all but one of these areas, more than half of the resident population was either black or Hispanic.

These mortality studies provide a grim picture of racial/ethnic disparities in the United States. As we presented earlier, these higher rates among racial/ethnic minorities may be partially attributable to differences in the quality of specific health care treatments they receive. In addition, the disparities may be partially attributed to certain greater health risk behaviors as described next.

Figure 3.8 shows several key findings in health risk behaviors by race/ethnicity. With obesity and overweight status fast becoming the leading contributors to mortality in the United States, it is important to examine differences in physical inactivity rates by race/ethnicity. While Asian and white adults have similar rates of inactivity (38 percent and 37 percent, respectively), meaning that these adults engage in absolutely no leisure-time physical activity during a given week, more than half of all blacks and Hispanics report no physical activity (National Center for Health Statistics, 2004). Considering that obesity contributes to heart disease, rates of stroke, diabetes, and potentially many cancers, there is good reason to focus future efforts on reducing racial/ethnic disparities in physical activity rates.

Cigarette smoking is also one of the most prevalent health risks in the U.S. population. American Indian and Native Alaskan males are more likely to smoke (39 percent) than males from other racial groups, putting them at increased risk of lung cancer, heart disease, and stroke, in addition to other health problems. Both black and white adults report similarly high rates of current smoking (27 percent and 26 percent, respectively) while Hispanics and Asians report slightly lower rates (22 percent and 20 percent, respectively). These slightly higher rates among blacks (compared to Hispanics and Asians) in conjunction with higher physical inactivity rates may be important influences in the higher rates of mortality among black adults from some of the most common health conditions.

Another interesting finding takes an environmental approach to assessing racial/ethnic disparities in health by reporting the percentage of each racial/ethnic minority group residing in an area not meeting air quality standards issued by the U.S. Environmental Protection Agency (EPA). Asians and Hispanics are more likely than other minorities to live in these areas (61 percent and 60 percent,

FIGURE 3.8. HEALTH RISK FACTORS BY RACE AND ETHNICITY, 2001

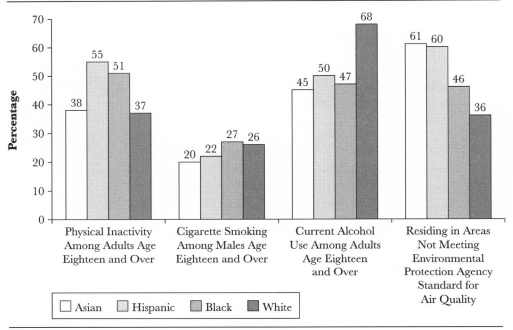

Source: National Center for Health Statistics (2003, 2004).

respectively), potentially putting them at risk for a higher **incidence** of asthma and other respiratory problems (National Center for Health Statistics, 2003).

Socioeconomic Status Disparities

Socioeconomic status is one of the most enduring contributors to disparities in health and health care. There have been many studies documenting the association of lower SES with poorer health status, barriers to accessing needed health services, and lower rates of using health care services (Adler, Boyce, et al., 1993; Feinstein, 1993). SES is defined by a combination of factors that typically include personal income, education, and occupational status.

Income represents the ability of an individual to acquire material resources and the potential to access different lifestyles, and it provides a sense of security. Education represents the potential to acquire knowledge and the ability to navigate through social institutions to meet one's desired ends, and it has also been found to be associated with health-related lifestyles and behaviors. Occupation reflects an ability to acquire resources, which influence feelings of **self-efficacy,** and reflects the societal prestige and privilege associated with one's occupation.

Despite the creation of numerous social welfare and safety net health care initiatives to compensate for lack of income, education, or occupation, the United States has not been able to effectively reduce these barriers to health care. For example, the U.S. Bureau of the Census reported that in 1997, 13.3 percent, or close to 36 million Americans, lived below the federal poverty level. In 2001, the estimated poverty rate was 11.7 percent (or 32.9 million people). The proportion of Americans living in poverty has remained relatively constant despite fluctuations in economic growth rates and expansion and retraction of government programs to help the poor (National Center for Health Statistics, 2003).

Health Care Access

With regard to accessing health care services, we intuitively find even greater differences associated with individual SES than with race and ethnicity. Overall, lower income, education, and occupational status are associated with reporting poorer access to care. Among these factors, income (measured by poverty and near-poverty status) appears to contribute most significantly to variations in access to care, though relatively few studies have examined the effects of education and occupation on this outcome. Consequently, the following review for access to care focuses mostly on the influences of income and poverty status.

Figure 3.1 showed the likelihood of lacking an RSC according to poverty status. The data source divided income into three groups: (1) poor (below the federal poverty line), (2) near-poor (between 100 percent and 300 percent of poverty), and (3) not poor (above 300 percent poverty). The figure shows that poor adults are more than twice as likely as nonpoor adults to lack an RSC (27.4 percent versus 12.4 percent). Interestingly, those with income levels between 100 and 300 percent of poverty were nearly as likely as those living in poverty to lack an RSC (25.3 percent), suggesting that there is not much of a benefit in terms of access to care for those with incomes just above the poverty line versus those in poverty.

Figure 3.9 presents the types of regular sources of care reported by adults according to income level. For this analysis, income levels were grouped in sets of approximately $10,000 to $15,000, beginning with those reporting incomes less than $10,000. The figure shows that higher income is associated with a greater likelihood of reporting a physician's office as the RSC. For example, individuals earning more than $50,000 per year were 33 percent more likely to report a physician's office than individuals earning less than $10,000 per year. Individuals with lower income rely more frequently on clinics and emergency departments as the RSC.

FIGURE 3.9. TYPE OF REGULAR SOURCE OF CARE BY INCOME, 2001

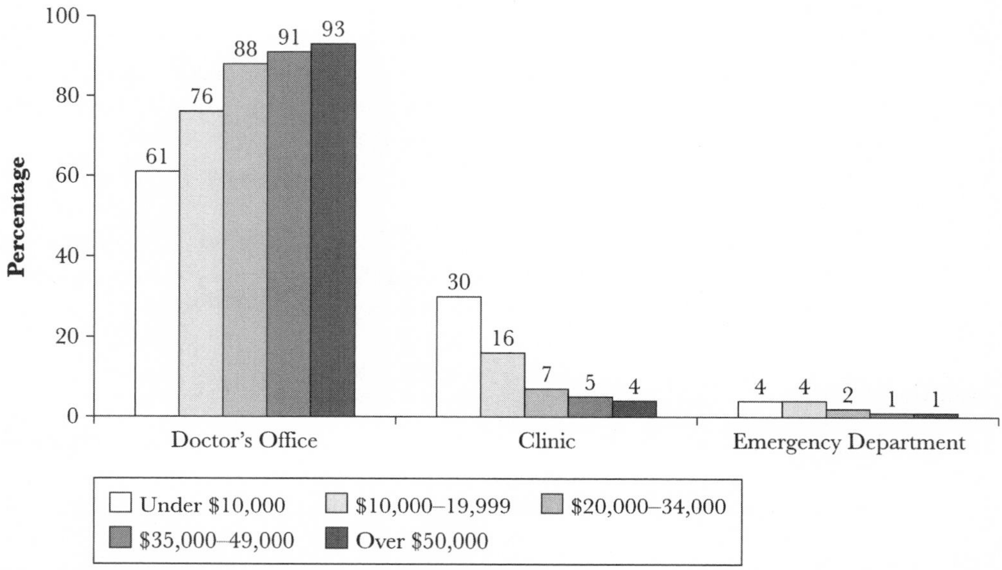

Source: National Center for Health Statistics (2003).

For example, 30 percent of individuals in the lowest income bracket reported a clinic for care as opposed to only 4 percent of those in the highest income bracket.

Individuals living at or below the federal poverty level also faced significantly more barriers to accessing their primary care site. Forrest and Starfield (1998) reviewed five barriers to access (long travel time to health center, no insurance, no after-hours care, long waiting time for scheduling an appointment, and long office wait time) and their effects on vulnerable populations. The most frequently reported barrier was a long wait time in the doctor's office (more than thirty minutes): 63.6 percent of the thirty-thousand respondents to the national survey had experienced at least one of the five barriers to access. Respondents living at or below the federal poverty line faced 34.7 percent more access barriers than those living above the poverty line (1.32 versus 0.98 mean number of barriers, $p < .001$).

Data from the three editions of the Community Tracking Study Household Survey (1996–1997, 1998–1999, and 2000–2001) reveal the likelihood of reporting a delay in seeking needed health care according to poverty status. In this analysis, poverty status was grouped using four categories: living in poverty, 100 to

199 percent of poverty, 200 to 399 percent of poverty, and above 400 percent of the poverty line. This study reveals a strong association for all years of the survey between lower income and more delays in obtaining medical care. In 2000–2001, for example, only 8.2 percent of adults living with incomes above 400 percent of poverty reported having delayed medical care in the past year, compared to 10 percent for those with 200 to 399 percent of poverty, 10.8 percent of those with 100 to 199 percent of poverty, and 10.0 percent of those living in poverty.

Health Care Quality

Socioeconomic status also strongly predicts the quality of health care that people receive. To examine the link between SES and health care quality, this section reviews evidence about SES and the receipt of preventive care, preventable hospitalizations, **qualitative experiences** in receiving health care, and satisfaction in the health care system.

The receipt of preventive services increases as SES increases. Data from *Health, United States* (National Center for Health Statistics, 2003) show the relationship between three preventive services for female adults and adult educational status (see Figure 3.10). Among mothers who did not complete high school, about 68 percent reported receiving prenatal care, compared to 82 percent of mothers who completed high school, 88 percent of mothers who received some college education, and 94 percent of mothers graduating college. The last two education levels are collapsed into a single category in the figure to reflect some college education or more, in line with how data for other preventive services is available.

Both receipt of a mammogram in the past two years for women ages forty years and over and receipt of a Pap smear in the past three years for women ages eighteen and over reveal similar patterns by educational status. Mammography rates increase from 58 percent among women with less than a high school education to 70 percent of women who graduate from high school and 76 percent of women with some college education. Pap smears are slightly more common overall, with 70 percent of women without a high school education reporting receipt in the past three years, compared to 80 percent of graduates from high school, and 88 percent of those with some college education. Overall, the difference in receipt of each of the services between the highest and lowest education levels is about 20 percent.

A recent longitudinal cohort study examined the receipt of preventive services according to SES and also found a significant association. Reviewing health service utilization data for twelve thousand female Medicare beneficiaries from 1991 to 1998, Earle, Burstein, et al. (2003) examined patient characteristics

FIGURE 3.10. RECEIPT OF PREVENTIVE SERVICES
BY EDUCATION LEVEL, 2000–2001

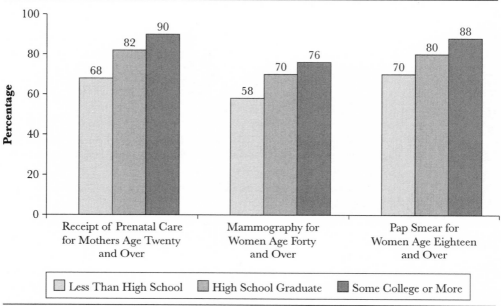

Source: National Center for Health Statistics (2003).

associated with receiving the following preventive services: influenza vaccination, lipid testing, cervical examination, colon examination, and bone densitometry. The study showed that among the study population, individuals received more preventive care with each quintile of higher socioeconomic status (OR=1.08; 95 percent CI: 1.04–1.12).

We recently analyzed data from the 2001 National Survey of Early Childhood Health (NSECH) to examine the influence of SES on the provision of anticipatory guidance to parents of young children ages three and under. **Anticipatory guidance** refers to the preventive counseling that physicians provide to parents on topics such as breast-feeding, sleeping positions to prevent sudden infant death syndrome, injury prevention, and healthy routines such as reading to children, having consistent bedtimes, and using appropriate discipline techniques. Our analyses showed that after controlling for age of child, health status, and health insurance, parents in the lowest income category had 2.42 higher odds ($p < .001$) than those in the highest income category of not receiving any anticipatory guidance item *and* saying the particular guidance would have been help-ful when it was not received. This latter factor indicates missed opportunities in receiving anticipatory guidance. In addition to income, mothers who had less than a high school education (compared to those with a college education or higher) had 2.51 higher odds ($p < .001$) of reporting any missed opportunity for guidance. These disparities reflect important deficits in preventive care in early childhood.

Using 1990 hospital discharge data, Billings, Anderson, et al. (1996) com-pared rates of preventable hospitalizations in both low- and high-income urban areas for those under age sixty-five in the United States, a market-driven health insurance system, and Canada, which offers universal health insurance. Pre-ventable hospitalizations are a marker for inadequate access to care, and also are an indicator of the quality of primary outpatient care. Receiving high-quality primary care may prevent hospitalizations for these ambulatory care sensitive conditions (ACS) including asthma, diabetes, and congestive heart failure.

Their analysis revealed a consistent pattern of higher ACS admission rates in low-income urban areas compared to high-income urban areas and an asso-ciation between the percentage of low-income residents and admission rates for ACS conditions. The associations of income and ACS admissions in Buffalo, New York, and Newark, New Jersey, were the strongest, where more than 80 percent of the variation across zip codes could be explained solely by the percentage of low-income residents. Although there remained income-based differences in the rates of ACS admissions, the differences were much narrower in Canada than in the United States, underscoring the importance of universal health insur-ance in decreasing SES disparities (Billings, Anderson, et al., 1996). These find-ings have also been reported in other studies (Djojonegoro, Aday, et al., 2000; Cable, 2002).

We further present the findings of a unique study by van Ryn and Burke (2000) of the perceived interpersonal relationships between physicians and pa-tients according to SES. The study examined physician perceptions of patients according to patient income grouped into three strata: low, middle, and high in-come (see Figure 3.11). The results reveal a strong bias in the perceptions of physi-cians against patients of lower SES. In general, physicians perceive patients of lower SES to be less independent, responsible, rational, and intelligent than patients of higher SES. The gaps are greatest for physician perceptions of pa-tient intelligence, where the difference between perceptions of lower- and higher-income patients is 17 percent, and the difference between middle- and higher-income patients is about 9 percent. These findings are important because they are likely to affect how physicians select treatments for patients.

FIGURE 3.11. PHYSICIAN-REPORTED PERCEPTIONS OF PATIENTS ACCORDING TO PATIENT SES

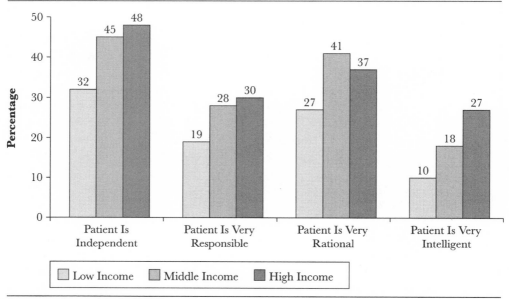

Source: van Ryn and Burke (2000).

There are several examples of how these treatment recommendations may differ by patient SES. Studies have shown that physicians are much less likely to recommend mammography to patients whom they think cannot afford the service or whom they perceive will not comply (Conry, Main, et al., 1993; Urban, Anderson, et al., 1994; Grady, Lemkau, et al., 1997). Consequently, low-income women and those with low educational attainment are less likely to be referred by their provider for a mammogram (O'Malley, Earp, et al., 2001). There is a need to better understand how widespread the effects of this physician-patient dynamic are, and to what extent such a bias influences recommendations for other preventive and acute services.

A final measure of quality that is often reported according to SES is patient satisfaction. One unique study examined how SES influences satisfaction with the health care system across five countries, including the United States. Using data from the Commonwealth Fund 2001 International Health Policy Survey (Collins, Hughes, et al., 2002), the study showed that across all countries, individuals with incomes below the median income level in each country were less likely to be highly satisfied with health care and more likely to report that "the health system is so bad that it should be rebuilt." Perhaps the most interesting part of this study is that the differences in satisfaction between high-income and low-income individuals were greater in the United States than in other countries. A likely reason for this finding is that all individuals in the other countries studied (United Kingdom, Australia, New Zealand, and Canada) are guaranteed universal coverage for access to health care (without regard to income), whereas in the United States no such universal guarantee exists (see Figures 3.12 and 3.13).

Health Status

Health risks and health status have been frequently compared across socioeconomic tiers. In fact, the relationship between socioeconomic status and mortality has been well documented since the 1960s (Antonovsky, 1967; Syme and Berkman, 1976). More recent research has shown that in addition to individuals with lower income, those with lower education and occupational status are more likely to report a range of health risks and poorer health status. In this section, we review evidence of these SES disparities in general health status, mortality, and health risks.

Figure 3.5 presented large disparities in how patients assess their own health according to poverty status. Using the same methodology as for the analysis of racial disparities in general health status, individuals in poverty report much worse health status than other income groups. The figure showed that just 6.2 percent of individuals who are not poor (incomes are above 200 percent of the FPL) were reported to be in "fair" or "poor" health. However, this percentage more than doubled (15.5 percent) for those living in near poverty (100 to 199 percent of the FPL), and more than tripled (21.0 percent) for those living in poverty. This means that among those living in poverty, more than one in every five individuals report having significantly impaired health (National Center for Health Statistics, 2003).

The prevalence of chronic health conditions has also been found to differ for children in poor families and children in nonpoor families. Newacheck (1994) found that poor children were more likely than nonpoor children to have severe chronic conditions (2.6 versus 1.5 per 100, $p < .05$). At the same time, nonpoor children had nearly 23 percent higher prevalence of mild chronic conditions compared to poor children (21.2 versus 17.2 per 100, $p < .05$). The study showed that poor children with severe chronic conditions were much less likely to have insurance and a regular source of care, suggesting that their health needs were not being met. The authors report that the higher rate of mild conditions among nonpoor children is probably due to better access to care, thus leading to better

FIGURE 3.12. PERCENTAGE REPORTING HIGH SATISFACTION WITH THE OVERALL QUALITY OF HEALTH CARE IN FIVE NATIONS BY INCOME, 2001

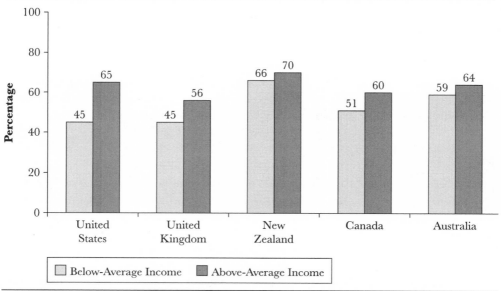

Source: Collins, Hughes, et al., 2002.

FIGURE 3.13. PERCENTAGE REPORTING THAT THE HEALTH SYSTEM IS SO BAD IT SHOULD BE REBUILT, IN FIVE NATIONS BY INCOME, 2001

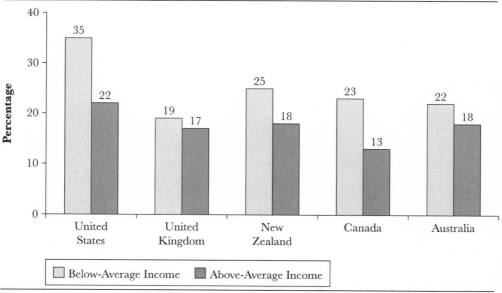

Source: Collins, Hughes, et al., 2002.

identification and diagnosis of chronic conditions (Newacheck, Jameson, et al., 1994; Newacheck, 1994).

Socioeconomic status is also associated with mental health status. Figure 3.14 simplifies several analyses conducted by the Centers for Disease Control of self-reported frequent **mental distress** according to SES factors, including income, education, and occupation. To present these data, we grouped the SES factors into three categories each: low, medium, and high. For income, the categories reflect incomes less than $15,000, between $24,000 and $49,000, and more than $50,000. For education, the categories reflect less than high school, some college or technical school, and college or graduate education. For occupation, they reflect unemployment, a part-time position, and a full-time salaried position. The analyses show that individuals with lower SES by any of these definitions are more likely to report frequent mental distress. The rates of frequent mental distress are generally two to three times higher for low-SES versus high-SES individuals.

Figure 3.15 reveals vast socioeconomic disparities in health risk behaviors among adults. Overall, individuals with lowest education level (less than a high school education) compared to those with the highest education level (a bachelor's

FIGURE 3.14. REPORTED FREQUENT MENTAL DISTRESS BY INCOME, EDUCATION, AND OCCUPATION, 1996

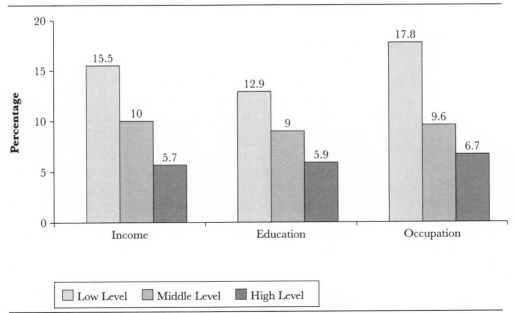

Source: Data from CDC Behavioral Risk Factor Surveillance System, 1993–1996.

FIGURE 3.15. ADULT HEALTH RISK BEHAVIORS
BY EDUCATIONAL STATUS, 1999–2001

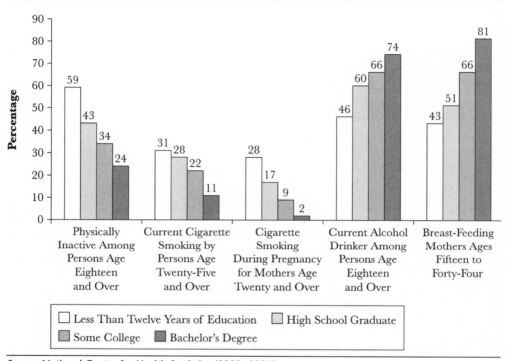

Source: National Center for Health Statistics (2003, 2004).

degree or higher) were more than two times as likely to report being physically in-active (59 versus 24 percent), about three times more likely to be current smok-ers (31 versus 11 percent), and, for mothers, were nearly fifteen times more likely to smoke during pregnancy (28 versus 2 percent), and half as likely to breast-feed (43 versus 81 percent). These gradients were apparent at each level of education in between. The only exception was for current alcohol drinking, where higher education levels were associated with a greater likelihood of being a current drinker (74 versus 46 percent).

Pappas, Queen, et al. (1993) used both the 1986 National Mortality Follow-back Survey and the 1986 National Health Interview Survey to replicate semi-nal analyses performed in the 1960s of overall all-cause mortality differentials for people ages twenty-five to sixty-four years by socioeconomic groups. They showed that the disparity in mortality rates between persons from lower- and higher-SES groups (defined by both income and education level) has persisted and even increased since the initial analysis in 1960. Moreover, blacks at every income and educational level continued to face a higher risk of death than their white counterparts.

Mortality differentials for specific health conditions have also been reported according to SES. According to data from *Health, United States* (National Center for Health Statistics, 1998, 2003), infant mortality rates, mortality from communicable diseases, and HIV mortality rates among men are related to education level. For example, the infant mortality rate increases from 5.1 deaths per 1,000 live births among mothers with thirteen or more years of education, to 7.4 deaths per 1,000 live births among mothers with twelve years of education, and to 8.0 deaths per 1,000 live births among mothers with less than a high school education. Similarly, **communicable disease** mortality for women jumps from 8.6 deaths per 100,000 for mothers with thirteen years of education, to about 25.0 deaths per 100,000 for mothers with twelve years of education and 36.0 deaths per 100,000 for those with fewer than twelve years of education. HIV mortality rates among men also show similar patterns, increasing by about 27 deaths per 100,000 (from about 37 to 64 deaths) for men with twelve years of education compared to those with thirteen years of education.

Using data from the National Longitudinal Mortality Study, Backlund, Sorlie, et al. (1999) found that income may influence mortality differently for people at different levels of SES. For example, for individuals with incomes at or below $22,500, the relative risk of mortality per $10,000 decrease in income is 1.21 for men and 1.15 for women, after adjusting for demographic and socioeconomic factors. For men and women above this income threshold, the relative risks of mortality are significantly less. This suggests that there is a minimum material standard that is necessary to prevent mortality. The study also concluded that mortality is more a function of education than income at the higher end of the socioeconomic spectrum.

The strong association of SES with overall mortality rates has also been demonstrated at the geographical level. Areas characterized by lower-SES indicators (for example, using median monthly rents of homes, median family incomes, and poverty levels of census tracts) have higher overall rates of mortality than areas characterized by higher-SES indicators. Using nine years of census data on residents (ages thirty-five and older) in Oakland, California, Haan, Kaplan, et al., (1987) found higher rates of mortality among residents of federally designated poverty areas. Adjusting for demographics, the overall mortality rates of residents in poverty areas remained 71 percent higher (RR = 1.71) than those in nonpoverty areas. Even after adjusting for other determinants of mortality such as health practices, social networks, and psychological impairment, these mortality differentials remained significant.

Health Insurance Disparities

Since the 1960s, the U.S. government has officially recognized the important role of health insurance coverage in ensuring adequate access to health care. The creation of public insurance programs like Medicare, Medicaid, and SCHIP has helped millions of low- or fixed-income citizens obtain needed health care services. Because these programs still do not guarantee coverage for every citizen, particularly excluding the working poor, researchers and advocates have continued to document and highlight the consequences of lacking insurance for health care access and health.

Such research informs the public and helps provide evidence for politicians and citizens to advocate for expansions of these programs. Because these programs have previously been closely linked with social welfare programs, advocates have been concerned about the quality of care delivered in these programs, often comparing the experiences of individuals in public programs to private health insurance plans. In addition, continued expansion of managed care plans (often criticized for restriction of both **patient autonomy** and physician autonomy through extensive cost-control measures) into public programs like Medicaid has led to greater concern about the quality of care provided to vulnerable populations. This section reviews the evidence for disparities in health care access and health outcomes among those with private insurance, public insurance, and no health insurance at all.

Health Care Access

Extensive work has been done to document the poorer access to health care experienced by people without insurance coverage. The cumulative evidence shows conclusively that people without health insurance are less likely to have a regular source of care, seek routine care from sites such as emergency departments, and delay or forgo needed health services.

Figure 3.1 demonstrated the consequences of lacking health insurance coverage on the likelihood of having an RSC for adults. Data from *Health, United States, 2003* (National Center for Health Statistics, 2003) show that privately and publicly insured adults are nearly equally likely to report not having an RSC (9.7 percent and 9.6 percent, respectively). Uninsured adults, however, are five times more likely than the insured not to have an RSC (46.3 percent), a difference that is substantially greater than any disparities by race/ethnicity or poverty status. Though not shown in the figure, uninsured children are about eight times more likely than insured children to lack an RSC (4 percent versus 31 percent). Other research has shown that these differences in the likelihood of having an RSC remain even after controlling for SES factors (Billings, 1999).

Lacking insurance coverage also affects the type of RSC that individuals report having. Privately insured individuals are more likely to report a physician's office as their source of care, while Medicaid-insured individuals are more likely to cite a clinic or emergency department as their source of care. Cunningham, Clancy, et al. (1995) found that even after adjustment for demographic variables and county-level use of emergency departments (EDs), nonurgent rates of ED use were much higher among those with public health insurance—Medicare, Medicaid, or other public insurance (OR 1.61, 1.47, 1.47, p <.01). Similar results were found by a study focusing on adolescents, where uninsured adolescents were more likely than insured adolescents to use an ED as their regular source of care (9 percent versus 5 percent, respectively, p <.01) (Klein, Wilson, et al., 1999).

The influences of lacking insurance coverage on access to care have been particularly well demonstrated for children. Newacheck, Stoddard, et al. (1998) analyzed 1993–1994 National Health Interview Survey (NHIS) data and demonstrated that children with health insurance were six times more likely to have a regular source of care (24 percent versus 4 percent) and less likely to receive care at community health centers (6 percent versus 18 percent) and in emergency departments (1 percent versus 2 percent) than children lacking insurance. After adjustment for demographics and other potentially confounding factors, health insurance coverage remained a substantial and significant **predictor** of access to and use of health care by children.

A later study by Newacheck, McManus, et al. (2000) examined the role of health insurance in access to care for children with special health care needs (those with chronic conditions, disabilities or other ongoing health problems) using 1994 NHIS data. The study found that 18 percent of children in the United States had a special health care need and that those with insurance were more likely to have a regular source of care (96.9 percent versus 79.2 percent), less likely to report unmet health needs (2.2 percent versus 10.5 percent), and more likely to have a physician contact in the past year (89.3 percent versus 73.6 percent). The effect of insurance remained significant after adjustment for SES, demographics, the level of health care need, and geographical residence.

Health insurance is further associated with delays in seeking health care services. Data from the 1996–1997, 1998–1999, and 2000–2001 Community Tracking Study Household Survey consistently show that uninsured adults are more likely than insured adults to report any delay in seeking needed health care. While 8.9 percent of all insured adults reported delaying care in the past year, almost one in five uninsured adults reported doing so. Medicaid recipients were less likely than privately insured individuals to report delays in care, most likely due to the Medicaid program not requiring significant copayments or premiums to obtain health services. This is a somewhat reassuring finding because Medicaid enrollees tend to be sicker than privately insured patients.

One particularly key study by Donelan, Blendon, et al. (1996) further showed that among the uninsured, 75 percent of those in poor health and 54 percent of those in fair health reported having difficulty getting needed care in the past year. This suggests that these delays are occurring most frequently for those who have the greatest need for medical care. The uninsured were also three times more likely to report having problems paying for medical bills than insured peers (36 percent versus 12 percent, $p < 0.05$).

Delays in obtaining health care also persist for newborns and very young children (age three and under). A study by Newacheck, Hung et al. (2002) using data on children from the 1997 National Health Interview Survey revealed that uninsured young children were much more likely to experience delays in care than insured young children, despite controlling for race/ethnicity, family income, health status, and other family and community factors. They showed that compared to insured children, uninsured children had 9.57 higher odds of not obtaining needed medical care, 6.10 higher odds of not obtaining needed prescription medications, and 5.35 higher odds of not obtaining dental care (all $p < .05$). This study also showed that uninsured young children had nearly seven times lower odds of having a regular source of care ($p < .05$).

A large number of studies have also shown that uninsured individuals are less likely than the insured to have annual medical visits (Freeman, Aiken, et al. 1990; Hafner-Eaton, 1993). One study demonstrated that these differences in physician visits are not attributable to differences in health status or health needs. Analyzing of the 1980 National Medical Care Utilization and Expenditure Survey (NMCUES) data, Howell (1988) found that uninsured persons reporting poor health had an average of about five visits per year compared with persons with poor health and private health insurance or Medicaid who reported about twelve visits per year.

Another measure of use, the use-disability ratio (UDR), adjusts the number of physician visits made by an individual by measures of disability between groups. The ratio is the number of physician visits made per 100 days of restricted activity reported by individuals with at least one restricted activity day. Comparing different groups of individuals with different types of insurance coverage, Howell (1988) found that Medicaid enrollees had a UDR of 18.1, which did not differ significantly from those with private insurance, who reported a UDR of 19.4. Uninsured individuals reported a UDR of 12.0, which suggests that access to care is not sufficient for the level of need among these individuals.

In an important analysis of Boston area hospital admissions during 1993, researchers found that self-pay or free care patients received fewer services and had shorter hospital stays than Blue Cross, privately insured patients. After adjusting for patient diagnosis, age, gender, number of diagnoses, presence of a mental illness as a secondary diagnosis, and weekend admission, self-pay or free care patients had on average 7 percent shorter stays (5.36 days versus 5.79 days) and underwent 7 percent fewer procedures (1.16 versus 1.25) than privately insured patients across all types of hospitals (Weissman and Epstein, 1989).

Health Care Quality

More recent attention has been given to evaluating how the quality of health care varies according to health insurance status and type. Health care plans provide an easily accessible sampling frame for research purposes; thus, much of the work on the more detailed experiences in quality of care is frequently conducted among various health plan types rather than comparing the insured and uninsured. There are, however, many studies documenting the consequences of lacking insurance coverage for utilization of health care and receipt of specific services.

Looking again at the receipt of preventive services as an important measure of quality of care, we present the results of a comprehensive study by Ayanian, Weissman, et al. (2000) that examines the lack of receiving recommended preventive care. Figure 3.16 shows a comparison of the receipt of clinically indicated preventive services across three insurance categories: those who were currently insured, those who were uninsured for less than one year, and those who were uninsured for more than one year. Examining both short-term and long-term lack of insurance, the study revealed previously unexplored deficits in the receipt of preventive care associated with the duration of noncoverage.

Insured women failed to receive a mammogram in the past year 11 percent of the time, while women who were uninsured for less than one year were almost twice as likely to not obtain a mammogram (21 percent). Women who were uninsured for longer were almost three times as likely as insured women to not have a mammogram (32 percent). This pattern of the inadequate receipt of care that is associated with the duration of noncoverage holds for all of the preventive services studied, including clinical breast exams, Pap tests, hypertension screening, cholesterol screening, receiving weight loss advice, and smoking cessation counseling.

Because uninsured individuals have substantially poorer access to primary care services, they consequently have different needs for and use of inpatient

**FIGURE 3.16. CLINICALLY INDICATED PREVENTIVE SERVICES
NOT RECEIVED IN THE PAST YEAR BY INSURANCE STATUS, 2000**

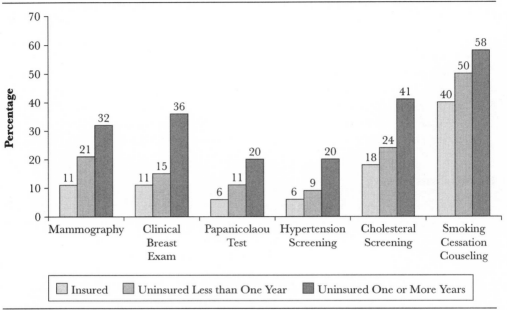

Source: Ayanian, Weissman, et al. (2000).

services. Researchers reviewed 1987 hospital discharge data in Massachusetts and Maryland to assess if both uninsured and Medicaid adults have higher rates of avoidable hospitalizations (Weissman, Gatsonis, et al., 1992). A panel of physicians identified twelve avoidable hospital conditions (including asthma, congestive heart failure, diabetes, immunizable conditions, and pneumonia) that can be averted if primary care is provided in a timely and high quality manner. After adjusting for age and gender, they found that uninsured and Medicaid patients were 71 percent more likely (RR = 1.71; 95 percent CI: 1.41–2.01) in Massachusetts and 49 percent more likely (RR = 1.49; 95 percent CI: 1.15–1.84) in Maryland than insured patients to be hospitalized for all avoidable hospital conditions combined.

In addition to differences in the utilization and receipt of health care services, differences exist according to health insurance status in more subjective quality experiences in health care. One study used nationally representative MEPS data to evaluate the **primary care experiences** of adults according to health insurance status and type (Shi, 2000). The study examined the likelihood of describing a positive primary care experience (for example, appointments were made rather than simply walking in for a visit, waiting times for appointments were shorter than thirty minutes, telephone contact could be made easily, and reporting satisfaction in obtaining care). The study found that most primary care quality measures were higher for insured individuals compared to the uninsured and for the privately insured compared to the publicly insured. For example, the odds of reporting a wait time of less than thirty minutes was 28 percent higher for the insured compared to the uninsured and 77 percent higher for the privately insured compared to those individuals covered by public insurance.

Figure 3.17 presents the results of another large study of primary care quality, this time examining differences across different types of health plans. The study compares traditional fee-for-service coverage to several types of common managed care plans that differ mainly in the degree to which they restrict patient autonomy and the methodology they use to reimburse their physicians. The study shows a consistent pattern of improved primary care performance in plans that are least restrictive for patients and contract with physicians on a more open basis

FIGURE 3.17. QUALITY OF PRIMARY CARE EXPERIENCE BY HEALTH INSURANCE PLAN TYPE, 2000

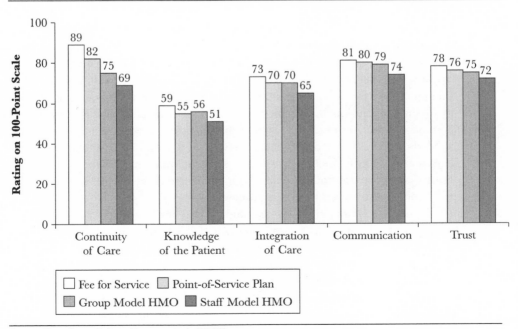

Source: Data from Safran, Rogers, et al. (2000).

(for example, contracting with physicians nonexclusively). For example, patients in fee-for-service plans reported better primary care performance across all aspects of care, and staff model HMOs (the most restrictive plans) generally received the lowest ratings.

Finally, Figure 3.18 shows differences in satisfaction with care according to health plan type (Reschovsky, Kemper, et al., 2000). The study compared the satisfaction of patients in HMOs and non-HMOs on a variety of factors, such as overall satisfaction, satisfaction with choice of primary care physicians, ratings of the last visit to a physician, and patient trust in the physician. The study revealed a consistent trend of lower satisfaction among patients in HMOs compared to those not in HMOs. Across all factors, HMO patients were between 4 and 7 percent less likely to be very satisfied or to have rated the factor highly than patients not in HMO plans. For example, 63 percent of HMO patients strongly agreed that the doctor puts the patient's medical needs first in making treatment decisions, while 69 percent of patients not in HMO plans strongly agreed with the statement. Although the differences are not very large in this study, the consistency of the findings here and across many other studies suggests the presence of real satisfaction problems (Miller and Luft, 1994, 1997, 2002; Lake, 1999).

Health Status

Insurance coverage is closely associated with health status and health risks through a range of possible pathways described in Chapter Two. Researchers have established an association between lacking insurance and lower health care utilization and, subsequently, lower health status (Rowland, Feder, et al., 1998; Billings, 1999). However, most studies use cross-sectional data that limit the ability to draw conclusions on whether lack of insurance actually causes worse health. It is still not clear, for example, whether the generally poorer health status of those in Medicaid (compared to being privately insured) could be attributable to problems with quality of health care rather than the inherently lower SES of those using that public program. We now highlight some of the key findings regarding the association between health insurance and health.

Figure 3.5 compared the self-assessed general health status of respondents according to health insurance status and type. Using data generated directly from the 2000 MEPS, we were able to compare the health status of those insured privately, insured by Medicaid, and uninsured. The figure shows that adults who were uninsured were more than twice as likely to report themselves in fair or poor health compared to those who were privately insured (11.6 percent versus 5.5 percent, respectively). Individuals in Medicaid, however, were more likely than the uninsured to report fair or poor health (19.2 percent), and this may be explained by

FIGURE 3.18. PATIENT SATISFACTION WITH CARE BY HEALTH INSURANCE PLAN TYPE, 1996–1997

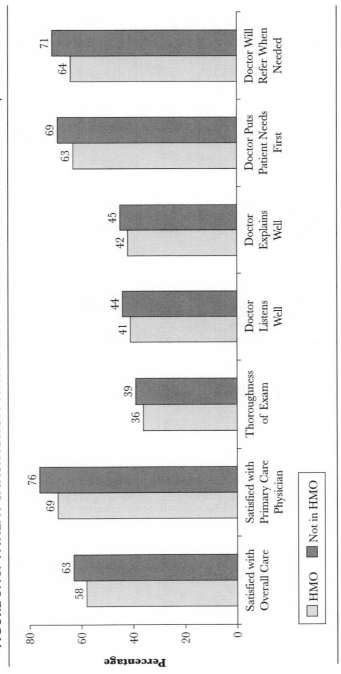

Source: Reschovsky, Kemper, et al. (2000).

the fact that Medicaid coverage is primarily for those living in poverty, and poverty status is associated with poorer health status. Those who are uninsured may in fact have higher incomes than those covered by Medicaid because of restrictive eligibility criteria.

Health risk behaviors are also higher among those without insurance coverage. About 39 percent of uninsured adults reported currently smoking compared to only 23 percent of insured adults. Similarly, adults without insurance coverage were more likely to report physical inactivity (31 percent) compared to only 25 percent of insured individuals. These findings are particularly important because they suggest that individuals with the greatest health risks (the uninsured and concomitant lower SES) are less likely to have good access to care to obtain preventive counseling, medical guidance and assistance on quitting a smoking habit, and health care for the consequences of these health risk behaviors (MMWR, 1998).

Not having insurance coverage is also associated with a greater likelihood of mortality in both the short and long terms. Individuals without insurance coverage are 1.25 times more likely to die in a one-year period than those who have insurance coverage. Moreover, the relative risk of death increases as the study period increases. After five years, uninsured individuals are 1.35 times more likely than insured individuals to die. Even more striking is that the uninsured are nearly twice as likely as the insured to have died during a longer seventeen-year period. Although these studies used data from the 1970s and 1980s, the results have withstood many years of substantial scrutiny (Franks, Clancy, et al., 1993; Sorlie, Johnson, et al., 1994).

Using hospital discharge data and the New Jersey Cancer Registry, Ayanian, Kohler, et al. (1993) studied 4,675 women ages thirty-five to sixty-four for whom invasive breast cancer was diagnosed between 1985 and 1987. They found that upon initial diagnosis, uninsured women had significantly more advanced breast cancer than privately insured women. The study showed that 12.3 percent of uninsured women compared to 7.3 percent of privately insured women were initially diagnosed with advanced breast cancer (or cancer than had spread beyond mammary lymph nodes, chest wall, subcutaneous tissue, or overlying skin; $p < 0.001$). Following women prospectively, the researchers compared chances of survival beyond diagnosis. After adjusting for age, race, marital status, household income, coexisting diagnoses, and disease stage, uninsured women faced a 49 percent higher risk of death than those privately insured. The results are explained by the likely greater frequency of delayed care and the associated **missed opportunities** for earlier detection of cancer among the uninsured.

Franks, Clancy, et al. (1993) using the National Health and Nutrition Examination Survey, a nationally representative prospective study, explored the causal association between lack of health insurance and higher risk of mortality. Study participants ($n = 5,218$) were between the ages of twenty-five and seventy-four years old and were followed from their initial interviews between 1971 and 1975 until 1987. Information on their demographic characteristics (race, gender, baseline age, income, education, employment status), self-rated health, risk behaviors (smoking status, leisure, exercise, alcohol consumption, obesity), and morbidity were collected from each participant through interviews, medical records, and death certificates. This study excluded those with public insurance and whose race was neither black nor white.

By the end of the study, 9.6 percent of the insured had died versus 18.4 percent of the uninsured. After adjusting for the above factors, the lack of health insurance was associated with a 25 percent increased risk of mortality (hazard ratio=1.25; 95 percent CI: 1.00–1.55). There was no significant interaction between insurance and other baseline variables; therefore, the risk of mortality associated with lacking insurance was independent of other risk factors. The effect of not having insurance on mortality was found to be as significant as that of education, income, and self-rated health. The researchers attribute this effect to the greater financial access barriers and lower quality of care faced by the uninsured.

Using a national sample of hospital discharge data for nearly 600,000 patients hospitalized in 1987, Hadley, Steinberg, et al. (1991) explored the association between insurance status and condition on admission to the hospital, inpatient resource use, and in-hospital mortality. The sample of discharged patients was divided into sixteen subsamples by age, sex, and race. In thirteen of the sixteen age-sex-race-specific cohorts, the uninsured had a 44 to 124 percent higher risk of in-hospital mortality at the time of admission than privately insured patients. When the researchers controlled for this baseline difference in mortality on admission, the in-hospital mortality remained higher for the uninsured in the majority of the cohorts. After adjustment, the actual in-hospital death rate was 1.2 to 3.2 times higher among uninsured patients in eleven of sixteen cohorts.

The effect of being uninsured on mortality is similar to its effects on morbidity. In a study conducted of the cutbacks to California's Medicaid program, Medi-Cal, researchers followed all indigent adults previously cared for by the University of California, Los Angeles, Medical Group practice who had lost their Medi-Cal insurance coverage (Lurie, Ward, et al., 1986). They were compared after one year to 109 patients in the same practice whose benefits had not been terminated. Health status was measured by an abbreviated General Health Perceptions Scale, and blood pressure measurements were obtained for all hypertensive patients.

The data showed that the general health of the medically indigent adults had declined 10 points on a 100-point scale ($p < 0.002$) after one year of follow-up. Among hypertensive patients, those who had lost health coverage showed serious deterioration in blood pressure levels compared with those who had stayed on the Medi-Cal program. The proportion of hypertensive patients with blood pressure under 90 mm (a healthy level) was 75 percent at baseline but only 51 percent by the end of the follow-up. The authors believe that the deterioration of health status among their adult indigent population is directly related to their loss of health care coverage and increased barriers to access and use of health services. Although the county was mandated to provide care to this population, there were no stipulations to provide free care, suggesting that the patients who lost coverage were not necessarily or easily finding care elsewhere.

Front-Line Experience: Helping Families One Community at a Time

Lila Guirguis, the early childhood program director of the Hathaway Family Resource Center in Los Angeles, discusses what can be done with minimal resources to help mobilize and strengthen communities that are dealing with a slippery slope of high unemployment, poverty, uninsurance, and the family social and health problems that result.

The Hathaway Family Resource Center is located in the community of Northeast Los Angeles, a densely populated, resource-deficient urban area just outside downtown LA. The area is mostly young, Latino, and living in poverty. Nearly half of the adults in this area never completed high school, and many speak limited English.

The center has been a leader in galvanizing tremendous community energy to promote community health and development at its unique location, a beautiful three-story home located on a large, tree-shaded property. In the late 1980s, the Hathaway Children and Family Services program that resided on the property decided to discontinue foster care services at this site and, in its place, developed one of the first family resource centers in the country. The purpose of this center is to serve as a catalyst for mobilizing the community to address social and health problems that accompany high levels of unemployment, poverty, and lack of insurance.

The center has served as a catalyst for the development of fledgling planning efforts throughout the community. This is often done by supporting ideas and projects from the community with resources, sometimes by leading new initiatives to address problems that have been identified by families, and sometimes simply by providing meeting space for groups to gather and plan. The success of the center is not the result of a top-down approach, but rather is the result of helping the community to address the concerns that members identify. It is a model of community building called asset-based community development.

The center is a one-stop resource in recognition of the interrelatedness of the health, educational, familial, environmental, economic, and social conditions that affect children and families. Our work is based on the premise that people are better served when they can access needed services in one convenient place, have a voice in what services they need, and feel empowered to help design these services. The center blends public and private financing to develop a variety of services that emphasize prevention and focus on the strengths of the community rather than its deficits. Members of the community are involved in the planning, governance, and volunteer work that are essential to operating the center.

The center is a major hub of community activity. It offers parenting and family support services that include family literacy strategies, a reading library for students and adults, parenting education in English and Spanish, English as a Second Language classes, computer training and career development, after-school activities for teenagers, and many other programs. Services assist families to achieve a healthy family life, self-empowerment, and leadership in the community.

With regard to health services, strong linkages have been made available with a local health clinic, community health center, hospital, and Planned Parenthood program. The center is a partner in Healthy Start and a site for a *Promotoras Comunitarias* program, a system designed to train women volunteers to become health educators. With the help of Planned Parenthood, high-risk, sexually active teens receive educational information and free or low-cost access to family planning services.

For young children and families, the center collaborates with local health providers to offer screenings for developmental risks and delays. It offers training for staff, parents, and child care providers to promote child development, such as how to provide effective learning experiences, monitor developmental milestones, and detect cues or alerts that may call for more formal developmental assessment by health providers. Referrals are made to medical providers, dental care, vision screening, and regional centers that offer specific state-funded services for children with special health needs.

The staff of the center recognizes the many challenges that families face. When children have been referred to health services or early intervention programs, many parents do not have an understanding of how these services work, how to obtain them, or how they will be paid for. Based on the suggestions of the community, we help parents through the process. We visit them at home—communicating with them in Spanish if necessary—help schedule initial visits, discuss what to expect from the provider and the range of services that they can receive, and then follow up with them throughout the process. When necessary, the staff mental health coordinator helps to advocate for families who are dealing with health and developmental problems by attending school meetings and supporting families to obtain the best school services for their child.

Overall, the center provides an essential, community-based, integrative health and social service to members of the community. The community members value the center because it reflects them, supports their interests and concerns, and champions their efforts to deal with the range of difficulties that families face.

Summary

This chapter has reviewed the extensive evidence of disparities in health and health care by three vulnerability characteristics: race and ethnicity, SES, and health insurance coverage. The literature provides abundant evidence that racial/ethnic minorities, lower-SES individuals, and the uninsured experience worse access to care, lower-quality care, and poorer health status than whites, higher-SES individuals, and those who are insured. Although we present only some of the highlights of the extensive research base, the comprehensiveness and consistency of the findings (with many approaches and data sources) offer policymakers an unprecedented foundation of knowledge to enhance efforts to eliminate disparities and enhance equity in both health and the American health care system.

Review Questions

1. Briefly describe the relationship between race/ethnicity and mortality. Which racial/ethnic group experiences the highest rates of mortality (overall and cause specific)? Which group experiences the lowest rates of mortality? Describe one nonmedical explanation, using what you learned from Chapter Two, for why the mortality rates for these groups are higher or lower.
2. Briefly describe the relationship between education and the receipt of preventive services for women. How strong is this relationship? Using what you learned from Chapter Two, what are two possible explanations for this relationship?
3. Briefly describe the relationship between health insurance status and access to primary health care for children. Describe how Medicaid-covered children differ from the privately insured in terms of access, and explain why differences might occur.

Essay Question

1. You are the director of a large managed care health insurance plan. You have a particular interest in reducing disparities in the receipt of preventive care among the large population of adults enrolled in your plan. Prepare a written presentation to the chief executives in your health plan to convince them of the importance of addressing this issue. Make sure to discuss what the benefits of preventive care are and where the disparities lie in terms of race/ethnicity and SES. Based on what you have learned from previous chapters, propose two possible courses of action for your organization that would help remedy these disparities.

CHAPTER FOUR

DISPARITIES IN HEALTH CARE ACCESS, QUALITY, AND HEALTH STATUS

The Influence of Multiple Risk Factors

As shown from the review of the literature in the previous chapter, there have been numerous studies exploring the independent influences of being a member of a racial/ethnic minority group, being low socioeconomic status, and lacking insurance coverage on health care access, quality, and health status. Each of these vulnerability characteristics is independently and strongly associated with disparities in both health and health care. Because these characteristics are so closely intertwined, however, having one risk factor increases the likelihood of having another, and it is this overlap of risk factors that is the focus of this chapter.

Perhaps one of the best ways to think about multiple risk factors is in terms of personal **risk profiles.** Each person in the United States may be characterized according to the presence or absence of certain risk factors that are generally considered vulnerable characteristics. A profile can then be developed for each person to describe the number and type of risk factors he or she has. In the United States, we know there is extensive overlap of the three main risk factors described in the previous chapter: minority race/ethnicity, low SES, and lack of health insurance coverage.

In Figure 4.1 we present the overlap of these three risk factors in the national adult and child populations using Venn diagrams. For both adults and children, the most common single risk factor is minority race/ethnicity, with 43.5 percent of the adult population and 50.4 percent of the child population being a racial/ethnic minority (with no other risk factors). The overlap of risk factors is the focus of these diagrams and reveals that about 24 percent of the adult population (nearly one in every four adults) has two risk factors.

The estimate can be derived by adding the 7.2 percent of the adult population that is minority and low income with the 12.7 percent of the population that is minority and uninsured and the 3.4 percent of the population that is uninsured and low income. For children, this estimate is slightly higher (about 26 percent), and that children are more than twice as likely as adults to be minority and low income (17.4 percent versus 7.2 percent), a result that is explained primarily by the higher rate of poverty among children. Adults, however, are more likely to be both minority and uninsured compared to children (12.7 percent versus 8.1 percent), which is explained by the greater availability of health insurance programs provided through public means for children compared to adults.

Of greatest interest is the proportion of both the adult and child population sharing all three risk factors, since these individuals are most likely to experience poor health status and inadequate health care access. These individuals with the maximum profile of three risks are less prevalent in the population (5 percent among adults and 4.2 percent among children), but still represent about 2.8 million adults and about 1 million children in the U.S. population. In total, about

FIGURE 4.1. INTERACTION OF THREE KEY RISK FACTORS AMONG U.S. ADULTS AND CHILDREN

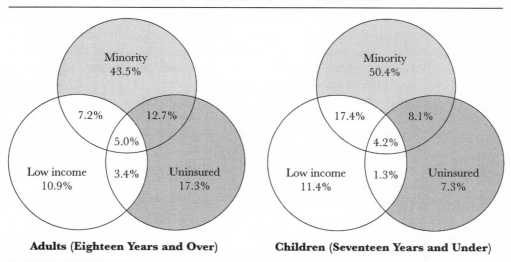

Adults (Eighteen Years and Over)   **Children (Seventeen Years and Under)**

Source: New Analysis of the 2002 National Health Interview Survey.

29 percent of adults and about 30 percent of children have any combination of multiple risk factors, meaning that between one-third and one-quarter of all individuals in the United States are at elevated risk. They are the focus of the data presented in this chapter.

While many studies have documented linkages of these risk factors, relatively few have examined the combined influence of these risks on health care access, quality of care, and health status. There are ultimately an endless number of potential risk factors that could be studied, many of which have a very specific or limited influence; for example, lack of transportation is directly related to the ability to arrive at medical visits. Although we present some studies addressing such other risk factors, this chapter focuses primarily on the interaction of race/ethnicity, SES, and health insurance coverage. Because most current studies examine the interactions of two risk factors at most, we conducted new analyses using a variety of national data sets, including the Medical Expenditure Panel Survey, the National Health Interview Survey, and the National Survey of Early Childhood Health, to present more complex models of vulnerability.

Front-Line Experience: It Takes a Village to Support a Family

Kynna Wright, a staff pediatric nurse practitioner in a community health center in an underserved area of southern California, describes how essential a multidisciplinary team is for providing medical and social services for underserved communities and how one of the greatest rewards is the acceptance and respect of the medical provider as part of the extended community.

Our community health center is located in a large, underserved area in southern California. We recognize that while families may live in a home, this home is part of a larger neighborhood, and that neighborhood is part of a larger community. In our experience, health providers must collaborate with other community-based organizations and become deeply involved with members of the community to be truly successful in improving the well-being of vulnerable populations, including health, child care, parenting, and educational development.

Underserved communities like ours are generally low income, have few social and professional resources, are culturally diverse, and face challenges and barriers to receiving optimal health care. Many families are uninsured, and clinics that serve families lacking insurance have limited business hours (for example, from 9:00 A.M. to 5:00 P.M.) that are not convenient for these families who are often working multiple jobs. Such clinics are often not centrally located and offer few ancillary services that would benefit families in these communities, like on-site health insurance enrollment and assistance with child care. These factors make it very challenging for families to obtain needed services. Lack of a culturally diverse medical staff and health practitioners who may not be culturally or community sensitive and may not understand the community and the role it plays in health care also create large barriers for families seeking care.

The biggest success of our community health center is involving ourselves deeply in the community. We began this process by recognizing that many patients were scheduling medical appointments, but few were keeping them. We started regularly asking patients why they were canceling and learned a few critical lessons. Families told us that we needed longer hours and appointments on Saturday, and most important, that we needed to take our services directly into the neighborhood. In response, our clinic expanded its hours and developed a mobile clinic program that is now one of the shining features of our community health center.

The process of launching this mobile clinic was not easy. Funding was an issue, but even more difficult was establishing the trust of the community to bring our services to the doorsteps of families. With the help of community health workers, we were able to assess the local resources; make connections with local community centers, schools, and child care providers; and ultimately bridge the gap between our medical providers and the people we were determined to help. Our mobile clinic started by serving families in local child care centers and quickly grew to family-based centers that were actually located in people's homes. Our services were primarily for children, but began serving the broader needs of families by offering parents a range of health education classes, referrals to our main community health center, and counseling services. We also provided tips on accessing local social services and encouraged their use of local libraries. Basically, we became a mobile resource center.

In the mobile clinic, we use a team of providers that includes me, a pediatric nurse practitioner, a licensed vocational nurse, nursing assistants, and community case managers. Collectively, we provide head-to-toe services. We offer physical exams, dental exams, vision and hearing screens, and developmental surveillance for younger children. We often encounter situations of domestic violence and have become a key player in referring men and women to the appropriate counseling and legal resources. While the focus of our mobile clinic is mostly on children, we aim to ensure that all family members get linked with a medical home, that is, a place they can easily go to get the health and social services they need.

Once families got to know and trust us, we received referrals to other child care sites (in centers, schools, or family child care), and soon neighborhoods were working together to coordinate miniature health fairs at several sites. I provided classes on health promotion to parents, including topics such as breast feeding and nutrition, stress reduction, and parenting skills. Because I became a familiar face in the neighborhoods and because I was young, bilingual in Spanish, and looked like many of the families I was serving, I was also asked to talk with teens. Among the many topics I was asked to address, perhaps the most important was teaching teens how to get back into school, since many were dropping out and many others were at risk of dropping out.

Serving African American communities has been particularly rewarding for me. In these families, I feel there is a sense of extended kin care, meaning that when someone outside the family (such as a nurse practitioner) truly cares for their family member, over time that person is viewed as an extension of the family. Having worked with many vulnerable families in the community, I feel fortunate that many of them now view me as part of their extended family, and this connection and continuity has facilitated the success and continued growth of our programs. Many families now affectionately refer to me and other providers in our mobile clinic as "aunt," and there is nothing more rewarding about the experience of serving the communities than to have a child say, "Thank you, aunt" even after having just received a series of no doubt painful shots.

This kind of connection that my colleagues and I have felt with the community has helped us to serve teenagers like Tanya, a pregnant fifteen year old. (Her name and other identifying information have been altered.) Tanya visited our clinic for the first time very late in her pregnancy. Because of her low-income status, she was eligible for Medicaid and other social services, and we quickly enrolled her. She delivered her baby nearly a month early, and during the bustle—and due to the extensive bureaucracy and paperwork required to maintain her enrollment in these public programs—she lost health insurance coverage for herself and her baby. We lost touch with Tanya but caught up with her several months later at one of our mobile clinic events. She had dropped out of school and was living with her grandmother, who was helping her raise her baby. The baby had not been examined since her delivery, did not have its immunizations, was not being breast-fed, and was not receiving adequate nutrition, and Tanya was not enrolled in many public programs designed to help her.

Like a trusted aunt does, I sat down with Tanya and her grandmother and talked about getting her life organized. We enrolled her in Medicaid; got her back into school with plans to complete her general equivalency diploma (GED); obtained food stamps, Women Infants and Children, and subsidized child care benefits for her; and enrolled both Tanya and her grandmother in parenting classes at the local community center. Getting all of these loose ends tied up for Tanya was difficult, but was made easier because of the close collaboration between our community health center staff, social services, local schools, and community centers. Our established presence in the community facilitated our obtaining the services she needed.

It has been a while since we have seen Tanya, but at our last visit, she reported that she had earned her GED and that her baby is doing fine (and has received some special services for a developmental delay we detected). Tanya is beginning a prenursing program at her local community college, following in the footsteps of her extended "aunt."

Health Care Access

Poverty status compounds the problems that minorities face in securing a regular source of health care. Figure 4.2 presents the combined effects of poverty status and race/ethnicity on the likelihood of having a regular source of care. This figure confirms the association between race/ethnicity and access, and it shows as well that the likelihood of lacking a regular source of care increases for each racial/ethnic group if living in poverty. For example, Hispanics who have incomes at 100 percent of the federal poverty level (FPL) or less are nearly twice as likely as Hispanics who are not living in poverty (201 percent of the FPL or higher) to report no regular source of care (44 percent versus 19 percent, respectively). Hispanics living in near poverty (101 to 200 percent of the FPL) are about 17 percent more likely than the nonpoor to lack a regular source of care. For blacks and whites, however, living in near poverty is similar to living in poverty with regard to lacking a regular source of care.

This figure also presents the combined influences of poverty status and health insurance coverage on the likelihood of having a regular source of care. The figure demonstrates that the likelihood of lacking a regular source of care increases for insured and uninsured individuals in poverty. Although the uninsured are already more likely than the insured to lack a regular source of care, uninsured adults who are also poor are even more likely to lack a regular provider (52 percent versus 41 percent, respectively).

FIGURE 4.2. NO REGULAR SOURCE OF CARE AMONG ADULTS EIGHTEEN TO SIXTY-FOUR YEARS BY RACE/ETHNICITY AND INSURANCE COVERAGE BY POVERTY STATUS, 2000–2001

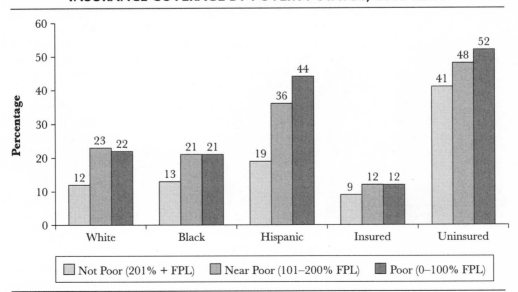

Source: National Center for Health Statistics (2003).

A study by Schoen, Lyons, et al. (1997) used data from a survey of 10,013 low-income adults in Minnesota, Oregon, Tennessee, Florida, and Texas to compare differences in access to health care for adults with private insurance coverage, Medicaid coverage, and no insurance coverage. All respondents had household incomes at or below 250 percent of the FPL. The study showed that among these low-income adults, the uninsured face greater barriers to care than those with Medicaid or private insurance coverage. The uninsured were more likely to report missing needed health care in the past year than either those covered by Medicaid or private insurance (22 percent versus 14 percent and 7 percent, respectively). The uninsured were also less likely to have a specific regular doctor (58 percent versus 34 percent for private insurance), any regular source of care (24 percent versus 8 percent for private insurance), or a physician visit in the past year (40 percent versus 24 percent for private insurance). Finally, about 21 percent of low-income adults reported that the quality of their overall health services was fair or poor, but among the uninsured, 31 percent reported fair or poor quality.

In a unique analysis of the National Health Interview Survey from 1983, 1984, and 1986, Freeman and Corey (1993) looked at the receipt of ambulatory services by insurance status for poor and near-poor adults. Individuals were categorized into four vulnerability groups based on their reported health status and SES, and mean number of **ambulatory visits** within the year were then reported for each of the four vulnerability groups by insurance status (private, Medicaid, or uninsured). The study showed that regardless of health status, among persons in poverty, those covered by Medicaid had ambulatory utilization rates 1.5 to 2.0 times those of persons without insurance, a pattern consistent for all vulnerability groups and all years. This was not the case with private insurance, however, suggesting something unique about Medicaid in encouraging the use of ambulatory services. The authors attribute this result to cost-sharing requirements in private plans that discourage use of services, but which is excluded by law from Medicaid.

If services are not received in ambulatory settings, vulnerable populations often will rely on emergency departments for basic services. While it has been relatively difficult to identify whether visits to an emergency department are due to true emergencies or for ambulatory care services, patterns vary by combinations of race/ethnicity, insurance coverage, and poverty status. Figure 4.3 shows that blacks are generally more likely than whites to receive emergency department services, but that use of emergency departments for both groups increases for those living in poverty or in near-poverty. For example, 5 percent of nonpoor whites reported an emergency department visit in the past year versus 14 percent of poor whites. The pattern was similar for black adults, with 7 percent not in poverty and 16 percent in poverty reporting use of the emergency department. Among insured patients, those living in poverty were over three times as likely as nonpoor individuals to report an emergency visit (5 percent versus 16 percent). Among uninsured

FIGURE 4.3. EMERGENCY DEPARTMENT VISIT IN THE PAST YEAR AMONG ADULTS EIGHTEEN TO SIXTY-FOUR YEARS BY RACE/ETHNICITY, INSURANCE COVERAGE, AND POVERTY STATUS, 2001

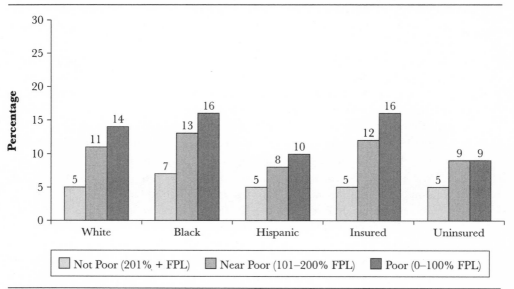

Source: National Center for Health Statistics (2003).

individuals, living in near-poverty and in poverty were the same in terms of emergency department use but higher than nonpoor uninsured adults (9 percent versus 5 percent)

Similar findings regarding multiple risk factors and access to care have been reported for children. Young minority children are more likely to report having no health care visits to an office or clinic in the past twelve months, and this problem is compounded when combined with the influence of poverty (see Figure 4.4; National Center for Health Statistics, 2003). For black children living in poverty, 16 percent report no health care visit compared to 12 percent of those living at 201 percent of the FPL or higher. Black children living in near-poverty (101 to 200 percent of FPL) were even more likely to report no health care visit (18 percent) because this group often earns too much to qualify for Medicaid and too little to purchase private health insurance, which would help to obtain a health care visit. The effect of poverty is even greater for Hispanic children, with nearly one-quarter (23 percent) of all poor Hispanics having no visit compared to 14 percent of those living at 201 percent of the FPL or higher. Similarly, poor white children are almost twice as likely as nonpoor whites to lack a health care visit in the past year (16 percent versus 9 percent).

FIGURE 4.4. NO HEALTH CARE VISITS IN THE PAST YEAR AMONG CHILDREN UNDER EIGHTEEN YEARS OF AGE BY RACE/ETHNICITY, INSURANCE COVERAGE, AND POVERTY STATUS, 2000–2001

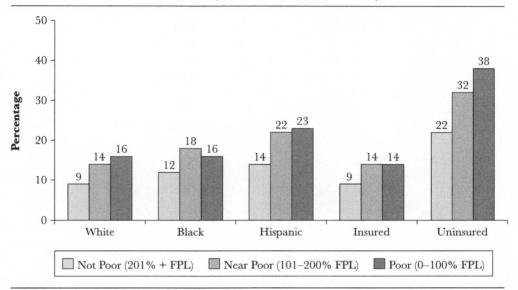

Source: National Center for Health Statistics (2003).

A similar story exists for the combinations of insurance coverage and poverty status. For insured children, living in poverty or near poverty increases the likelihood of no health care visit (14 percent versus 9 percent among nonpoor children). Among uninsured children, the influence of poverty is even more striking, with 22 percent of nonpoor children lacking a health care visit, increasing to 32 percent for those children living in near poverty and 38 percent for those living below the poverty line.

For American adolescents aged ten to seventeen years, health insurance has a differential impact by race/ethnicity on health care visits and compliance with recommended preventive visits. The study by Lieu, Newacheck, et al. (1993), using the child health supplement to the 1988 National Health Interview Survey, examined physician visits in relation to preventive guidelines issued by the American Academy of Pediatrics (AAP). The study found that for both whites and blacks, not having insurance was associated with a decrease of about 0.8 in the mean number of annual visits, from 2.8 to 2.0 for whites and from 2.2 to 1.4 for blacks. For Hispanics, lack of insurance decreased the mean number of visits by half, from 2.2 per year among the insured to just 1.1 among the uninsured. Although there was no significant effect of lacking insurance on visit compliance with AAP-recommended visits for whites, it was associated with a lower compliance for blacks (83 percent versus 70 percent, $p < .05$) and Hispanics (78 percent versus 63 percent, $p < .01$).

A study by Klein, Wilson, et al. (1999), using nationally representative data from 1997, examined combinations of socioeconomic status and insurance as determinants of health care use among America's adolescent population. The study found that adolescents who had no family financial problems were equally likely to have a regular primary care physician regardless of insurance status, but that those without insurance were more likely to report a clinic (as opposed to a specific doctor) as their regular source of care than those with insurance (33 percent versus 19 percent, $p < .03$). Among those with family financial problems, however, uninsured adolescents were less likely than those with insurance to have a regular primary care physician (74 percent versus 85 percent, $p < .01$). The study also found that a number of highly educated families had recently found themselves in hard times due to parents' losing their jobs or becoming disabled. The authors stress the vulnerability of newly financially troubled families who may be less familiar with available public support services.

Most studies of access to care examine the interactions of at most two risk factors. To develop a more complex model, we examined combinations of three risk factors (race/ethnicity, income, and education level) using the nationally representative 1998–1999 Community Tracking Study developed and conducted by the Center for Studying Health System Change. The vulnerability model we present reveals clear **gradients** associated with multiple risk factors in having a regular source of care and any health care visit in the past twelve months (see Table 4.1). The study shows that racial/ethnic adult minorities, low-income adults, and those with less than a high school education (and most combinations of these risk factors) more often lack a regular source of care. While this pattern does not hold in every instance (for example, in some combinations, graduates of high school are as or more likely than adults with less than a high school education to report not having a regular source of care), it appears to be consistent for both measures of access to care.

In another new analysis, we assembled even more complex models of vulnerability and examined their relation to primary care access. We operationalized the concept of vulnerability using profiles that reflect both predisposing factors (race/ethnicity) and enabling factors (income, health insurance, and regular source of care) that are associated with access to care. Risk profiles were composed of the enabling risk factors and examined by race/ethnicity so that differences in the influences of risk factors across racial/ethnic groups could be readily detected. These profiles were examined in relation to four unmet health care needs: missed or

TABLE 4.1. MULTIPLE VULNERABILITIES AND ACCESS TO HEALTH CARE AMONG ADULTS

Race/ Ethnicity	Income	Education	Sample size[a]	No Regular Source of Care	No Health Care Visit in Past Year
White (N = 36,782)	High income (N = 19,248)	College and above	7,858	10.1%	16.7%
		High school and less than college	10,653	9.3	19.5
		Less than high school	737	12.5	22.3
	Middle income (N = 14,960)	College and above	2,864	16.0	20.5
		High school and less than college	10,112	13.2	22.7
		Less than high school	1,984	14.0	21.4
	Low income (N = 2,574)	College and above	323	16.3	18.1
		High school and less than college	1,466	19.4	25.6
		Less than high school	785	16.3	28.8
Minority (N = 11,835)	High income (N = 4,132)	College and above	1,407	15.4	21.8
		High school and less than college	2,383	17.5	25.6
		Less than high school	342	22.2	30.5
	Middle income (N = 5,286)	College and above	781	21.5	27.6
		High school and less than college	3,268	23.2	28.8
		Less than high school	1,237	27.8	35.9
	Low income (N = 2,417)	College and above	166	36.8	42.3
		High school and less than college	1,191	23.5	33.4
		Less than high school	1,060	29.5	36.3
Total sample size[a]			48,617		

[a]Sample sizes are shown for analyses of regular source of care, but are approximately the same for analyses of health care visits.

Source: New analyses of 1998–1999 Community Tracking Study.

delayed medical care, prescriptions, mental health, and dental care. The analyses were adjusted for demographic and community factors.

These analyses used data on 26,208 adults from the 2000 National Health Interview Survey (NHIS). Risk factors included having low income, being uninsured, and not having a regular source of care, and were summed to create a risk profile. Individuals with profiles of one, two, and three risk factors were compared with those having zero risk factors as the reference group, and analyses were conducted by racial and ethnic group.

These analyses reveal that regardless of race/ethnicity, having low income, lacking insurance coverage, and not having a regular source of care independently and in combination create substantial barriers to accessing needed health care (see Tables 4.2 to 4.4). A substantial proportion of U.S. adults (about one in five) have

TABLE 4.2. SELECTED NATIONALLY REPRESENTATIVE RISK FACTORS BY RACE/ETHNICITY

Study Variable	Asian (N = 724)	African American (N = 3,711)	Hispanic (N = 1,380)	White (N = 20,393)
Vulnerability risk factors				
Income***				
Low income (<200% FPL)	25.44%	44.67%	52.32%	28.69%
High income (200%+ FPL)	74.56	55.33	47.68	71.31
Health insurance***				
Private coverage	62.92	59.67	46.69	73.68
Public coverage	10.99	20.54	15.23	9.85
Uninsured	12.59	19.78	38.08	16.48
Have RSC or not***				
Have RSC	86.68	84.88	69.45	81.71
No RSC	13.32	15.12	30.55	18.29
Demographic factors				
Health status***				
Poor health	10.92	16.71	13.84	6.01
Good health	89.08	83.29	86.16	93.99
Risk profiles				
0 risk factors	59.58‡	41.41‡‡‡	27.21‡‡‡	53.86
1 risk factor	28.10‡	39.94‡‡‡	36.81‡‡‡	28.42
2 risk factors	9.02‡	14.3‡‡‡	24.45‡‡‡	13.43
3 risk factors	3.30‡	5.3‡‡‡	11.53‡‡‡	4.29

[a]The number of vulnerabilities a person has (having low income, no insurance coverage, and lacking a regular source of care).

*p < .05, **p < .01, ***p < .001 for the chi square across racial/ethnic groups.

‡ p < .05, ‡‡‡ p < .001 for the chi square of each racial/ethnic group compared to whites.

TABLE 4.3. LOGISTIC REGRESSION OF INDEPENDENT RISK FACTORS PREDICTING DELAYED OR MISSED HEALTH CARE: ODDS RATIOS AND CONFIDENCE INTERVALS ($N = 26,208$)

	Delayed Needed Medical Care	Did Not Get Needed Medical Care	Delayed Filling a Prescription	Delayed Mental Health Care	Delayed Dental Health Care
Race/ethnicity (ref: white)					
African American	0.61***	0.82*	0.81*	0.62**	0.72***
	(0.53, 0.71)	(0.70, 0.96)	(0.69, 0.95)	(0.45, 0.84)	(0.61, 0.84)
Hispanic	0.53***	0.57***	0.63***	0.42**	0.57***
	(0.41, 0.70)	(0.43, 0.75)	(0.48, 0.82)	(0.23, 0.75)	(0.44, 0.73)
Asian	0.51**	0.45**	0.53*	0.31*	0.44***
	(0.33, 0.79)	(0.26, 0.76)	(0.32, 0.86)	(0.11, 0.93)	(0.29, 0.68)
Risk factors					
Low income (ref: high)	1.46***	1.56***	2.11***	1.84***	1.65***
	(1.26, 1.68)	(1.33, 1.83)	(1.76, 2.54)	(1.37, 2.48)	(1.43, 1.90)
Health insurance (ref: private)					
Public coverage	1.69***	2.00***	1.56***	1.17	1.80***
	(1.40, 2.04)	(1.61, 2.49)	(1.26, 1.93)	(0.80, 1.73)	(1.50, 2.16)
Uninsured	5.78***	6.92***	3.98***	4.10***	4.12***
	(4.88, 7.46)	(5.81, 8.24)	(3.27, 4.83)	(3.02, 5.58)	(3.56, 4.76)
No RSC (ref: having an RSC)	1.25**	1.26**	1.10	1.02	1.40***
	(1.07, 1.46)	(1.07, 1.49)	(0.93, 1.30)	(0.75, 1.38)	(1.22, 1.60)

Note: Models are adjusted for age, gender, marital status, education, employment, health status, MSA, and geographical region.

*$p < .05$, **$p < .01$, ***$p < .001$.

TABLE 4.4. MULTIPLE RISK FACTORS ASSOCIATED WITH DELAYED OR MISSED HEALTH CARE: ODDS RATIOS AND CONFIDENCE INTERVALS (N = 26,208)

	Delayed Needed Medical Care	Did Not Get Needed Medical Care	Delayed Filling a Prescription	Delayed Mental Health Care	Delayed Dental Health Care
Total (ref: zero)					
1 risk factor	2.87***	3.58***	3.06***	2.91***	2.37***
	(2.49, 3.31)	(3.02, 4.25)	(2.59, 3.62)	(2.17, 3.91)	(2.05, 2.73)
2 risk factors	7.14***	9.36***	6.44***	5.93***	5.68***
	(6.05, 8.42)	(7.66, 11.44)	(5.32, 7.79)	(4.29, 8.21)	(4.87, 6.61)
3 risk factors	7.39***	10.98***	7.36***	6.24***	7.00***
	(5.92, 9.24)	(8.55, 14.10)	(5.76, 9.42)	(4.26, 9.12)	(5.62, 8.73)
White (ref: zero)					
1 risk factor	2.97***	3.52***	3.10***	3.04***	2.43***
	(2.54, 3.46)	(2.90, 4.26)	(2.57, 3.75)	(2.23, 4.16)	(2.07, 2.85)
2 risk factors	8.03***	9.93***	6.95***	6.32***	6.14***
	(6.62, 9.74)	(7.84, 12.58)	(5.59, 8.64)	(4.43, 9.00)	(5.18, 7.29)
3 risk factors	7.53***	11.33***	7.41***	6.40***	7.33***
	(5.70, 9.94)	(8.36, 15.35)	(5.51, 9.96)	(4.12, 9.96)	(5.65, 9.51)
African American (ref: zero)					
1 risk factor	2.76***	4.34***	2.94***	2.60*	1.72**
	(1.84, 4.14)	(2.85, 6.63)	(1.97, 4.41)	(1.10, 6.17)	(1.23, 2.39)
2 risk factors	7.52***	11.41***	6.26***	6.36***	4.62***
	(4.99, 11.34)	(7.08, 18.40)	(4.04, 9.70)	(2.71, 14.92)	(3.17, 6.74)
3 risk factors	10.84***	14.52***	9.20***	10.00***	7.19***
	(6.65, 17.68)	(8.43, 25.02)	(5.36, 15.78)	(3.82, 26.18)	(4.54, 11.40)

(continued)

TABLE 4.4. MULTIPLE RISK FACTORS ASSOCIATED WITH DELAYED OR MISSED HEALTH CARE: ODDS RATIOS AND CONFIDENCE INTERVALS ($N = 26,208$) (continued)

	Delayed Needed Medical Care	Did Not Get Needed Medical Care	Delayed Filling a Prescription	Delayed Mental Health Care	Delayed Dental Health Care
Hispanic (ref: zero)					
1 risk factor	2.59*	7.25***	2.91**		5.12***
	(1.16, 5.81)	(2.29, 22.97)	(1.32, 6.38)		(2.23, 11.75)
2 risk factors	4.89***	16.78***	4.22**		7.77***
	(2.21, 10.85)	(5.26, 53.58)	(1.72, 10.34)		(3.82, 15.79)
3 risk factors	6.47***	17.78***	4.95***		8.22***
	(2.78, 15.08)	(5.39, 58.66)	(1.97, 12.45)		(3.63, 18.60)
Asian (ref: zero)					
1 risk factor	3.30**	4.28*	4.97*		6.75***
	(1.43, 7.60)	(1.18, 15.50)	(1.19, 20.67)		(2.69, 16.96)
2 risk factors	4.05**	6.13**	11.19**		13.98***
	(1.41, 11.59)	(1.62, 23.21)	(2.19, 57.03)		(4.63, 42.27)
3 risk factors	8.85***‡	6.04***‡	38.33***‡		39.46***‡
	(2.62, 29.85)	(4.81, 141.05)	(7.09, 207.16)		(10.56, 147.36)

Note: Models are adjusted for age, gender, marital status, education, employment, health status, MSA, and geographical region. Empty cells were not estimable due to very small sample sizes. Cells with ‡ are not likely to be stable estimates because of the small number of Asians ($n = 38$) with three vulnerability factors.

*$p < .05$, **$p < .01$, ***$p < .001$.

multiple risk factors for unmet health care needs, and these combined risk factors create up to fivefold differences in reported rates of unmet needs (such as delayed medical care) between the most vulnerable and least vulnerable profiles, regardless of race/ethnicity. The results for receipt of dental care are presented in Figure 4.5. This view of vulnerability is even more striking when we consider that adults who were most likely to report unmet needs are also those most likely to be in poor health.

Interestingly, our analyses show that after adjusting for the study **covariates,** whites were more likely than other racial and ethnic groups studied to report delayed or missed care for each type of health service. After controlling for other risk factors, minorities had 0.40 to 0.80 lower odds of reporting delayed or missed care than whites. Since minorities have lower income, are more likely to be uninsured, are less likely to have a regular source of care, and have poorer health status than whites, it is difficult to believe that whites are truly more likely to have delayed or missed needed care.

One possible explanation for this finding is that whites may have different ideas or perceptions of health needs or a greater belief in their ability to access

FIGURE 4.5. DELAYED DENTAL CARE BY NUMBER OF VULNERABILITIES

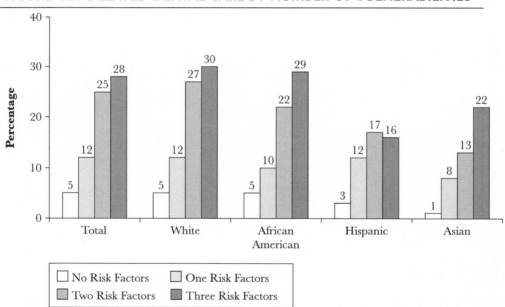

Source: Shi and Stevens (in press a).

care than other racial and ethnic groups. This may contribute to greater reporting of delayed or missed care because whites may feel more empowered to obtain care and speak up or report delays when their health needs are not being met. Whites may be overreporting unmet needs, but given that racial and ethnic minorities generally have poorer health status (a consequence of inadequate access to care), it may be that minorities are underreporting unmet needs.

Overall, these analyses suggest that the potential determinants of delayed or missed care are multifactorial. Reducing disparities in obtaining needed health care services for vulnerable populations will therefore likely require multiple clinical or policy strategies. To ensure that racial/ethnic minorities obtain needed health care services, health systems may need to address language difficulties, cultural beliefs and practices, and ensure that all adults feel empowered to obtain care. Reducing disparities associated with SES will require attention to factors such as level of education (which are related to health care behaviors and seeking) and occupation (which may limit the flexibility in where and when health care services can be sought).

Quality of Health Care

Multiple risk factors are also associated with the quality of health care. While relatively few analyses of health care quality have examined the combined influence of multiple risks, the studies that exist provide some strong initial evidence that should be expanded in future research.

The most commonly reported quality measure in analyses of multiple risk factors is the receipt of preventive care. In a recent study, DeVoe, Fryer, et al. (2003) examined the receipt of adult preventive services associated with combinations of health insurance coverage and the presence of a regular source of care. The study used nationally representative data to show that individuals with both insurance and a regular source of care were more likely to receive each service, compared to those without insurance and a regular source of care. For example, 85 percent of adults who had both insurance and a regular source received a blood pressure check in the past year versus only 46 percent of those without either insurance or a regular source. Similarly, while 57 percent of women aged forty to sixty-nine years with both insurance and a regular source of care received a mammogram in the past year, just 16 percent of uninsured women without a regular source did so. This pattern was the same for each preventive service studied (cholesterol check, physical exam, dental checkup, Pap test, and breast exam). Those with either a regular source of care or insurance had intermediate levels of preventive services.

Poor preventive care often results in the advancement of undiagnosed disease. One study has examined the influence of community income, education levels, and race on diagnoses of advanced-stage breast cancer among thirty-eight thousand breast cancer patients in New York City (Merkin, Stevenson, et al. 2002). The study demonstrated that while lower community income and education levels were associated with late-stage diagnoses of breast cancer, the combination of these SES measures with race/ethnicity was associated with even higher rates of these late diagnoses. For white women living in areas with the lowest education levels and lowest income levels, the rates of advanced-stage breast cancer diagnoses were 10.6 percent and 11.2 percent, respectively. For black women with lowest education and living in the lowest income areas, the rates were 34.8 percent and 43.8 percent, respectively .

Avoidable hospitalizations are also often used as indicators of not receiving high-quality primary and preventive care. Hospitalizations for some conditions such as pneumonia, diabetes, cellulitis, and congestive heart failure can be successfully avoided if they are diagnosed, treated, and managed in primary care settings. In one study, Pappas, Hadden, et al. (1997) examined the difference in rates of avoidable hospitalizations between black and white adults across different income levels. The greatest racial disparity existed at the lowest levels of income. Among those with a median income of less than $20,000, for example, blacks had an avoidable hospitalization rate of over 90 per 1,000 hospitalizations. This is a conspicuous rate compared to whites in the same income bracket, who had an age-adjusted rate of just 50 per 1,000 hospitalizations. At each income level, blacks had a higher rate of avoidable hospitalizations than whites. The disparity in black-white rates, however, was much smaller at the highest income level studied (just under $50,000), where blacks had a rate of about 50 avoidable hospitalizations per 1,000 compared to whites with just 30 per 1,000.

The influence of multiple risk factors in quality of care is evident not only in preventive care and diagnoses, but also in the qualitative experiences in health care. In one recent study, Shi, Forrest, et al. (2003), using data from the 1996–1997 Community Tracking Study Household Survey, examined the influence of several risk factors (race/ethnicity, poverty status, and health status) on the reported quality of adult interpersonal relationships with their health care providers. The interpersonal **patient-provider relationship** was based on responses to seven questions about interpersonal trust, communication, and competence. The study grouped individuals into profiles of risk and demonstrated reductions in patient-provider relationship ratings associated with increasing vulnerability profiles (see Figure 4.6). The study also demonstrated gradients in office wait times by number of risks, such that 73 percent of whites with high income and good health waited thirty minutes or less to be seen compared to the lowest rate of 41 percent among Hispanics with low income and poor health.

FIGURE 4.6. RATINGS OF INTERPERSONAL PATIENT-PROVIDER
RELATIONSHIPS AMONG ADULTS, BY RACE/ETHNICITY,
INCOME, AND HEALTH STATUS

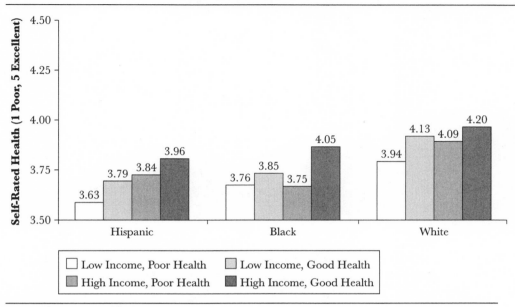

Source: Shi, Forrest, et al. (2003).

To continue to examine more complex models of risk, we examined three risk factors (race/ethnicity, income, and education level) using the nationally representative 1998–1999 Community Tracking Study in relation to primary care experiences. The models we developed demonstrate gradients associated with multiple risk factors in adult reports of patient-provider interpersonal quality (an index scored from 0 to 20, based on four questions about interpersonal trust and communication), and in continuity of care (see Table 4.5). The results for interpersonal relationship ratings suggest gradients across combined profiles of race/ethnicity and income but not educational status. For example, whites with high income rated their interpersonal patient-provider relationships most highly (a mean of approximately 17) compared to low-income whites (about 16.5), high-income minorities (16.0), and low-income minorities (15.5). Within these groups, educational status did not appear to matter.

With regard to primary care continuity, gradients were also apparent across racial/ethnic and income profiles, and educational status again appeared to matter less. For example, only about 11 percent of whites with high incomes reported

TABLE 4.5. MULTIPLE VULNERABILITIES AND QUALITY OF HEALTH CARE AMONG ADULTS

Risk Factors			Sample Size	Interpersonal Quality Rating Mean (SE)	No Continuity of Care
Race/Ethnicity	Income	Education			
White (N = 27,976)	High income (N = 14,809)	College and above	6,242	17.1 (0.04)	11.5%
		High school and less than college	8,033	17.0 (0.04)	12.6
		Less than high school	534	16.8 (0.17)	10.9
	Middle income (N = 11,311)	College and above	2,226	16.7 (0.13)	13.4
		High school and less than college	7,601	16.8 (0.05)	13.9
		Less than high school	1,484	16.7 (0.10)	15.8
	Low income (N = 1,856)	College and above	248	16.0 (0.24)	16.5
		High school and less than college	1,057	16.6 (0.11)	18.8
		Less than high school	551	6.2 (0.12)	21.4
Minority (N = 8,011)	High income (N = 2,932)	College and above	1,043	16.1 (0.12)	12.5
		High school and less than college	1,667	16.0 (0.10)	16.5
		Less than high school	222	15.4 (0.25)	10.4
	Middle income (N = 3,587)	College and above	546	15.8 (0.17)	17.2
		High school and less than college	2,274	15.9 (0.09)	20.7
		Less than high school	767	15.6 (0.16)	21.8
	Low income (N = 1,492)	College and above	97	15.4 (0.48)	30.2
		High school and less than college	785	15.4 (0.16)	28.8
		Less than high school	610	15.5 (0.23)	26.9
Total sample size[a]			48,617		

[a]Sample sizes are shown for analyses of interpersonal quality, but are larger for continuity-of-care analyses.

Source: New analyses of the 1998–1999 Community Tracking Study.

no continuity of care compared to about 19 percent of low-income whites, roughly 14 percent of high-income minorities, and 28 percent of low-income minorities. The educational status breakdowns within these categories appeared to matter less, though there may be differences by education among low-income whites. Among low-income whites, only 17 percent of adults with a college education reported no continuity compared to 19 percent of high school graduates and 21 percent of those without a high school education.

To expand on analyses of preventive services using more complex vulnerability risk profiles, we conducted our own analyses of nationally representative data (Shi and Stevens, in press b). Risk factors in these analyses included predisposing (educational status) and enabling factors (income, health insurance, and regular source of care). Profiles were examined by race/ethnicity, so differences in the influence of risk factors across racial/ethnic groups could be detected. We examined five preventive services recommended by the U.S. Preventive Services Task Force (USPSTF): receipt of blood pressure and cholesterol screening, flu shot, Pap smear, mammogram, and dental check. These analyses controlled for demographics, geography, and managed care that are strongly associated with access to care.

We analyzed data on 15,604 adults from the Household Component of the 1996 Medical Expenditure Panel Survey (MEPS), which was cosponsored by the Agency for Healthcare Research and Quality and the National Center for Health Statistics. Profiles reflected low education status, low income, lack of health insurance coverage, and no regular source of care, and were examined by race and ethnicity. The profiles were examined as each unique possible combination and as a count of the total risk factors a person has.

These analyses confirm the results of many other studies demonstrating the independent associations of these key risk factors with lower receipt of preventive services. In contrast to other studies (Hegarty, Burchett, et al., 2000; Williams, Flocke, et al., 2001; Stewart and Silverstein, 2002; Doty and Weech-Maldonado 2003), our analyses suggest that racial/ethnic disparities in some preventive services are not fully explained by SES and access to care factors. Most important, this study demonstrates that a substantial proportion of U.S. adults (about one in five) has multiple risk factors (see Table 4.6) and that these risk factors create up to fivefold differences in preventive services received between the highest and lowest profiles, regardless of race/ethnicity (see Tables 4.7 and 4.8). Clear gradients were also seen when examining the various combinations that were used to create the profiles (see Figure 4.7).

These findings are particularly salient when we consider that multiple risk factors are disproportionately found in African American and Hispanic populations. Approximately 78 percent of Hispanics and 68 percent of African Americans have

TABLE 4.6. CHARACTERISTICS OF THE U.S. POPULATION BY RACE/ETHNICITY (N = 15,604)

Study Variables	Asian (N = 418)	African American (N = 1,973)	Hispanic (N = 2,883)	White (N = 10,330)
Risk factors				
Low income[F] (vs. high: 200% or over FPL)	26.9%	49.0%***	53.6%***	24.4%
Education	***	***	***	
Less than high school[F]	14.2	23.5	42.8	14.1
High school	39.5	58.0	43.4	54.0
College degree or higher	46.3	18.5	13.9	32.0
Health system factors				
Insurance coverage	**	***	***	
Private	68.0	59.6	50.5	81.5
Medicaid	11.4	17.0	16.1	4.4
Medicare	2.8	4.7	2.4	4.8
Uninsured[F]	17.8	19.1	31.1	9.4
No regular source of care[F] (vs. yes)	24.8*	23.7***	37.7***	18.0
Vulnerability profile[a]	*	***	***	
0 risk factors	47.1	31.6	22.3	54.7
1 risk factor	29.7	34.4	26.3	29.1
2 risk factors	17.2	23.0	25.4	12.6
3 risk factors	4.7	9.3	17.2	3.3
4 risk factors	1.3	1.6	8.9	0.4

(continued)

TABLE 4.6. CHARACTERISTICS OF THE U.S. POPULATION BY RACE/ETHNICITY (N = 15,604) *(continued)*

Study Variables	Asian (N = 418)	African American (N = 1,973)	Hispanic (N = 2,883)	White (N = 10,330)
Preventive services in past year				
Dental checkup‡	31.8	26.0	31.9	38.7
Flu shot‡‡‡	23.4	18.4	21.1	27.3
Blood pressure screening‡‡	67.0	76.2	79.9	78.8
Cholesterol screening‡	43.7	52.3	49.3	46.4
Pap smear‡‡	51.6	62.1	69.6	56.9
Mammogram‡	39.2	46.8	71.2	49.0

Note: A F denotes the category of the variable that was considered a risk factor and included in the risk profile.

[a]Number of vulnerabilities based on low income, less than high school education, uninsured, and no regular source of care.

*$p < .05$, **$p < .01$, ***$p < .001$ for the chi square of the racial/ethnic group compared to white.

‡$p < .05$, ‡‡$p < .01$, ‡‡‡$p < .001$ for the chi square across all racial/ethnic groups.

TABLE 4.7. INDEPENDENT ASSOCIATIONS OF RACE/ETHNICITY AND RISK FACTORS WITH THE RECEIPT OF PREVENTIVE SERVICES

	Dental Checkup	Flu Shot	Blood Pressure Screening	Cholesterol Screening	Pap Smear	Mammogram
Sample size	14,667	14,477	13,691	5,551	6,274	3,368
Race/ethnicity (ref: white)						
Asian	0.71*	0.89	0.60**	1.16	0.64*	0.65
	(0.54, 0.94)	(0.59, 1.34)	(0.43, 0.84)	(0.72, 1.86)	(0.44, 0.93)	(0.40, 1.04)
African-American	0.62***	0.70***	0.87	1.43**	1.27*	1.00
	(0.53, 0.73)	(0.59, 0.84)	(0.74, 1.03)	(1.14, 1.79)	(1.04, 1.56)	(0.78, 1.28)
Hispanic	0.79**	0.76**	0.81*	1.30*	0.95	1.15
	(0.68, 0.92)	(0.63, 0.92)	(0.68, 0.96)	(1.06, 1.60)	(0.80, 1.14)	(0.89, 1.49)
Risk factors						
Low income (ref: high)[F]	0.55***	0.88	0.93	0.79*	0.98	0.80*
	(0.49, 0.62)	(0.77, 1.01)	(0.82, 1.05)	(0.66, 0.95)	(0.83, 1.15)	(0.65, 0.99)
Education less than high school	0.49***	0.70***	0.77**	0.92	0.68***	0.75*
(ref: high school graduate)[F]	(0.42, 0.56)	(0.61, 0.80)	(0.66, 0.90)	(0.74, 1.13)	(0.58, 0.81)	(0.58, 0.97)

(continued)

TABLE 4.7. INDEPENDENT ASSOCIATIONS OF RACE/ETHNICITY AND RISK FACTORS WITH THE RECEIPT OF PREVENTIVE SERVICES

	Dental Checkup	Flu Shot	Blood Pressure Screening	Cholesterol Screening	Pap Smear	Mammogram
Risk factors						
Health insurance (ref: private)						
Medicaid	0.55***	0.83	1.12	0.84	1.12	0.84
	(0.44, 0.68)	(0.66, 1.04)	(0.89, 1.41)	(0.58, 1.22)	(0.91, 1.39)	(0.61, 1.17)
Medicare	0.57***	0.83	0.75	1.17	1.27	0.63
	(0.44, 0.73)	(0.66, 1.03)	(0.54, 1.05)	(0.66, 2.07)	(0.55, 2.93)	(0.39, 1.04)
Uninsured[F]	0.38***	0.61***	0.45***	0.44***	0.38***	0.38***
	(0.32, 0.46)	(0.49, 0.77)	(0.38, 0.52)	(0.35, 0.56)	(0.37, 0.52)	(0.27, 0.53)
Other	0.61	1.09	1.27	0.80	0.94	1.00
	(0.35, 1.08)	(0.63, 2.54)	(0.48, 1.32)	(0.51, 1.72)	(0.43, 2.30)	
No RSC (ref: having an RSC)[F]	0.65***	0.53***	0.38***	0.32***	0.62***	0.45***
	(0.58, 0.74)	(0.45, 0.62)	(0.33, 0.43)	(0.27, 0.38)	(0.53, 0.73)	(0.35, 0.58)

Note: Blood pressure screening is limited to ages twenty-one and over, cholesterol screening to women ages forty-five to sixty-four and men ages thirty-five to sixty-four, Pap smear to women ages eighteen to sixty-four, and mammogram to women ages forty to sixty-nine. The model is adjusted for age and gender (when appropriate), health status, marital status, MSA, employment status, and managed care enrollment. The [F] denotes that the category of the variable was considered a risk factor and included in the risk profile. The numbers in the tables are odds ratios (OR), followed by the 95 percent upper and lower confidence intervals (CI) for the estimate.

$*p < .05$, $**p < .01$, $***p < .001$ for the odds ratio estimate.

TABLE 4.8. VULNERABILITY PROFILES BY RACE/ETHNICITY PREDICTING PREVENTIVE SERVICES: MULTIVARIATE LOGISTIC REGRESSIONS

	Dental Checkup	Flu Shot	Blood Pressure Screening	Cholesterol Screening	Pap Smear	Mammogram
Sample size						
Total (ref: zero)	14,845	14,649	13,846	5,599	6,351	3,400
1 risk factor	0.56***	0.73***	0.54***	0.70***	0.54***	0.65***
	(0.50, 0.62)	(0.65, 0.82)	(0.47, 0.61)	(0.46, 0.62)	(0.60, 0.80)	(0.53, 0.79)
2 risk factors	0.29***	0.51***	0.36***	0.26***	0.59***	0.30***
	(0.25, 0.35)	(0.43, 0.61)	(0.30, 0.43)	(0.20, 0.33)	(0.48, 0.71)	(0.23, 0.40)
3 or more risk factors	0.13***	0.24***	0.12***	0.12***	0.26***	0.16***
	(0.10, 0.17)	(0.17, 0.34)	(0.10, 0.15)	(0.08, 0.17)	(0.19, 0.35)	(0.10, 0.25)
White (ref: zero)						
1 risk factor	0.58***	0.71***	0.53***	0.48***	0.71***	0.61***
	(0.51, 0.65)	(0.63, 0.81)	(0.46, 0.61)	(0.41, 0.57)	(0.59, 0.85)	(0.49, 0.76)
2 risk factors	0.28***	0.48***	0.36***	0.20***	0.56***	0.28***
	(0.23, 0.34)	(0.38, 0.61)	(0.29, 0.44)	(0.15, 0.28)	(0.44, 0.72)	(0.20, 0.40)
3 or more risk factors	0.12***	0.16***	0.15***	0.12***	0.30***	0.14***
	(0.08, 0.19)	(0.10, 0.27)	(0.11, 0.20)	(0.07, 0.20)	(0.19, 0.46)	(0.07, 0.29)
African American (ref: zero)						
1 risk factor	0.56***	1.19	0.57**	0.66	0.80	0.80
	(0.40, 0.78)	(0.84, 1.68)	(0.38, 0.84)	(0.43, 1.00)	(0.56, 1.15)	(0.45, 1.40)
2 risk factors	0.40***	1.13	0.30***	0.30***	0.65	0.28**
	(0.24, 0.64)	(0.68, 1.90)	(0.17, 0.51)	(0.16, 0.56)	(0.39, 1.10)	(0.12, 0.68)
3 or more risk factors	0.21***	0.63	0.11***	0.07***	0.24**	0.16**
	(0.10, 0.45)	(0.31, 1.29)	(0.06, 0.19)	(0.02, 0.18)	(0.09, 0.60)	(0.04, 0.59)

(continued)

TABLE 4.8. VULNERABILITY PROFILES BY RACE/ETHNICITY PREDICTING PREVENTIVE SERVICES: MULTIVARIATE LOGISTIC REGRESSIONS (continued)

	Dental Checkup	Flu Shot	Blood Pressure Screening	Cholesterol Screening	Pap Smear	Mammogram
Hispanic (ref: zero)						
1 risk factor	0.57***	0.97	0.56**	0.89	0.50***	1.32
	(0.42, 0.77)	(0.66, 1.41)	(0.39, 0.81)	(0.50, 1.58)	(0.34, 0.73)	(0.71, 2.46)
2 risk factors	0.39***	0.70	0.38***	0.41**	0.47***	0.74
	(0.25, 0.57)	(0.41, 1.21)	(0.25, 0.57)	(0.22, 0.76)	(0.30, 0.72)	(0.34, 1.59)
3 or more risk factors	0.15***	0.39*	0.11***	0.16 ***	0.19***	0.39*
	(0.09, 0.25)	(0.18, 0.83)	(0.07, 0.17)	(0.08, 0.33)	(0.12, 0.32)	(0.17, 0.87)
Asian (ref: zero)						
1 risk factor	0.54	0.40**	0.60	0.80	0.49	0.13*
	(0.29, 1.02)	(0.21, 0.75)	(0.32, 1.11)	(0.30, 2.12)	(0.20, 1.19)	(0.02, 0.71)
2 risk factors	0.21*	0.31	0.68	0.63	0.47	0.05**
	0.12–0.81	0.09–1.08	0.30–1.55	0.15–2.63	(0.12, 1.79)	(0.01, 0.33)
3 or more risk factors	0.16*	0.16*	0.27	0.24	0.09*	
	(0.04, 0.67)	(0.03, 0.77)	(0.07, 1.05)	(0.03, 2.39)	(0.01, 0.76)	

Note: Blood pressure screening is limited to ages twenty-one and over, cholesterol screening to women ages forty-five to sixty-four and men ages thirty-five to sixty-four, Pap smear to women ages eighteen to sixty-four, and mammogram to women ages forty to sixty-nine. The model is adjusted for age and gender (when appropriate), health status, marital status, MSA, employment status, and managed care enrollment. The empty cell was not stable due to very small sample size and thus not reported. The numbers in the tables are odds ratios (OR), followed by the 95 percent upper and lower confidence intervals (CI) for the estimate.

*p < .05, **p < .01, ***p < .001 for the odds ratio estimate.

FIGURE 4.7. ALL COMBINATIONS OF RISK FACTORS AND THE PERCENTAGE OF INDIVIDUALS REPORTING RECEIPT OF A FLU SHOT IN THE PAST YEAR

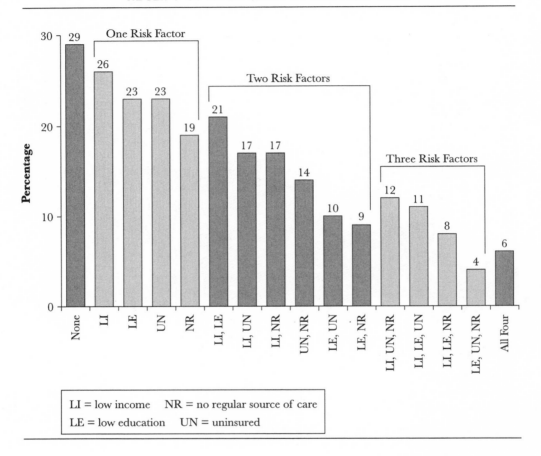

one or more risk factors, compared to about 50 percent of Asians and whites. Perhaps even more striking is that Hispanics are four times and African Americans are three times more likely than whites to have the maximum risk factors (three or more) in this study. This suggests that addressing multiple risk factors will be essential not only to meeting national prevention goals but to reducing the prevalence of racial/ethnic disparities in mortality associated with preventable diseases.

Suggestive of some improvement is the finding that before and after adjustment for SES and potential access factors, African Americans and Hispanics were more likely than whites to report having a cholesterol screening, and African Americans were more likely to receive a Pap smear. These findings are corroborated by other research (Martin, Calle, et al., 1996; Jones, Caplan, et al., 2003; Sambamoorthi and McAlpine, 2003) that shows higher Pap smear screening and mammograph rates among African American and Hispanic women. In these studies, the higher rates have been attributed to the effectiveness of targeted education and screening programs or to perceived higher risk for disease among these groups, creating a greater awareness among providers of the need for screening this population. Similar to other studies (Calle, Flanders, et al., 1993; Tu, Taplin, et al., 1999; Goel, Wee, et al., 2003), Asians were least likely to report receiving most preventive services despite fewer risk factors. This has been attributed to low perceived risk of disease, language issues, and acculturation (Han, Williams, et al., 2000; Tang, Solomon, et al., 2000; Yu, Hong, et al., 2003).

Overall, improving the receipt of preventive services for vulnerable populations will require multifaceted clinical and policy interventions. While research is needed to determine how to intervene for particular risk groups most effectively, a range of efforts that might be adopted could simultaneously include identifying the risk groups, providing education regarding obtaining preventive services, linking vulnerable populations with accessible providers who are experienced in serving these populations, and reducing cost sharing for these services. Such an approach addresses these potentially interactive influences of multiple risks and may help reduce disparities among vulnerable populations in preventable diseases.

Health Status

Multiple vulnerabilities have perhaps their most clearly observed influences on health status. Data from *Health, United States 2003* (National Center for Health Statistics, 2003) show that lack of health insurance and being low income combine to increase the likelihood of being in fair or poor health status. Among adults who have private insurance, having low income increased the likelihood of being in fair or poor health from 6 percent to 19 percent. Among those with public insurance, poverty similarly increased the likelihood of being in fair or poor health from 18 percent to 40 percent, and for the uninsured this jump was from 11 percent to 32 percent. While the uninsured appeared to be in slightly better health than those with public insurance, the increase associated with poverty status among the uninsured was much greater compared to among the publicly insured (three times higher versus about two times higher).

Using data from the 1997 National Survey of America's Families (NSAF; Staveteig and Wigton, 2000), the Urban Institute assessed differences in perceived health status by race and ethnicity and income. Racial and ethnic disparities in perceived health status varied across both low- and higher-income groups, as shown in Figure 4.8. Low income is defined as below 200 percent of the federal poverty level, and higher income is at or above 200 percent of the federal poverty level. Low-income Hispanic adults, in particular, were most likely to report being in fair or poor health. One out of three low-income Hispanic adults (33 percent) reported being in fair or poor health compared to 13 percent of higher-income Hispanics. Twenty-three percent of African Americans and 20 percent of Native Americans and whites in the low-income bracket reported fair or poor health status. Low-income Asian adults were the least likely to be in fair or poor health (12 percent), a rate significantly lower than that for low-income whites. Whites had the lowest percentage of higher-income adults reporting fair or poor health (7 percent) though not much lower than Asians (8 percent). Only 10 percent of higher-income blacks and Hispanics reported fair or poor health status.

Figure 4.9 shows the combined effects of race, ethnicity, and maternal education on **infant mortality rates.** The figure demonstrates very large disparities in infant mortality across racial and ethnic groups, and shows the figure demonstrates the added effects of low maternal education on infant mortality for each racial and ethnic group. For example, the black infant mortality rate increases by about 4 deaths per 1,000 live births for mothers with less than a high school education compared to those with greater than a high school education (thirteen or more years of education). The same pattern in infant mortality rates holds for American Indian and Alaskan Native individuals, increasing roughly 25 percent (about 3 deaths per 1,000) for mothers with less than a high school education. The interactive effects of education and race are most obvious for the racial groups that have the highest infant mortality rates.

To better understand the effects of race and poverty on patterns of mortality, Geronimus, Bound et al. (1996) analyzed 1990 **standardized mortality rates** (SMR) for black and white, poor and nonpoor adults, ages fifteen to sixty-four, living in eight areas around the country. In each area, data were analyzed from residents of one area of persistent poverty and another of higher income. The mortality rates for each of the eight groups were compared to national standardized 1990 death rates for whites; the results for men and women are shown in Table 4.9. **Multivariate analysis** of the data showed that the likelihood of a fifteen-year-old black girl in Harlem surviving to forty-five years of age was the same as a typical white girl anywhere in the United States surviving to sixty-five years. For black boys in Harlem, the likelihood of surviving to age forty-five was even lower.

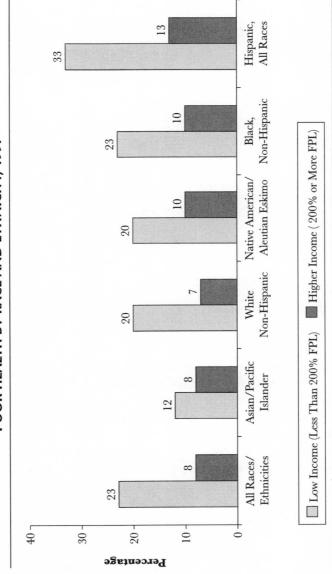

FIGURE 4.8. NONELDERLY ADULTS REPORTING FAIR OR POOR HEALTH BY RACE AND ETHNICITY, 1997

Percentage

40 — 30 — 20 — 10 — 0

All Races/Ethnicities: 23, 8
Asian/Pacific Islander: 12, 8
White Non-Hispanic: 20, 7
Native American/Aleutian Eskimo: 20, 10
Black, Non-Hispanic: 23, 10
Hispanic, All Races: 33, 13

☐ Low Income (Less Than 200% FPL)   ■ Higher Income (200% or More FPL)

Source: Staveteig and Wigton (2000).

FIGURE 4.9. INFANT MORTALITY BY RACE/ETHNICITY AND MATERNAL EDUCATION, 1998–2000

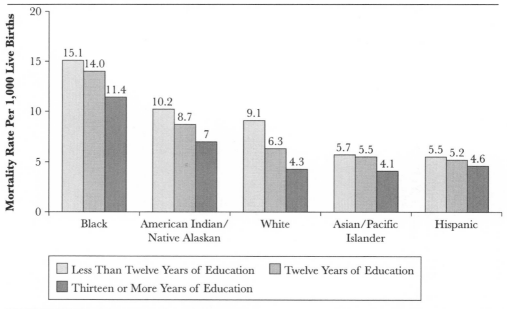

Source: National Center for Health Statistics (2003).

Several studies have shown that when SES is taken into account, the disparities between African Americans and whites for various health measures may diminish but are not eliminated. Researchers examined the association of race and social class with stroke mortality among a ten-year cohort of North Carolina men ages thirty-five to eighty-four. They defined social class by occupation in four categories: primary white collar (executive, managerial, administrative), secondary white collar (sales and clerical), primary blue collar (production, craft, and repair), and secondary blue collar (services, machine operators, transportation, and farming). The researchers concluded that both lower social class and being a minority placed individuals at greater risk for premature stroke mortality. For all races, the highest rates of premature stroke mortality occurred among the lowest social classes. Black men in the lowest social class were 2.6 times more likely to die than black men in the highest social class, and for whites this relative risk was about 2.3. Illustrating the influence of multiple risk factors even further, the study showed that within each social class group, there were significant differences in rates of premature stroke mortality between black and white men. The black-to-white

TABLE 4.9. MORTALITY RATES AMONG BLACK AND WHITE POPULATIONS IN SELECTED U.S. AREAS, 1989–1990 (PER 100,000 RESIDENT POPULATION)

	Annual Male Death Rates	Annual Female Death Rates	Male SMR (95% CI)	Female SMR (95% CI)
Whites	417	225	1.00	1.00
Low-income area				
Lower East Side	625	250	1.50 (1.40–1.61)	1.11 (0.99–1.26)
Detroit	838	428	2.01 (1.88–2.15)	1.90 (1.73–2.09)
Appalachia	574	311	1.38 (1.27–1.49)	1.39 (1.24–1.55)
High-income area				
Queens	363	190	0.87 (0.80–0.95)	0.84 (0.76–0.94)
Sterling Heights	172	121	0.41 (0.36–0.47)	0.54 (0.45–0.64)
West Kentucky	360	203	0.86 (0.78–0.95)	0.91 (0.80–1.03)
Blacks	791	439	1.90	1.95
Low-income area				
Harlem	1,713	759	4.11 (3.91–4.32)	3.38 (3.15–3.62)
Central Detroit	1,163	580	2.79 (2.67–2.92)	2.58 (2.42–2.75)
Watts	1,216	584	2.92 (2.77–3.07)	2.60 (2.43–2.79)
High-income area				
Queens-Bronx	491	242	1.18 (1.10–1.26)	1.08 (0.98–1.26)
Northwest Detroit	691	335	1.66 (1.56–1.76)	1.49 (1.37–1.62)
Crenshaw	781	347	1.87 (1.75–2.00)	1.87 (1.75–2.00)

Note: SMR = standardized mortality ratio.

Source: Geronimus, Bound et al. (1996).

stroke mortality ratio ranged from 4.0 in the highest social class to 4.9 in the lowest social class (Casper, Barnett, et al., 1997). This increasing mortality ratio across social classes suggests that race, ethnicity, and social class combine to strongly influence mortality above and beyond the effects of either race or social class alone.

Using the same population, researchers also found that the decrease in mortality from coronary heart disease seen in the past few years has not benefited black men of lower social class to the same degree as white and black men of higher social classes, controlling for age. For all social classes, the age-adjusted mortality rates from coronary heart disease were higher for black men compared to white men. Although there was a clear decline in heart disease mortality rates for white men across all social classes, only black men in the highest social class had any decline. The researchers point to the importance of targeting public health efforts to vulnerable subgroups, and this further highlights the needs of addressing multiple vulnerabilities at the same time (Barnett, Armstrong, et al., 1999). Similar findings have been reported with regard to asthma prevalence among adults and children (Grant, Lyttle, et al., 2000; Miller, 2000).

Several previous studies among children have shown that the accumulation of risk factors influences health status and child development. Studies by Starfield, Robertson, and Riley have demonstrated a strong association between higher social class (measured as a combination of parent education and employment levels) and several domains of both child and adolescent health status (Starfield, Riley, et al., 2002; Starfield, Robertson, et al. 2002). In addition, Sameroff and colleagues, and later Furstenberg and colleagues (Sameroff, Seifer, et al., 1987; Furstenberg, Cook, et al., 1999), demonstrated strong associations of the number of risks and adolescent social-emotional health, psychological adjustment, academic performance, and IQ scores. The selected risk factors were chosen to reflect risks related to family processes (parent investment and discipline), parent characteristics (education, mental health status), family structure (marital status, welfare receipt), community factors (social resources and neighborhood SES), and peer networks (antisocial versus prosocial). These studies showed risks in each domain that were associated with child health and developmental outcomes. Thus, it is not only parent or family factors that have an influence on child health, but also peer group, neighborhood, and community factors.

Using data from the Center for Studying Health System Change's 1998/1999 Community Tracking Study (2001), we analyzed the relationship between multiple risk factors and self-perceived physical and mental health status among adults (see Table 4.10). Both health status and mental health status declined for minorities, low-income individuals, and those with low education and increasing combinations of these risk factors. For example, among whites with no other risks, just 4.6 percent reported being in poor health. Among blacks with low income and low education, this risk increased to about 44 percent, ten times higher than whites with no risk factors. Moreover, it is important to note that for adults with the greatest level of vulnerability (all three risk factors), nearly half have poor health status. A similar pattern is found for mental health status, with 14.6 percent of whites with no other risk factors reporting poor mental health status, compared to 37.3 percent of blacks with both other risk factors.

New analyses using more complex vulnerability profiles were conducted to examine the health status of children in California. These new analyses create a vulnerability profile for each child that accounts for the combined influences of race/ethnicity, income, parent education, insurance coverage, citizenship, and language. The analyses used parent-reported data on 12,592 children from birth to eleven years of age from the 2001 California Health Interview Survey. While each risk factor was examined separately, a vulnerability profile was constructed as a count of six possible risk factors: (1) minority race/ethnicity, (2) family income less than 200 percent of the FPL, (3) parent education less than high school, (4) child uninsured, (5) noncitizen, and (6) primary language other than English among parents.

These analyses (see Table 4.11) suggest that 45 percent of children have three or more risk factors, with 16.5 percent with three risks, 12.9 percent with four risks, 9.8 percent with five risks, and 5.3 percent with six risk factors. Each risk factor was independently associated with child health status, and the vulnerability profile revealed a strong association between the number of risk factors and child health status. The **relative risk** (RR) of being in good, fair, or poor health compared to excellent or very good health increased for each additional risk: one risk (RR = 1.68), two risks (RR = 2.89), three risks (RR = 4.52), four risks (RR = 8.70), five risks (RR = 17.48), and six risks (RR = 29.39) compared to zero risks (all $p < .001$).

In another new analysis (see Table 4.12), substantial gradients were found in health and developmental status for even the youngest children according to profiles of risk factors. These analyses used data from the 2000 National Survey of Early Childhood Health (NSECH) conducted by the National Center for Health Statistics. The NSECH is a cross-sectional, nationally representative survey of the parents of 2,068 children four to thirty-five months of age, in which parents report on their child's health and health care (Halfon, Olson et al. 2002).

The vulnerability profile in these analyses encompasses three risk factors: (1) nonwhite child race/ethnicity, (2) less than high school maternal education, and (3) lack of child health insurance. General health status was measured with a five-point Likert-type scale (from "poor" to "excellent"). Risk for developmental problems was measured with a shortened Parents' Evaluation of Developmental Status instrument that assesses parent concerns regarding child development and

TABLE 4.10. MULTIPLE VULNERABILITIES AND HEALTH STATUS AMONG ADULTS

Race/ Ethnicity	Income	Education	Sample size	Poor Physical Health Status	Poor Mental Health Status
White (N = 36,845)	High income (N = 19,272)	College and above	6,242	4.6%	14.6%
		High school and less than college	8,033	8.5	17.7
		Less than high school	534	20.2	26.0
	Middle income (N = 14,992)	College and above	2,226	9.6	18.4
		High school and less than college	7,601	14.3	21.8
		Less than high school	1,484	33.7	28.5
	Low income (N = 2,581)	College and above	248	12.7	29.0
		High school and less than college	1,057	24.5	33.2
		Less than high school	551	45.7	36.9
Minority (N = 11,879)	High income (N = 4,148)	College and above	1,043	8.2	17.4
		High school and less than college	1,667	11.5	19.6
		Less than high school	222	29.5	21.8
	Middle income (N = 5,308)	College and above	546	10.9	21.4
		High school and less than college	2,274	16.6	24.3
		Less than high school	767	34.1	31.0
	Low income (N = 2,423)	College and above	97	19.6	37.3
		High school and less than college	785	29.2	37.0
		Less than high school	610	43.9	37.3
Total sample size[a]			35,987		

Risk Factors

[a]Sample sizes are about the same for analyses of health status and mental health status.

Source: New analyses of the 1998–1999 Community Tracking Study.

TABLE 4.11. LOGISTIC REGRESSION PREDICTING CHILD HEALTH STATUS (*N* = 11,000)

Children Ages 0–11	Excellent or Very Good Health Status Odds Ratio
Individual vulnerabilities	
Child race/ethnicity (ref: white)	
Asian/Pacific Islander‡	0.52***
African American‡	0.65***
Latino‡	0.53***
Other‡	0.74**
Poverty level (ref: 300% or more)	
Less than 100% FPL‡	0.45***
100–199% of FPL‡	0.57***
200–299% of FPL	0.68***
Insurance coverage (ref: private)	
Uninsured‡	0.71***
Medi-Cal	0.84**
Healthy Families	0.85
Other	0.98
Education of respondent (ref: college graduate)	
Less than high school	0.34***
High school graduate	0.70***
Some college	0.49***
Citizenship status (ref: child and parent both citizens)	
Parent noncitizen‡	0.49***
Child and parent noncitizen‡	0.65***
Non-English language at home‡ (ref: English)	0.65***
Risk profiles (ref: zero)	
1 risk factor	0.60***
2 risk factors	0.35***
3 risk factors	0.22***
4 risk factors	0.11***
5 risk factors	0.06***
6 risk factors	0.03***

Note: Model is adjusted for child age and gender.

*$p < .05$, **$p < .01$, ***$p < .001$ for the variable category versus the reference group. ‡Indicates the risk factors included in the combined vulnerability risk profile.

Source: New analyses of the 2001 California Health Interview Survey.

TABLE 4.12. LOGISTIC REGRESSION MODELS PREDICTING CHILD HEALTH STATUS AND DEVELOPMENTAL RISK (N = 2,068)

	Excellent or Very Good Health Status Odds Ratio (CI)	High Risk for Developmental Delay Odds Ratio (CI)
Individual risk factors		
Child race/ethnicity (ref: white)		
African American‡	0.56 (0.36–0.90)**	1.32 (0.88–1.97)
Hispanic‡	0.48 (0.31–0.74)***	1.63 (1.14–2.33)**
Other‡	0.54 (0.24–1.19)	1.34 (0.63–2.86)
Maternal education (ref: any college)		
Less than high school‡	0.48 (0.30–0.78)***	1.58 (1.01–2.51)*
High school graduate	0.84 (0.54–1.30)	1.31 (0.91–1.91)
Insurance coverage (ref: private)		
Uninsured‡	0.40 (0.21–0.76)**	2.83 (1.63–4.90)***
Public (Medicaid/SCHIP)	0.65 (0.41–1.03)	1.22 (0.80–1.87)
Other	1.04 (0.64–1.69)	1.46 (0.91–2.36)
Risk profile (ref: zero)		
1 risk factor	0.36 (0.24–0.55)***	1.66 (1.19–2.31)***
2 risk factors	0.23 (0.15–0.36)***	2.26 (1.52–3.37)***
3 risk factors	0.09 (0.04–0.17)***	5.62 (2.98-10.61)***

Note: Both models are adjusted for child gender and parent mental health status. *$p < .05$, **$p < .01$, ***$p < .001$ for the variable category versus the reference group. ‡Indicates the risk factors that were included in the combined vulnerability risk profile.

Source: New analyses of the 2001 California Health Interview Survey.

accurately identifies children at high risk of developmental delays (Glascoe, 2003). **Logistic regressions** predicting these outcomes are presented controlling for child gender and maternal mental health status that has been previously associated with reported child health status.

These new analyses suggest that child minority race/ethnicity, low maternal education, and being uninsured were independently associated with poorer health and higher risk of developmental problems. Lack of insurance was the strongest predictor of both outcomes (OR = 0.40, CI: 0.21–0.76 for being in excellent/very good health and OR = 2.83, CI: 1.63–4.90 for high **developmental risk**). There was a combined additive association of the risk factors with both outcomes. Young children with one vulnerability had 0.36 lower odds of being in excellent or very good health status than children with zero vulnerabilities ($p < .001$). Children with two and three vulnerabilities were even less likely to be in excellent or very good health with odds ratios of 0.23 and 0.09 respectively (both $p < .001$). Similarly, the odds of being at high risk for developmental delays increased to 1.66 for children with one risk, 2.26 for those with two risks, and 5.62 for those with three risks (all $p < .001$). The results for health status are presented in terms of adjusted percentages in Figure 4.10. This shows the percentage of children with each vulnerability profile who are in excellent/very good health status, adjusted for age, gender, and maternal mental health. The gradients found in this study are particularly important because they are evident in the first few years of life and may threaten future **health trajectories** and outcomes.

Summary

This chapter has reviewed the existing evidence and presented new data regarding the markedly negative influence of multiple co-occurring risk factors on health care access, quality of care, and health status. Once we acknowledge that vulnerable individuals with multiple risk factors are common in the population (and would be even more common if we could account for all of the known risk factors in existence), and recognize the synergistic influences of these co-occurring

FIGURE 4.10. RELATIONSHIP BETWEEN NUMBER OF VULNERABILITIES AND CHILDREN IN EXCELLENT OR VERY GOOD HEALTH ($p < .0001$)

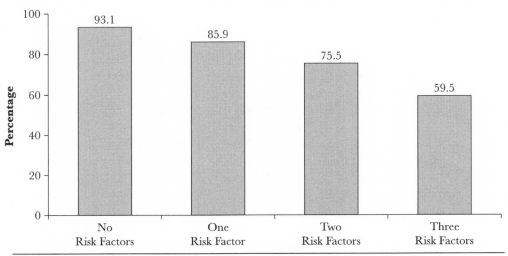

Source: New analyses of the 2000 National Survey of Early Childhood Health.

risk factors on health and health care experiences, there is a clear call for assisting these vulnerable populations in more comprehensive ways.

Review Questions

1. Describe the distribution of multiple risk factors (using race/ethnicity, income, and health insurance coverage) within the national population. How does this distribution vary between adults and children. Based on what you have learned so far, why does this distribution vary?
2. When considering other risk factors such as income, insurance, education, and having a regular source of care, how does the distribution of multiple risks vary by race/ethnicity? Which groups are most at risk, and which are least at risk?
3. Briefly describe how race/ethnicity, SES, and health insurance profiles are associated with health care access, quality of care, and health status. If you were asked to present some of these data to a group concerned with children's health, what would you say are the biggest gaps in knowledge about multiple risks?

Essay Questions

1. Why do risk factors tend to cluster within groups of individuals? Select three risk factors in addition to non-English language, and describe how they are related and how they increase the likelihood of each other. Draw a model with arrows linking these risks. How do these risk factors have the potential to be replicated across generations? Where are the most and least feasible places to intervene to interrupt these relationships? What would likely happen to each of the risk factors once the pathways were disrupted?
2. You have been awarded a large research grant to study the implications of multiple risk factors on access to care, quality, or health status. What three risk factors would you study, and in relation to what outcomes? Justify your decision by considering the previous research on the risk factors and outcomes you select, the feasibility of collecting and measuring this information, and what gaps in knowledge this research will fill. What are the results you would expect to find?

CHAPTER FIVE

CURRENT STRATEGIES TO SERVE VULNERABLE POPULATIONS

The previous two chapters have presented a range of evidence showing the relationships between individual and multiple risk factors and poor access to care, poor quality of care, and poor health outcomes. Recognizing the growing importance of these factors as determinants of health and health care experiences, both government and private organizations have developed a variety of policies and programs to help mitigate the adverse consequences of vulnerability. This chapter reviews the most sophisticated programs currently in place, discusses the mechanisms of vulnerability addressed by each, and systematically critiques their potential to improve the health of vulnerable populations.

The discussion of the programs is organized according to each vulnerability factor addressed by the program (race and ethnicity, SES, and health insurance coverage). Many programs address multiple vulnerability factors, in which case we categorize programs according to the vulnerability factor most explicitly targeted by the program. Within these large categories, the programs are further grouped according to financial sponsorship: federal government, state and local government, or private agency. We review the history, purpose, budget, and current activities of each program.

Programs were identified through correspondence with, and the Web sites of, many sources, including government agencies, congressional committees, national associations for legislators and health care professionals, and private health policy organizations. We supplemented our discussion with information gathered from the peer-reviewed literature. It is important to note here that our review of existing programs is again not intended to be exhaustive but rather illustrative of the major programs available to assist vulnerable populations. A complete listing of the program Web sites and other contact information is provided in Exhibit 5.1.

We critique the potential impact of the programs according to four criteria. First, we examine the validity of the programs and whether they address the most appropriate mechanisms (discussed in the previous chapter) contributing to the disparities targeted by the programs. Second, we examine the scope of the programs, including the number of vulnerable people served and whether the programs reach their intended populations. Third, we explore the sustainability of the endeavors, including the stability of their funding sources and revenues, and the ability of the programs to adapt to and integrate with changes in financing of the health care system. Fourth, we examine the **effectiveness** of the programs and, when possible, incorporate into our analyses the findings of prior studies and evaluations. The chapter concludes with a summary of the major strengths and weaknesses of existing programs and identifies gaps in serving vulnerable populations.

Programs to Eliminate Racial and Ethnic Disparities

There has been growing recognition by both government and private organizations of the importance of race and ethnicity as determinants of health and health care experiences. Recent seminal reports on racial and ethnic disparities issued by the Institute of Medicine and the Commonwealth Fund have further crystallized the importance of these issues among health policy professionals and call for the development of new initiatives to eliminate these disparities (Smedley, Stith, et al., 2002; Collins, Hughes, et al., 2002). While programs and policies to address racial disparities have been in place for many years, only recently has an extensive effort been made to comprehensively address the nonsocioeconomic pathways of racial and ethnic disparities.

Federal Initiatives

The federal government has implemented several broad-sweeping programs that include the development of national governmental agencies, offices, task forces, and health provider recruitment and training programs. These federal initiatives have generally served to bring attention to racial disparities in health, centralized efforts to monitor and reduce these disparities, and provided health services to underserved minority communities.

EXHIBIT 5.1. CONTACT INFORMATION FOR CURRENT MAJOR PROGRAMS TO SERVE VULNERABLE POPULATIONS

The program name, in italics, is followed by the address, telephone number, and URL.

California Endowment Focus on Multicultural Health
California Endowment
21650 Oxnard St., Suite 1200
Woodland Hills, CA 91367
800-449-4149, www.calendow.org

Center for Health and Health Care in Schools
Center for Health and Health Care in Schools
1350 Connecticut Ave., Suite 505
Washington, DC 20036
202-466-3396, www.healthinschools.org

Commonwealth Fund Program on Quality of Care for Underserved Populations
Commonwealth Fund
One East 75th St.
New York, NY 10021
212-606-3800, www.cmwf.org

Community Health Centers
Division of Community and Migrant Health
Bureau of Primary Health Care
4350 East-West Highway, 7th Floor
Bethesda, MD 20814
301-594-4300, www.bphc.hrsa.gov/chc

Health Care for the Homeless
Bureau of Primary Health Care
4350 East-West Highway, 9th Floor
Bethesda, MD 20814
301-594-4430, www.bphc.hrsa.gov/homeless

Healthy Schools, Healthy Communities
Center for School-Based Health
Bureau of Primary Health Care
4350 East-West Highway, 9th Floor
Bethesda, MD 20814
301-594-4470, www.bphc.hrsa.gov/hshc

Indian Health Services
Indian Health Services Headquarters
801 Thompson Ave., Suite 400
Rockville, MD 20852-1627
301-443-1083, www.ihs.gov

(continued)

EXHIBIT 5.1. CONTACT INFORMATION FOR CURRENT MAJOR PROGRAMS TO SERVE VULNERABLE POPULATIONS *(continued)*

Indiana American Indian Health Program
Indiana State Department of Health
Office of Minority Health
2 North Meridian St.
Indianapolis, IN 46204
317-233-7596, www.in.gov/isdh

Kansas City TeleKidcare
Center for TeleMedicine and TeleHealth
University of Kansas Medical Center
2012 Wahl Annex, 3901 Rainbow Blvd.
Kansas City, KS 66160-7171
913-588-7162
www2.kumc.edu/telemedicine/tkc.html

Lincoln-Lancaster Mobile Health Clinic
Lincoln-Lancaster County Health Department
Division of Health Promotion
3140 N St., Lincoln, NE 68510
402-441-8011, www.ci.lincoln.ne.us/city/health

MassHealth Family Assistance Program
www.state.ma.us/dma/

Migrant Health Centers
Division of Community and Migrant Health
Bureau of Primary Health Care
4350 East-West Highway, 7th Floor
Bethesda, MD 20814
301-594-4303, www.bphc.gov

National Health Service Corps
Bureau of Health Professions
5600 Fishers Lane
Rockville, MD 20857
1-800-221-9393, http://nhsc.bhpr.hrsa.gov

DHHS Initiative to Eliminate Racial and Ethnic Disparities in Health. In February 1998, President Clinton announced a new initiative to prioritize the elimination of racial and ethnic disparities in health at the top of the nation's agenda. The main strategy of the initiative was for the U.S. Department of Health and Human Services (DHHS) to reduce disparities in six key topic areas: infant mortality, cancer screening and management, cardiovascular disease, diabetes, HIV

EXHIBIT 5.1. CONTACT INFORMATION FOR CURRENT MAJOR PROGRAMS TO SERVE VULNERABLE POPULATIONS *(continued)*

Office of Minority Health
Office of Minority Health Resource Center
P.O. Box 37337, Washington, DC 20013
1-800-444-6472, www.omhrc.gov

Public Housing Primary Care Program
Bureau of Primary Health Care
4350 East-West Highway, 9th Floor
Bethesda, MD 20814
301-594-4420, www.bphc.hrsa.gov/phpc

Racial and Ethnic Approaches to Community Health
Centers for Disease Control and Prevention
National Center for Chronic Disease Prevention and Health Promotion
Mail Stop K-45
4770 Buford Highway, N.E.
Atlanta, GA 30341-3717
770-488-5269, www.cdc.gov/reach2010

South Carolina Commun-I-Care Program
Commun-I-Care Program
P.O. Box 186
Columbia, SC 29202-0186
803-933-9183, www.commun-i-care.org

Strengthening Primary Care Providers for the Poor
Health Foundation of Greater Cincinnati
Rookwood Tower
3805 Edwards Rd., Suite 500
Cincinnati, OH 45209
888-310-4904, www.healthfoundation.org

and AIDS, and immunizations. The DHHS provides leadership for this initiative by supporting research, expanding and improving programs to purchase or deliver high-quality health services, funding programs to reduce the effects of poverty and provide children with safe and healthy environments, and expanding prevention efforts. The initiative also provides the foundation for an important change in Healthy People 2010 from a goal of *reducing* to one of *eliminating* health disparities. While the DHHS initiative and Healthy People 2010 are separate endeavors, they share a common principle of national equity in health and health care and a common goal to eliminate disparities in the six target areas.

U.S. Office of Minority Health. The Office of Minority Health (OMH) was created within the DHHS in 1985. It was proposed as part of the *Report of the Secretary's Task Force on Black and Minority Health* (Task Force on Black and Minority Health, 1985), and its stated mission is to "improve the health of racial and ethnic minority populations through the development of effective health policies and programs that help eliminate disparities in health." Under the direct supervision of the deputy assistant secretary for minority health, OMH advises the secretary of the DHHS on public health issues affecting minorities.

The OMH plays an important role in the development and coordination of federal health policy by promoting minority health issues in Congress and ensuring that the government is actively accountable to the needs of disadvantaged and minority populations. Specifically, the OMH continues to collect and analyze data on the health of racial and ethnic minority populations and monitors national efforts to achieve the goals set forth in Healthy People 2010, which prioritizes the elimination of racial and ethnic disparities in health and health care.

In addition, the OMH has taken an active role in designing and implementing the DHHS Initiative to Eliminate Racial and Ethnic Disparities in Health. The OMH assisted the surgeon general in identifying and promoting the six minority health target areas. The OMH serves on target area work groups and collaborates with the Centers for Disease Control and Prevention to award and monitors grants supporting initiatives to reduce racial disparities in community health. The OMH also coordinates a wide variety of smaller programs operating from the White House and the DHHS to improve the health of minority Americans.

The OMH regularly funds cooperative agreements and grants that support many research and demonstration programs. The grant programs are intended to facilitate **community linkages** and strategies that use scarce resources efficiently and across organizational lines. Examples of grant programs are the Minority Community Health Coalition Demonstration, the Bilingual and Bicultural Service Demonstration Grants, the Information Technology Infrastructure Grant Program, and multiple grant programs for minorities with HIV and AIDS.

In 1987, OMH established the Office of Minority Health Resource Center to meet the public's need for reliable, accurate, and timely information and technical assistance on issues affecting the health of minority populations. Since that time, the resource center has become one of the nation's largest sources of minority health information. Some of its services are referrals to minority providers and programs, publications on minority health issues, and publication of a newsletter, *Closing the Gap*, that reports on national, state, and local activities related to minority health.

Racial and Ethnic Approaches to Community Health. The Racial and Ethnic Approaches to Community Health (REACH 2010) program was launched by the Centers for Disease Control in 1999 to support the goals of Healthy People 2010 to eliminate racial disparities in health and health care. REACH is a five-year demonstration grant program that supports community coalitions in designing, implementing, and evaluating efforts to eliminate health disparities. Each coalition comprises a community-based organization and three other organizations, such as local or state health departments, a research university, or a research organization. These programs address one or more of the six target topics identified as part of the presidential initiative.

In 2001, the program was appropriated $37.8 million to support thirty-one REACH projects, $5 million of which was contributed by the National Institutes of Health. Supported projects were designed to test the effectiveness of programs to improve the health of racial and ethnic minority populations. Examples of funded programs are the Cambodian Community Health program in Massachusetts, which aims to improve prevention and management of diabetes and heart disease among Cambodian refugees. Another example is the Reach Out program in Chicago, which draws on leadership in churches to encourage black and Hispanic low-income women to seek breast and cervical cancer screening.

Minority Health Initiative. In 1992, the Office for Research on Minority Health at the National Institutes of Health (NIH) launched the Minority Health Initiative (MHI) to improve the national research agenda on minority health issues and strengthen the national commitment and responsiveness to the health and training needs of minority Americans. The research agenda, prompted by Congress, includes biomedical and behavioral research studies that build on existing NIH efforts to improve the overall health of minorities and to train additional minority researchers. Training programs have been implemented for minorities at all education levels, ranging from K-12 science training to postdoctorate fellowships for minority researchers.

Through the initiative, the NIH has also taken steps to include more minorities in clinical trials and other research studies. The NIH has identified barriers to the participation of minorities in clinical research and has developed several programs and activities designed to eliminate these barriers. Efforts include improving community outreach to minority groups, strengthening provider communication with minority patients about participation in clinical trials, and developing a patient recruitment and referral center for minority patients. The MHI was funded at $80 million in FY 1999.

Indian Health Service. The Indian Health Service (IHS) is an agency within the DHHS with the mission to be the principal advocate for and provider of health services to American Indians and Alaska Natives. These populations have higher rates of death from accidents, homicides, suicide, and alcoholism than the general U.S. population. Tribes often lack adequate public health infrastructure, including safe water supplies and adequate waste disposal. To compound the problem, their communities also are often located in isolated areas, making it difficult to access health services.

The IHS currently provides health services to about 1.5 million of the nation's 2 million American Indians and Alaska Natives. There are more than 560 federally recognized tribes in the United States, and their members live mainly on reservations and in rural communities in thirty-five states, mostly in the western United States and Alaska. Federal recognition is reserved for tribes that signed treaties with the federal government between 1787 and the late 1800s. It is important to note that not all tribes are federally recognized and therefore are not included in the IHS.

The stated goals of the IHS are to "ensure that comprehensive, culturally acceptable personal and public health services are available and accessible to all American Indian and Alaska Native people" and to "raise the physical, mental, social, and spiritual health of American Indians and Alaska Natives to the highest level." To achieve these goals, the IHS provides tribes with comprehensive health services and helps tribes develop their own health programs, coordinate health planning, and obtain available health resources.

Comprehensive medical care is provided in nearly fifty hospitals and over four hundred health care centers and **school-based clinics** owned and operated by the IHS. In locations where the IHS does not have its own facilities, it contracts with local hospitals, state and local health agencies, tribal health institutions, and individual health care providers to deliver needed care. Services provided by the IHS include preventive, acute, and emergency medical services; environmental health and engineering; mental health services; health education and promotion programs; and pharmacy, dental, and laboratory services. It also has special initiatives in injury control, alcoholism, maternal and child health, and mental health.

The IHS was part of the Bureau of Indian Affairs from 1924 to 1955, when it was transferred from the Department of the Interior to DHHS. In 1975, Congress passed the Indian Self-Determination and Education Assistance Act, giving tribes the option of staffing and managing the health services in their communities and providing funding for training tribe members to do so. Tribes can decide whether to provide all of their own health care, only a portion of it, or none at all, with the IHS remaining their provider of choice. Almost 60 percent of the IHS clinics are now administered and operated by tribes.

Migrant Health Center Program. **Migrant and seasonal farm workers,** who are primarily Hispanic and African American, face a number of health risks due to poverty and poor living and working conditions. Problems including malnutrition, tuberculosis and other infectious diseases, and exposure to pesticides are compounded by nearly universal lack of insurance coverage and poor access to health care. The Migrant Health Act of 1962 established the migrant health program, which provides medical and support services to migrant farm workers and their families.

Within the program, migrant health centers (MHCs) have become the main health care delivery mechanism, helping more than 125 nonprofit organizations to deliver comprehensive and culturally competent primary care services in more than four hundred clinic sites. The MHC program is administered by the Bureau of Primary Health Care (BPHC) within the DHHS. In fiscal year 2001, the MHC program was appropriated almost $99 million to serve about 600,000 workers and dependents each year.

The MHCs offer primary care and preventive services, transportation, patient outreach, pharmaceutical services, dental care, occupational health and safety, and environmental health. They also provide prevention-oriented and pediatric services such as immunizations, well-baby care, and **developmental screenings.** To ensure comprehensive access to health services, MHCs also partner with state and local health departments, hospitals, specialty providers, social service agencies, and other providers. In order to tailor the services to migrant farm workers, the MHCs rely on bilingual and bicultural outreach workers and health personnel and emphasize culturally sensitive protocols.

State and Local Initiatives

States and counties have independently established programs to address the needs of racial and ethnic minorities. Initiatives established in each state and county reflect the differing racial/ethnic composition, needs, and resources of their areas. States frequently address problems that federal programs fail to address adequately, and these state programs often become models and prototypes for future federal efforts. Because of the vast number of programs operating at the state and local levels, we highlight and discuss only a few key examples. More comprehensive listings of these programs are available in compilation documents produced by trade and professional organizations such as the Association of State and Territorial Health Officials and the National Association of City and County Health Officials and the Bureau of Primary Health Care through the Models That Work program.

Indiana State American Indian Health Program. In 1999, the Indiana State Department of Health, with funding from the Indiana Minority Health Coalition, launched the American Indian Health Program to address the health needs of Native Americans residing in Indiana. The State of Indiana did not qualify for reservation status, which would have allowed Native American residents to obtain health care from the federal Indian Health Service, and thus a large proportion of the estimated fifteen thousand Native Americans living in the state did not have adequate access to health services.

The goals of the program are to increase access to health promotion services in a manner that is culturally appropriate, increase access to health screenings and link patients needing care with providers offering free or low-cost services, facilitate a network of providers who can offer services to meet the needs of Native Americans, and systematically collect health data on this population to develop new programs and improve existing activities. Most services are provided on-site at the American Indian Health Care Center in Indianapolis and through a network of local clinics and at cultural gatherings of Native Americans.

Lincoln-Lancaster County Mobile Health Clinic Services. In 1997, the Lincoln-Lancaster County Health Department in Nebraska created a mobile health clinic system to provide medical and dental services to underserved racial and ethnic minority populations and to non-English-speaking populations. To identify areas of the county experiencing the greatest barriers to accessing health services, the health department employed a unique geographical information system to determine which areas had high rates of poverty, above-average death rates, particularly high housing deterioration, and, most important, a large nonwhite population. In addition, door-to-door surveys were completed to identify neighborhood needs, and focus groups were conducted in the identified underserved areas to develop targeted and culturally appropriate health services.

The health department uses a local television station and local newspapers to advertise the location and services of the mobile health clinic. Information is also disseminated through neighborhood churches, schools, businesses, cultural centers, and outreach workers. The mobile clinic is staffed by community providers and medical students and has had some of its greatest impact through delivering dental screenings and providing dental follow-up services to children in nearly fifty elementary and middle schools. Medical and dental services are provided through the mobile clinic to those with the greatest barriers to accessing services, but referrals to many community providers are given when the need for care is not as pressing.

Private Initiatives

A number of nonprofit organizations, philanthropies, and private collaboratives have developed innovative programs to address problems overlooked or inadequately addressed by federal, state, and local initiatives. Often these organizations are capable of providing substantial funding to develop demonstration programs that may become models for government programs and policies. Because of the large number of such programs, we present only a few examples.

Commonwealth Fund Program on Quality of Care for Underserved Populations. In 2000, the Commonwealth Fund established a program of grants for demonstrations and research to address disparities in health, access to care, and utilization across racial/ethnic and socioeconomic groups. The program aims to improve the understanding of disparities in health care quality for minorities and to identify and support the implementation of practices that will lead to better quality of care and reduced disparities. The program funds initiatives and research in four areas: quality measurement, patient experiences with health care, clinical care outcomes, and the role of Medicaid and safety net providers. The program has allocated nearly $11 million to fund over forty research and demonstration projects to date, including the ongoing collaborative minority fellowship program with Harvard University to train minority health care providers to become effective physician leaders, researchers, and advocates for minority communities.

California Endowment Focus on Multicultural Health. Created in 1996, the California Endowment is the state's largest health care foundation, with $3.4 billion in assets. Since its inception, the organization has awarded more than twenty-eight hundred grants, totaling over $900 million, to community-based organizations throughout the state. Many of the grants are targeted toward improving multicultural health and access to health care, and most are awarded through an open grant application program, requests for proposals, funding partnerships, and program-related investments. The endowment adopted a regional approach to awarding its grants, and this regional orientation assists decision makers in better understanding the unique needs of California's culturally diverse populations and communities. Recent grants have been made to develop health and wellness clinics for Native Americans, expand patient advocate training and support services for Latina breast cancer patients, and support a mobile health clinic in Latino communities.

Front-Line Experience: Managed Care Investing in Vulnerable Populations

Lily Quiette and Phinney Ahn, respectively the manager and management specialist of medical administration and special projects at L.A. Care Health Plan, describe how one managed care organization, designed to serve vulnerable populations, has made substantial investments in reducing financial and linguistic barriers to care. It has reached deep into the community to address the wide range of risk factors that contribute to poor health.

L.A. Care Health Plan is a nonprofit, Medicaid managed care organization serving over 700,000 Los Angeles County residents who participate in the Medi-Cal, Healthy Families (SCHIP), and Healthy Kids public insurance programs. The goal is to promote health and emphasize prevention by providing quality health care services to vulnerable populations. Our members face many barriers to obtaining health care, including being low income, lacking health literacy, and having limited English proficiency. To address these barriers, we are committed to outreach and seek to integrate with the community to provide the most culturally competent care through providers who understand and respect the community they serve.

In this racially and ethnically diverse community, approximately 85 percent of members are nonwhite, and 52 percent prefer to speak a language other than English. The ability to understand and communicate effectively with members is crucial to ensuring that they access health services. We work with both members and providers to help them connect in a common language by providing interpreter services and language training to providers and office staff. We also try to provide an environment for patients that is culturally sensitive by training providers to acknowledge and respect cultural differences and by preparing health education materials in ways that are appropriate for different cultures. Most programs and services are offered at no charge to providers or members.

In order to stay connected to our members, we go out into the communities where they live. Every year, we sponsor a number of community health fairs in various geographical areas to raise awareness of health and safety issues. These events feature free blood pressure screenings, mammograms, eye exams, and Medicaid eligibility screening and enrollment. We have partnered with our local professional soccer team to raise public awareness of the availability of health care coverage for vulnerable populations. Activities like these have enabled us to extend outreach into the community and get to know our members' needs.

The L.A. Cares for Kids program conducts specific outreach to high-risk children who have multiple physical, mental, and social needs, including children under the supervision of the Los Angeles County Department of Children and Family Services. We identify those who are eligible for Medicaid coverage and make special efforts to assess their unique health care needs. A nurse coordinator develops personalized care plans and coordinates essential services with physicians to help the family navigate the health care system. This program is especially vital to families that are uninsured, have limited English-speaking ability, or distrust traditional public or county agencies. The outreach team also visits homeless shelters to identify families that may be eligible for health insurance and distribute health information.

Since positive change can also come from within the community, we work with eleven regional community advisory committees that are composed of L.A. Care members, advocates, and providers who organize community events and advise us on local health care needs. Some of the recent community events developed by these committees have focused on diabetes, asthma, heart disease, osteoporosis, and obesity. L.A. Care also reserves two spaces on the board of governors for a member and a member advocate to ensure that we stay accountable to the community. The board of governors allocates specific funds to support nonprofit and public health care providers to maintain and expand health services in areas of critical and immediate need, including dental care services and asthma self-management.

Once members are enrolled, we have programs in place to encourage them to receive the care they need. Several incentive programs are targeted to different preventive care and chronic conditions. One, for example, focuses on increasing the number of well-care visits among children and adolescents and encourages conducting initial health assessments in a timely manner. For each completed series of well-care visits, we offer financial incentives to providers and gift certificates and movie tickets to members. In the past two years, due to these incentives and other quality improvement activities, we have dramatically improved our rates of child and adolescent well-care visits.

These multiple strategies work together to break down and overcome the multiple barriers members face in navigating an increasingly complex health care system. L.A. Care is constantly working directly with the community to develop innovative programs that cater to the multiple needs of members and will promote access, quality, and, most important, health.

Strengths and Weaknesses of Programs Addressing Racial Disparities

Addressing racial/ethnic disparities in health and health care experiences is no easy task. The success of programs and initiatives that have been developed is based on many factors (among them are validity, scope and reach, sustainability, and effectiveness). Here, we review some of the major strengths and weaknesses of these programs.

Validity. The majority of federal initiatives have served primarily to generate national attention on racial disparities in health care. The creation of the OMH was particularly important because it plays a coordinating role for other federal agencies and the minority health initiatives they support. The programs offering services at both the federal and state levels provide extensive services that address some of the key pathways leading to racial disparities in Hispanic and Native American health and health care. These pathways include improving access to care through low- or no-cost services, the creation of local clinics, and mobile vans to enable patients to identify and develop a relationship with a regular source of care. These federal programs also address some cultural barriers by making services and outreach available in a culturally and **linguistically appropriate** manner. Future programs may wish to consider other mechanisms by which racial disparities may operate, including aspects of provider training and setting, and both patient and provider expectations for care.

Scope and Reach. The programs we have presented address a broad range of issues and serve extensive populations. The federal Indian Health Service and Migrant Health Center programs alone reach well over 2 million minorities (and about 75 percent of the entire Native American population), and the combination of the various state and local programs serves tens of thousands more. While these service programs are designed to address specific needs of the minorities in their target populations, they nonetheless reflect a somewhat fragmented approach to addressing disparities in minority health and health care. The creation of the federal OMH may overcome this problem by coordinating future efforts to improve health, access to health care, and quality of health services. Yet it will remain important to balance national efforts to improve racial/ethnic equity in health and health services delivery with the ability to address the specific cultural barriers and unique needs of each minority group.

Sustainability. Most federal programs addressing racial disparities in health have been well funded to meet the aims of Healthy People 2010 to eliminate racial and socioeconomic disparities in health. For example, President Bush's Initiative to Expand Access to Health Care in May 2004 substantially expands funding to strengthen the safety net for those most in need by extending the availability of primary care services to new patients. It is expected that the budget initiative will allow safety net health centers, including migrant health centers, to reach an additional 6 million people over the next five years. Similarly, the budget for the Indian Health Service is expected to increase by about 2 percent, or roughly $60 million, in the next year. State, local, and private initiatives are generally financially dependent on grants and reimbursement by enrolling clients in programs like Medicaid, but the sustainability of each is dependent on local supporters, federal and state policies to expand insurance coverage for the indigent, and the economy.

Effectiveness. Relatively few **evaluations** have been completed on national efforts to reduce racial disparities in health care. Migrant health centers are likely providing an effective safety net to migrant farm workers, of whom only 4 percent have private medical insurance. A study by the National Association of Community Health Centers showed that 63 percent of farm workers had a regular source of care and that 95 percent of those reported health centers as that source of care. Patient experience has been positive in the health centers with almost 100 percent of farm worker patients responding to a questionnaire that they were either satisfied or very satisfied with the quality of their care at their center. Because community health centers were included in the study in addition to MHCs, it is difficult to isolate the exact benefit from the MHCs (Zuvekas, 2002). In general, the MHC program has not been well studied in comparison to the larger sister community health center program.

Studies of the IHS suggest that it has had a drastic impact on the health of Native Americans and Alaska Natives. The program is reported to have helped contribute to a life expectancy increase of 12.2 years, and a decrease in infant mortality by 50 percent, tuberculosis mortality by 74 percent, and gastrointestinal mortality by 81 percent among Native Americans since 1973 (Indian Health Service, 2003). Studies of the Indian Health Service suggest that they have had a drastic impact on the health of Native Americans and Alaska Natives.

Though still evaluating many new initiatives, the REACH 2010 program has demonstrated some success. A REACH-sponsored South Carolina coalition to improve diabetes outcomes in the state's African American population met its goal ahead of deadline to increase the number of diabetics receiving A1C tests by 20 percent (Centers for Disease Control, 2003). The other programs we have presented have not been as rigorously evaluated to date, though studies are or may soon be under way for many of the Commonwealth Fund projects.

Programs to Eliminate Socioeconomic Disparities in Health

Many programs have also been developed to address SES disparities in health and health care experiences. Most of these have focused on income-related factors such as providing free or low-cost health services to lower-income individuals, but few have focused on other aspects of SES, such as education and occupation. We review these programs next.

Federal Initiatives

An equally large number of federal initiatives have been created specifically to assist low-income individuals and families to access high-quality health services. These programs are generally what health policymakers consider to be the nation's health care safety net and range from programs targeted to low-income populations broadly defined, to specific groups of vulnerable populations, such as homeless individuals.

Community Health Centers. The community health center (CHC) program was established by the federal government in 1969 to improve access to health care services to low-income families. CHCs were created under the Economic Opportunity Act and are currently operated by the BPHC. To qualify for federal funds under the CHC program, a clinic or health center must be located in a medically underserved area, operate as a nonprofit, have a board of directors consisting of area consumers, provide culturally competent and comprehensive primary care services to all age groups, offer a **sliding-fee scale,** and provide services regardless of ability to pay.

The CHC program provides family-oriented primary and preventive health services for people living in rural and urban underserved communities. It was designed to serve areas where economic, geographical, or cultural barriers limit access to primary care for a substantial portion of the population. Most CHC patients have either Medicaid coverage or are uninsured (about 40 percent and 38 percent, respectively). The health centers tailor services to the specific community needs and provide essential **ancillary services** including prenatal care, laboratory and pharmacy services, health education, transportation to visits, and language translation services. The CHC program links clients with welfare programs, Women Infants and Children (WIC) services, mental health and substance abuse treatment centers, and a full range of specialty care services.

The BPHC received about $1.2 billion in 2000 to administer CHC grants to over seven hundred community-based nonprofit organizations that deliver health services in over three thousand service sites. The allotment reflected an increase of nearly $400 million in the federal investment in CHCs in the past six years alone. In 2002, $165 million was added to the budget to expand health care services in an additional 260 clinical sites, enabling them to serve an additional 1.25 million people annually. The recipients of these funds were primarily CHCs, but other recipients included programs operated under the Consolidated Health Center Program, which incorporates grant programs for providing health care to the homeless, in public housing settings, and in school-based health centers (U.S. Department of Health and Human Services, 2002).

National Health Service Corps. More than three thousand federally designated health professional shortage areas exist across the nation. Individuals living in these shortage areas have little or no access to primary care services because the demand for services exceeds the available resources, the services are located a great distance away, or they are inaccessible because of culture, language, and other barriers. The National Health Service Corps (NHSC) works with communities and health care facilities to provide medical care to individuals living in these underserved areas.

The NHSC assists medically underserved communities with the recruitment and retention of health care professionals, including physicians, nurses and nurse practitioners, and physician assistants. The program links both providers and medical residents who are interested in serving vulnerable populations with existing medical groups in shortage areas. In addition, it attracts providers to serve in shortage areas by offering scholarship and loan repayment programs on a competitive basis to students and clinicians committed to serving the neediest communities. Participating providers are offered training in cultural competency to meet the particular needs of the vulnerable communities they are serving.

Public Housing Primary Care Program. The Public Housing Primary Care (PHPC) Program was created under the Disadvantaged Minority Health Improvement Act of 1990, was reauthorized in 1996 under the Public Health Service Act, and is currently administered by the BPHC. This program supports health centers and other community providers to deliver care, either on-site or at a nearby location, to residents of public housing, low-income individuals living near public housing, and anyone benefiting from public rent subsidies. As of 2001, the program received an allocation of $15.7 million to support twenty-nine active centers that serve over seventy thousand clients annually.

The PHPC provides primary health care services including direct medical care, dental and preventive care, prenatal care, health screening, health education, and case management. The sites conduct outreach to inform residents about services and also help residents to obtain federal assistance for health insurance coverage and social services. The PHPC programs have established partnerships with public housing authorities and resident organizations to facilitate the delivery of services. Residents are actively involved in the design and governance of PHPC programs, and residents are routinely trained and employed in the programs as outreach workers, health educators, and case managers.

Health Care for the Homeless Program. The Health Care for the Homeless (HCH) Program was established by the McKinney Homeless Assistance Act of 1987 and is administered by the BPHC. The program was modeled after the successful four-year demonstration project developed and operated by the Robert Wood Johnson Foundation and the Pew Charitable Trust. The program currently supports 135 grantees from CHCs, local health departments, community coalitions, and other nonprofit organizations to provide services to homeless individuals. Appropriations for the HCH program grew from $65 million in 1994 to $100 million in 2001 and support services for about 500,000 clients annually.

The HCH program has the sole federal responsibility for addressing the primary health care needs of homeless persons. Programs combine aggressive street outreach with integrated primary care delivery systems and substance abuse services located in places easily accessible for homeless individuals. The HCH programs ensure around-the-clock access to emergency care, provide or refer clients to mental health services, conduct outreach to homeless individuals, and assist clients with obtaining health insurance coverage and assistance through social services.

A complementary component of the HCH program is the Outreach and Primary Health Services for Homeless Children Program, also operated within the HCH program by the BPHC. More commonly known as the Homeless Children's Program (HCP), it was established in 1992 as an amendment to the McKinney Homeless Assistance Act. Grants have been awarded to ten community-based organizations and provide care to more than twenty-two thousand patients annually. The HCP addresses the needs of homeless children and their families by providing, or arranging for, services to address their health care and social service needs. Like the larger HCH program, the HCP conducts outreach to identify homeless children and children at risk of homelessness and inform them about the health services available, and it provides comprehensive primary care services, including dental care.

Healthy Schools, Healthy Communities. For more than thirty years, the BPHC has supported and promoted the concept of school-based health centers. The Center for School-Based Health at the BPHC currently administers grants to support the operation of 512 school-based health center programs, of which about one-quarter are funded through the Healthy Schools, Healthy Communities (HSHC) program. The HSHC program, established in 1994, became the first federal program to encourage the development of new, comprehensive, full-time, school-based primary care programs that serve vulnerable children.

The program funds seventy-six nonprofit organizations to establish the 130 health clinics in schools and deliver comprehensive primary care services, mental health counseling, dental health services, and nutrition and health education to more than 160,000 children annually. Funding for this program has more than quadrupled since its founding, increasing from $4.25 million in 1996 to $17 million in 2001. Using multidisciplinary staff and a **family-centered** approach to care, the programs tailor services to their unique communities. In addition to direct medical care, the centers emphasize targeted health education projects such as violence prevention activities, fitness programs, parenting groups, self-esteem enhancement, and home medical and health education visits.

State and Local Initiatives

State and local health departments have implemented a vast array of initiatives, aside from insurance programs, to address socioeconomic disparities in access to health care. These programs often receive funding as demonstrations or funds are funded in conjunction with private organizations. The example programs we present here have received recognition for their achievements from several organizations, including the Models That Work Campaign sponsored by the BPHC, which awards innovative programs and publishes them as models for reproduction elsewhere.

South Carolina Commun-I-Care Program. Commun-I-Care, based in Columbia, South Carolina, is a statewide program that provides free primary care, prescription medication, laboratory services, and pediatric dental care to uninsured people living in poverty. It provides services in communities through a network of volunteer health professionals offering free or low-cost services in their offices and clinics during regular working hours. Volunteers include physicians, pharmacists, pharmaceutical companies, hospitals, labs, and other providers who donate their resources to persons in need.

Currently there are nearly three thousand patients from forty-six counties enrolled in the program, and services are available from more than eighteen hundred providers. Patients call a toll-free number to apply for the program, and operators determine if their annual income qualifies them for any other government programs, such as Medicaid. Once approved, patients can use the same toll-free number to obtain a referral to any participating provider in their area. If medications are prescribed, over two hundred participating pharmacies will fill prescriptions at no cost to the patients. The list of corporate and community partners is extensive and includes foundations and endowments, hospitals, clinics, colleges, pharmaceutical companies, and many businesses and corporations.

Kansas City TeleKidcare. TeleKidcare of Kansas City, Kansas, is a unique health care delivery system that has successfully removed obstacles to obtaining medical care encountered by medically underserved children of Wyandotte County, Kansas. In 1998, the Kansas University Medical Center partnered with the city school system to launch the country's first **telemedicine** delivery system in schools to address the lack of access to medical care services. Currently, twelve schools serving fifty-five hundred children in medically underserved communities participate in the system, and all children at the schools are eligible to receive health care services.

When a school nurse or other school professional identifies a child who needs medical assistance, the nurse schedules a telemedicine appointment. The system transmits real-time information to a physician over specialized telephone lines using videoconferencing technology. Electronic stethoscopes and otoscopes allow the remote physician to conduct physical exams and diagnose health problems.

Since the creation of the telemedicine program, over twelve hundred visits have been made for consultation.

The program has been designed for replication across Kansas because the inexpensive and user-friendly technology is readily available for implementation in urban and rural areas. The creators of the program have developed a training program for interested school districts, and continue to develop partnerships with medical schools, school districts, foundations, and phone service providers.

Private Initiatives

While many of the private initiatives to address socioeconomic disparities in health are delivered through medical organizations, groups of providers, and community organizations, a vast majority receives their funding through national and regional philanthropies. A growing trend is the creation of philanthropic organizations through the conversion of health plans from nonprofit to for-profit status. Law requires that profit from the conversion supports health care initiatives consistent with the original mission of the health plan, and the assets of the newly created philanthropies are used to improve the health for low-income families in the community (*Assets for Health,* 2002).

Center for Health and Health Care in Schools. The Center for Health and Health Care in Schools (CHHCS) is a program resource center located at the George Washington University School of Public Health and Health Services. The center has been a leader in the development of school-based health center programs for children for the past twenty years and is the current incarnation of the Making the Grade program that began funding the demonstration of school-based health centers in the early 1980s. The center receives the majority of its funding from the Robert Wood Johnson Foundation (supplemented by funds from the BPHC) to continue to test model programs to expand medical, dental, and mental health services to children in schools.

The CHHCS also serves as a leading advocate for school-based health centers. The center analyzes options for organizing and financing health programs in schools, advises government leaders and health care institutions on how to provide cost-effective and accountable health care programs in schools, and synthesizes research on school-based health centers to inform policymakers and the public about the best approaches to delivering health care in schools. Among the priority issues for the CHHCS are efforts to improve the financial stability of school-based health centers by collaborating with publicly sponsored health insurance programs. CHHCS also aims to increase access to dental and mental health services through school-based health centers, and integrate systems of care with community-based health programs to improve access to health services and eliminate duplication of effort.

In support of these priorities, the CHHCS has created a new grant program to develop and support sustainable models of dental and mental health services in school-based health centers. The grant program, known as Caring for Kids, is an initiative of the Robert Wood Johnson Foundation and provides $3.4 million to support fifteen projects to enhance access to dental care or mental health services for a period of up to three years. Grant recipients are geographically diverse and range from private organizations to departments of public health and universities that operate school-based health centers.

Strengthening Primary Care Providers to the Poor. The Health Foundation of Greater Cincinnati is a social welfare organization dedicated to improving community health and has developed, as one of its initiatives, a program of grants aimed at strengthening primary care systems for the poor in Cincinnati and twenty counties in Ohio, Kentucky, and Indiana. In 1998, an advisory group to the foundation identified two community-focused strategies to target funding toward strengthening the capacity of primary care providers. The first strategy is to strengthen the primary care infrastructure and improve the resources and networks of information available to primary care physicians serving the poor. The second strategy is to improve the **integration of care** among primary care providers and service providers for special needs individuals, including gerontology, mental health, substance abuse, and health literacy. The foundation has assets of over $260 million and since its inception has awarded fifty or more grants to improve primary care for the poor.

Johnson & Johnson Community Health Care Program. Founded in 1987 as part of Johnson & Johnson's corporate commitment to social responsibility, the Community Health Care Program's goal is to provide support to community-based, nonprofit organizations that propose innovative ways to measurably improve access to quality health care for the impoverished and medically underserved. The program's support is financial; qualifying organizations receive a two-year, nonrenewable $150,000 grant. Grants are primarily awarded to health, education, and human services organizations. Since the program's inception sixteen years ago, $9.5 million in community health care support has been awarded to 103 distinguished health care organizations from thirty states and Puerto Rico.

In 2003, Johnson & Johnson awarded more than $1.85 million in grants to thirteen community health care organizations. The program also grants a leadership award of $50,000 each year to an outstanding individual whose progressive ideas and efforts in the community health field have substantially improved the health status of medically underserved populations.

Strengths and Weaknesses of Programs Addressing Socioeconomic Disparities

Addressing socioeconomic disparities in health is perhaps one of the most challenging health-related tasks before the United States. These programs have met with varying levels of success, and we review the strengths and weaknesses of these programs next.

Validity. Most federal safety net initiatives are administered by the BPHC. Centralizing the administration of these programs, along with relatively recent legislation combining their funding in a single legislative bundle, has led to a greater capacity for coordination and cooperation among programs. The programs at the federal, state, local, and private levels generally address disparities in access to health care. The programs frequently establish or expand comprehensive health clinics or service delivery units (mobile vans and school-based health centers, for example) in underserved areas, or assemble networks of providers willing to provide vulnerable populations with free or low-cost services. Although these programs address socioeconomic disparities through an access-to-care mechanism (see the previous chapter), they tend to overlook even greater (though less amenable to intervention) contributors to disparities in health, including education, occupation, and community social cohesion factors.

Scope and Reach. The safety net programs we have discussed serve a large number of vulnerable individuals and address the needs of several unique populations, including children, residents of public housing, and the homeless. The CHC program is by far the largest safety net program in the country. It operates in nearly every state and annually serves over 11 million low-income individuals. Another large program, Healthcare for the Homeless, has served over 500,000 individuals since its inception. Even the smaller state and local initiatives we have highlighted have provided almost 10,000 individuals with access to primary care services in South Carolina and Kansas. Moreover, national programs such as school-based health centers are expanding with increased federal funding and are gaining wider recognition among policymakers at both the state and local levels interested in replicating the successes of the program in their localities.

Sustainability. President Bush's Initiative to Expand Access to Health Care builds on a recent history of funding increases for safety net programs. This funding increase is expected to allow safety net programs, including CHCs and school-based health centers, to reach an additional 6 million people by 2004. Nonetheless, there remain several substantial threats to the financial stability of these programs, including the need to remain competitive service providers for Medicaid-eligible clients to obtain reimbursement, collaborating with managed care organizations, and adapting to changes in the financing of health care, while maintaining the financial ability to offer supportive services like transportation and case management to indigent clients (Lewin and Altman, 2000). Becoming successfully competitive in the health care market, however, helps ensure the stability of these programs regardless of changes in periods of unstable grant funding.

Effectiveness. In comparison to programs addressing racial disparities, several safety net programs have been relatively well evaluated. CHCs have been studied frequently because of their predominance in caring for vulnerable populations. Studies have demonstrated substantial cost-effectiveness and an ability to help reduce costs to the Medicaid program. They have also been shown to reduce infant mortality, lower hospital admissions and length of stay, and deliver high-quality care for vulnerable populations (Forrest and Whelan, 2000; Dievler and Giovannini, 1998; Starfield, Powe, et al., 1994; Zuvekas, 1990; Lefkowitz and Todd, 1999; Okada and Wan, 1980). School-based health centers have been similarly evaluated and successful at improving access to medical and dental care, decreasing emergency room visits for primary care and mental health services, and leading to greater satisfaction compared to other community clinics (Key, Washington, et al., 2002; Kaplan, Brindis, et al., 1998, 1999; Anglin, Naylor, et al., 1996; Young, D'Angelo, et al., 2001; Adams and Johnson, 2000; Terwilliger, 1994). Still, many school-based health centers face difficulties educating parents about the availability of services, collaborating with managed care organizations, and reassuring users of the confidentiality of services (Pastore, Juszczak, et al., 1998; Kaplan, Calonge, et al., 1998).

The Public Housing Primary Care program reported (2002) that it increased medical contacts for public housing residents to over 175,000 per year and increased immunization rates for young children to well over 95 percent in most sites, and 100 percent in some. An evaluation of the South Carolina Commun-I-Care program (2002) suggests that the program has successfully reduced emergency room visits and hospitalizations, saving an estimated $3.5 million for the state. Additional evaluations estimate that the program has further saved the state over $20,000 in Medicaid eligibility screening costs.

Programs to Eliminate Disparities in Health Insurance

Health insurance coverage is an essential enabler for individuals to obtain health care services and maintain good health. Since the mid-1960s, there have been extremely large public and private investments to afford low-income individuals, who are generally unable to obtain private insurance easily, with adequate coverage through several public insurance programs. Although these programs cover large numbers of individuals, there remain over 38 million Americans without any form of insurance coverage. Thus, there remains substantial need for greater public and private investment to ensure greater equity in coverage.

The main federal and state health insurance initiatives are Medicare, Medicaid, and the State Children's Health Insurance Program (SCHIP; discussed in detail in Chapter Two). Together, they cover nearly 40 percent of the U.S. population. To assist the remaining uninsured population, states and private organizations have developed their own initiatives to provide these individuals with health insurance coverage. Because there are a large number of state programs, we will highlight and discuss only a few examples. More complete listings of state efforts are available through the National Academy for State Health Policy (Riley and Yondorf, 2000) and the National Conference of State Legislators.

State and Local Initiatives

States are exploring ways to expand the coverage of the uninsured and underinsured, while still leaving the current system of employer-based insurance intact. These programs are most often directed toward covering the working poor: individuals and families who cannot afford to purchase health insurance coverage but earn too much to qualify for public assistance through Medicaid or SCHIP (Silow-Carroll, Anthony, et al., 2000; Silow-Carroll, Waldman, et al., 2001).

MassHealth Family Assistance Program. In 1998, the Massachusetts Division of Medical Assistance established the MassHealth Family Assistance Program. The program is designed to make employment-based coverage affordable to low-income employees and self-employed individuals in the state and to encourage and assist small employers in offering health insurance to low-income workers. The program offers subsidies to families and employers regardless of whether they have been previously insured or providing coverage. The program is financed in part with federal funds and in part with state money, and it offers participants a straightforward, seamless subsidy program.

The program has two components. The Premium Assistance program offers subsidies to help low-wage workers, with incomes up to 200 percent of the federal poverty line, to pay their shares of employer-based insurance premiums. For individuals and families with incomes below 133 percent of poverty, the program covers the cost of the entire premium. For those above 133 percent of poverty, the program covers most of the cost and requires only a maximum monthly contribution of $30 per family. Before enrolling a person in the program, the state must determine it is more cost-effective to cover him or her through premium assistance rather than through Medicaid or SCHIP. Currently, over twelve thousand individuals receive subsidies for coverage through the program.

The Insurance Partnership, the second component, offers subsidies directly to small businesses to help pay for health insurance premiums for low-wage workers and low-income, self-employed individuals. This subsidy of up to $1,000 per family is financed almost entirely through state funds, and currently assists about sixteen hundred employers to provide insurance policies to about five thousand individuals. This program is unique because it does not require employers to be offering coverage for the first time in order to be eligible for subsidies. The risk of this policy is that public dollars might merely substitute for private dollars spent for health coverage, without necessarily increasing the number of insured people. However, the benefit is that firms that have provided coverage in the past are not penalized for acting responsibly.

Healthcare Group of Arizona. In 1988, the Healthcare Group (HCG) of Arizona was established by the state legislature to offer prepaid medical coverage to small businesses and the self-employed through a group of three health maintenance organizations (HMOs). While most insurance companies market their group insurance plans only to businesses with more than five employees, this program was made available to very small firms with two or more employees and to self-employed individuals. Although the state mandates HMOs to make this option available to employers, it does not subsidize any of the costs of coverage, and employers are responsible for the entire insurance premiums. There are no income limits for employee enrollment and no requirement that the enrollees must have been uninsured previously or that the employer did not offer coverage previously. Participating health plans are required to accept all full-time workers in small firms and to charge a community rate. Although the program has undergone some difficult changes, including implementing more sophisticated **reinsurance** programs to protect the HMOs from losses due to individuals with high medical costs, it has managed to stabilize while providing thirty-six hundred small businesses with coverage for nearly twenty thousand insured lives.

Private Initiatives

While there are many foundations and other private organizations that are involved in improving access to care for vulnerable populations, few directly support health insurance programs or subsidize premiums for individuals and families. Although we present one private health insurance initiative, the primary role for private groups has been to inform policymakers and the public of the problem of the uninsured. Organizations such as the Kaiser Family Foundation, the Commonwealth Fund, and the Robert Wood Johnson Foundation have invested extensive energy to conduct, synthesize, and publish high-quality research on the uninsured.

Healthy Kids Program in Santa Clara County. To provide all children with better access to health coverage, the Santa Clara County, California, board of supervisors, in partnership with several local and statewide private entities, created the Children's Health Initiative in 2001. The initiative seeks to make health insurance available to 100 percent of children in families with incomes up to 300 percent of poverty, including children who are undocumented immigrants. What makes this goal realizable is the development of a new local health insurance plan for children who are not eligible for existing public insurance programs. This new plan, the Healthy Kids program, is similar to the state's Healthy Families SCHIP program, but all initial funding has been provided through local funds to fill the gap for children who do not qualify for either Medicaid or CHIP.

Healthy Kids is a low-cost comprehensive health, dental, and vision insurance program with monthly premiums ranging from four dollars per child to a maximum of eighteen dollars per family. Premium assistance is available for families experiencing financial hardship. Families may pay three months in advance and receive the fourth month free, or pay for nine months in advance and receive the next three months free. There are no copayments for preventive services and a small five dollar payment for other visits. Families eligible for this program enroll in the Santa Clara Family Health Plan and can choose their own health, dental, and vision providers. The program currently provides health insurance coverage for about one thousand children who were not able to obtain coverage from other private or public programs. This program has now been replicated in a handful of other counties in California, and many other counties have plans for implementation.

Strengths and Weaknesses of Programs Addressing Health Insurance

Programs that focus on insurance coverage have perhaps the longest legacy in the United States. These programs have been created in distinct initiatives at different levels of government and community, and often in a piecemeal fashion. Nevertheless, together they reflect a movement that is leading toward more comprehensive national coverage. We review some of the major strengths and weaknesses of these programs next.

Validity. Health insurance coverage is one of the largest determinants of access to care for a population. Countries that provide universal insurance coverage have ensured their citizens access to at least a basic set of primary care services. Although the federal government has not yet elected to provide this benefit universally, many federal and state programs like those discussed are in place to ensure that most older individuals and many low-income families and children receive some form of health insurance coverage. Even among those who have coverage, there are still limitations and financial barriers to care. In addition to restricted Medicare services such as long-term care, those eligible for Medicare under age sixty-five have a two-year waiting period before they can enroll. Privately insured individuals are often underinsured for conditions of mental illness or substance abuse and are under financial pressure to pay increasingly high premiums or copayments for care.

Of the 38 million or so Americans who lack health insurance, many can access care through grant-funded safety net health programs or in emergency departments. In a strikingly obvious way, even though the government has not funded universal insurance coverage, federal and state dollars still finance the care of uninsured individuals through these safety net programs or through the rising costs of health services to make up for the costs of uncompensated care. Until health services are available to every citizen through some form of universal coverage, lacking health insurance will remain an important contributing factor to disparities in health and health care.

Scope and Reach. The impact of federal programs such as Medicare, Medicaid, and SCHIP has been tremendous. Medicare provides insurance coverage for nearly every citizen over the age of sixty-five, and Medicaid now covers one of every four individuals in the United States. Although SCHIP had a relatively slow start, increased outreach and enrollment efforts have assisted the program to enroll over 4.6 million children. However, early studies of the SCHIP program have shown concurrent declines in the number of low-income, uninsured children and the number of privately insured low-income children, suggesting that a significant percentage of SCHIP beneficiaries were not previously uninsured but switched from private insurance to the less expensive public program (Cunningham, Hadley, et al., 2002). This is contrary to the intended goal of the SCHIP program to include only children who were not previously covered by public (Medicaid) or private insurance plans. However, it is likely that in many cases of private-to-public substitution, SCHIP is still serving the role of safety net by giving low-income families relief from the expensive premiums often paid by low-wage workers for private coverage (Cunningham, Schaefer, et al., 1999). Nevertheless, there are still uninsured children eligible for SCHIP programs, and despite easing the enrollment process, organizational and social barriers to enrollment remain (Kenney and Haley, 2001).

Considering the 38 million individuals still lacking insurance coverage, these state, local, and private initiatives serve an extremely important role in filling gaps in coverage. State and local initiatives have deftly designed insurance plans to encourage the availability of insurance coverage for the working poor. Most states have expanded Medicaid coverage to individuals above the poverty level (though with some small form of copayment or premium), and many states have expanded insurance coverage for children up to 250 percent of poverty (and some as high as 300 percent). Already in place among many states, and under consideration by many others, is expanding health insurance coverage to parents of SCHIP-enrolled children, noting that parent insurance coverage affects access to care for children regardless of children's coverage.

Sustainability. Although consistent federal funding of Medicare, Medicaid, and SCHIP is ensured for the near future, concerns about financing these programs—primarily Medicare—have been widely discussed in Congress and in the media and have not been fully solved. For states, economic downturns have made it difficult to fully finance their share of Medicaid program costs. As of January 2002, forty states reported budget shortfalls totaling an estimated $40 billion. Although increasing revenues from state taxes are expected to help many states rebound in the coming years, virtually every state will be considering spending cuts. Because Medicaid makes up a large portion (about 15 percent) of state budgets, it is a central focus for reducing state spending. Moreover, Medicaid costs are increasing on average by 8 to 9 percent per year, and physicians in many states are leaving Medicaid because of extremely low payment rates. In an effort to curb rising costs, more states are turning to managed care to consolidate resources and reclaim greater control over the health care marketplace. By 2002, more than 58 percent of Medicaid beneficiaries were receiving care through managed care arrangements (Hurley and Somers, 2003). If costs cannot be controlled, new state health insurance expansions may be retracted, enrollment may be limited or reduced, and plans for new expansions may be derailed indefinitely. Finally, due to the way the original federal legislation was enacted and because of slow program start-up, an estimated $3.2 billion in unused federal SCHIP funds was required to be returned to the federal treasury. Unless Congress acted to remedy this, the expected result was a decrease in enrollment of about 900,000 children between 2003 and 2006 (Mann, 2002). Congress did revise the rules to allow states to keep most of their allocated funds through 2003, though some money was reverted to the Treasury and some was redistributed to states with greater need. Due to effective lobbying on the part of many states, the administration's budget for 2003 included a plan to extend the availability of unspent funds until 2006.

State and local initiatives to improve health status for the uninsured are also facing difficult times in the current economic climate. After ten successful years of providing low-cost health insurance to small businesses and self-employed individuals, the Healthcare Group of Arizona (HCG) is struggling with potential financial losses that exceed insurance premiums. A large percentage of the population covered by HCG that was directed to the state program was unable to afford or have access to coverage elsewhere as a result of high-risk conditions. Over time, the combined risk of the HCG population has become higher than the general population and thus much more expensive to care for. In 2001, one of the three health plans providing care to HCG beneficiaries terminated its contract after significant financial losses. HCG has requested $5 million from the state legislature for 2004 to help sustain the program and may receive only $3.5 million. Even with help from the state, HCG members are likely to see significant increases in their premiums and co-payments in 2004 (Erikson, 2003; Gonzales, 2002; Academy for Health, 2001).

Massachusetts' MassHealth Family Assistance Program has been facing similar fiscal problems due to a state budget crisis in 2002 that forced the state legislature to reduce spending on public programs. Until 2001, Massachusetts was steadily adding people to its MassHealth plan and lowering the number of uninsured citizens. Decreased state spending has resulted in limited eligibility, reduced benefits, and increased cost sharing for MassHealth programs (Cooney, 2003; Lawrence, 2002; Sacks, Kutyla, et al., 2002).

In contrast, despite statewide budget cuts, the Healthy Kids program in California, has expanded to include several more counties. Based on the success of the Santa Clara program and with the help of $6.4 million in state tobacco tax money, the expanded Healthy Kids Initiative will provide comprehensive health and dental care to thirty-one thousand or more uninsured children (Kurtzman, 2003; Gold, 2003).

Effectiveness. The impact of health insurance programs has been discussed previously. A number of studies have been completed on the benefits of Medicaid insurance coverage to vulnerable populations, ranging from demonstrating improved access to care to improved health status (Iglehart, 1999; Lurie, Ward, et al., 1984, 1986). Because the SCHIP program is relatively new, very few studies have been completed, although there has been substantial discussion of what these evaluations should include (Shi, Oliver, et al., 2000; Halfon, Inkelas, et al., 1999a, 1999b; Starfield, 2000). Evaluations of programs similar to SCHIP, however, have shown benefits including improved access to care, improved receipt of preventive services, and a reduction in emergency department use (Feinberg, Swartz, et al., 2002; Lave, Keane, et al., 1998; Szilagyi, Rodewald, et al., 2000; Holl, Szilagyi, et al., 2000).

Although there are few evaluations of health status available to assess the effectiveness of state and local initiatives, more adults and children are insured in Arizona, Massachusetts, and California since the inception of these programs and thus are likely to be receiving the basic benefit of access to care. Compared to the national average, the uninsured population in Massachusetts is significantly smaller and awareness of new public health care programs is far greater than in other states.

Nevertheless, there remains important work to be completed on comparisons of quality of care received by patients in publicly sponsored insurance plans, given the low reimbursement rates for physicians serving patients in programs such as Medicaid and SCHIP.

Summary

In this chapter, we have discussed many federal, state, local, and private initiatives to address racial, socioeconomic, and insurance coverage disparities in the United States. While many of the programs have made substantial contributions to reducing these disparities, there remains a great need to develop new, more sophisticated, and creative approaches to addressing some widening gaps in access to health care, experiences with care, and quality of care.

Prevention may be the best, most cost-efficient way to reduce the effects of vulnerability on health status; however health care in the United States continues to be dominated by highly technical, treatment-oriented medical care. Consequently, the majority of money spent to care for vulnerable populations goes to treatment instead of making the investment earlier with preventive services. Providers need to be better trained in prevention-oriented procedures and appropriately reimbursed and rewarded with financial incentives for integrating them into their practice. Furthermore, the physical, psychological, and social functioning problems often associated with the poor health status of vulnerable populations are difficult to address in a treatment-oriented medical care system because these conditions and their causes can fall outside the current clinical domain.

Vulnerable populations require a broad spectrum of care, from clinical to social services. However, care for vulnerable populations tends to be fragmented. Funding that targets certain illnesses or very specific subgroups of vulnerable populations contributes to this fragmentation. Programs such as Health Care for the

Homeless, the Indian Health Service, and the Indiana State American Indian Health Program offer integrated systems of care, and thus a more effective safety net.

Finally, it is important to consider the complex sociopolitical origins of vulnerability. While initiatives such as the Office of Minority Health develop health policy to promote minority health issues and strive to ensure that the federal government is accountable to the needs of minority populations, it is essential to identify and continue to address the fundamental social and political influences that allow vulnerability to persist (Aday, 2001).

As greater knowledge becomes available on the determinants of disparities, newer programs will tailor their efforts to intervene in the contributing pathways. In the final chapter, we synthesize the complexities of eliminating disparities in health care and consider the next steps to achieving this goal.

Review Questions

1. Describe the national efforts to address racial/ethnic disparities in health. What agencies and organizations are the main participants, and which government agency provides the coordinating role? How do these initiatives support the goals of Healthy People 2010?
2. The Bureau of Primary Health Care is the home of many federal efforts to address health care disparities for lower-SES individuals and other vulnerable populations. Describe two initiatives of the BPHC, discuss their purpose and scope, and identify what level of overlap there is between these programs in terms of their design and purpose. Does either program address multiple risk factors?
3. Describe the State Children's Health Insurance Program. Identify those it serves, whether the program varies by state, and its current and potential effectiveness. How is the program different from Medicaid in terms of its target population. Describe the sustainability of the program.

Essay Questions

1. Identify one health-related program in your community or state that is designed to address health disparities for racial/ethnic minorities, lower-SES individuals, or the uninsured. Describe the program, how and when it was started, what its target disparity is, and its current activities. Assess whether the methods by which this program is aiming to reduce disparities are valid (using what you learned in Chapter Two), whether its scope is sufficient given the size

of the problem, the current and future sustainability of the program, and its effectiveness. Describe what kinds of outcomes you would use to determine whether the program is effective, and briefly summarize what kinds of evidence of effectiveness exist and what kinds of information are still needed.

2. You are in charge of a health clinic for low-income individuals in your community. The clinic has just received a five-year grant to fund a small intervention to reduce disparities in asthma among local Hispanic and African American children and teenagers. Based on what you have learned in the previous chapters and using the programs described in this chapter as examples, design a small program or initiative to address this disparity. Examples could include some type of health education offered in local schools, free screenings, efforts to improve air quality in the area, or something more creative. For your program, make sure to describe its purpose and methods (validity), the scope of services and who will be reached, how it will be sustained after five years, and how you will assess its effectiveness.

CHAPTER SIX

RESOLVING DISPARITIES
IN THE UNITED STATES

Throughout this book, we have analyzed disparities in access to medical care, quality of care, and health status using a conceptualization of vulnerability that captures the combined influences of race/ethnicity, SES, and health insurance. We have reviewed the deep social, political, economic, and medical roots of vulnerability and presented a wealth of evidence linking vulnerability risks, both individually and in combination, to poor health care experiences and health outcomes. These relationships convey a high level of health and health care inequality within U.S. society.

These inequalities are not surface deep or easily remedied, but it is our intent in this final chapter to assemble and synthesize the most progressive theory- and evidence-based strategies for preventing, treating, and eliminating national disparities in health. We begin with an overview of the Healthy People Initiative that provides the imperative and direction to resolve these health disparities. In support of this initiative, we then present a unifying solutions-focused framework for resolving these disparities, synthesizing models presented in Chapters One and Two.

Guided by this framework, we highlight and discuss examples of the most progressive and effective strategies for reducing disparities associated with vulnerability risk factors—race/ethnicity, SES, and health insurance—individually and in combination. We discuss specific examples of interventions at the policy, community, medical care, and individual levels, and explore the challenges in adopting these interventions. Finally, we propose a specific course of action, accounting for practical challenges and barriers.

The Healthy People Initiative

Disparities in health have become conspicuous enough in the United States to merit placement as one of two major goals selected by the U.S. Department of Health and Human Services (DHHS) Healthy People 2010 initiative. The ongoing **Healthy People Initiative** has spanned the past twenty-five years and represents the most comprehensive national effort to improve the health of American in this new century. The initiative has produced four reports, beginning with the original 1979 publication, *Healthy People: The Surgeon General's Report on Health Promotion and Disease Prevention*. Then came three more reports produced decennually that outlined national health objectives to be completed during the following ten-year period: *Healthy People 1990* (released in 1980), *Healthy People 2000* (released in 1990), and most recently, *Healthy People 2010* (released in 2000).

Past initiatives have made important strides toward accomplishing their stated objectives. Healthy People 2000, for example, surpassed the goals set for reducing coronary heart disease and cancer and succeeded in decreasing the incidence of AIDS and syphilis. Today, more children than ever before are receiving vaccinations in a timely and comprehensive manner, and infant mortality has declined significantly since 1979, in line with two ongoing Healthy People indicators. Many goals have also been missed (examples are physical activity and obesity levels), and are of continuing concern.

National Goals and Objective for 2010

Healthy People 2010 has two main goals: to increase the quality and years of healthy life and to eliminate health disparities. The first goal targets the general population, noting that U.S. life expectancy is ranked just eighteenth in the world despite much higher health care spending than other developed countries. The second goal targets the disproportionate burden of poor health that exists by gender, race/ethnicity, education, income, and geographical location. Figure 6.1 presents the framework for these goals as key components in the strategy to improve the public's health by 2010.

To gauge progress toward the two main goals, Healthy People 2010 identified 28 focus areas and 467 specific measurable targets or objectives to be achieved over the next ten years. The objectives and focus areas address an array of influences on individual health as shown in the Healthy People initiative framework for health

FIGURE 6.1. GOALS OF THE HEALTHY PEOPLE 2010 INITIATIVE

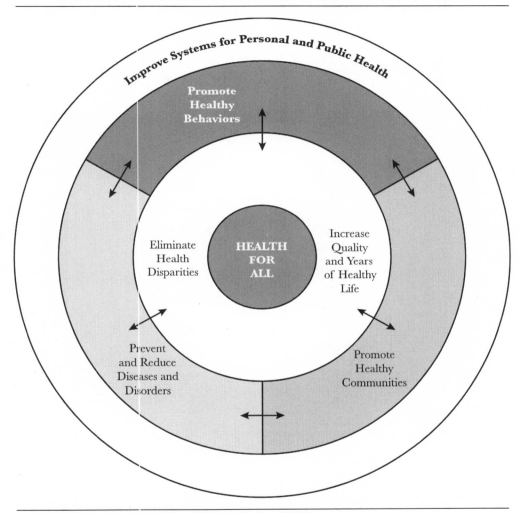

Source: U.S. Department of Health and Human Services (2002).

improvement (Figure 6.2). Identifying the determinants of health reveals opportunities for intervention, and the model depicts the influence of biology, behaviors, and environment on health, and how these can be modified by public policy and access to medical care. Led by the U.S. surgeon general, experts from federal agencies used this model to select focus areas and objectives, with input from the Healthy People Consortium, state organizations, and community groups.

FIGURE 6.2. CONCEPTUAL FRAMEWORK FOR THE HEALTHY PEOPLE INITIATIVE TO IMPROVE HEALTH

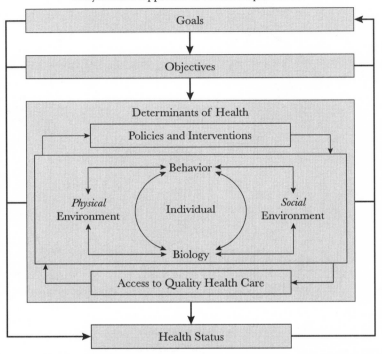

Healthy People in Healthy Communities

A Systematic Approach to Health Improvement

Source: U.S. Department of Health and Human Services (2002).

The resulting focus areas and objectives also reflect a changing national demographic and evolving health care system. The U.S. population is becoming older and more racially/ethnically diverse, and the resulting different health needs necessitate a reallocation of resources to provide better age-appropriate and culturally specific care. Changes in the health care system include new technologies, advanced preventive and curative care, better vaccines and pharmaceuticals, and improved health surveillance. New threats to public health, such as emerging infectious diseases and bioterrorism, have also arisen and are accounted for in Healthy People 2010. The focus areas and objectives also reflect the growing recognition of the importance of community-level health influences, and the report assigns a significant role to community partners in civic, professional, and religious organizations, to care for local populations.

Strategies and Partnerships to Achieve National Objectives

The general strategy of the Healthy People 2010 initiative is to motivate diverse groups to combine efforts in accomplishing the national objectives. The initiative objectives are designed to be easily used and exchanged by federal and state governments, and community and professional organizations, to improve national health. Although the federal government maintains much of the responsibility for achieving the national goals, the initiative formed a diverse network of partnerships to delegate some responsibility among state governments and interested local public and private parties. This strategic collaboration reduces redundant efforts at the national, state, and local levels and takes advantage of the unique competencies of each partner.

One of the most important Healthy People 2010 partnerships is with the Healthy People Consortium, an alliance of organizations dedicated to meeting the national goals and objectives. The consortium's membership is an assembly of all state and territorial public health agencies and representatives from advocacy and business sectors. Members have contributed in many ways, including defining the goals and objectives of the initiative, developing national health promotion projects, and incorporating objectives into their mission statements.

Because the objectives identified in Healthy People 2010 are not necessarily relevant to every region of the country, state-specific plans were established that identify and address unique regional public health needs. In this way, objectives are accomplished more efficiently when prioritized by state or regional relevance. Historically, involvement at the state level has been impressive. Nearly all states and territories created a state-level Healthy People 2000 plan, and twenty-three states have created and published Healthy People 2010 plans.

To facilitate the achievement of Healthy People 2010 objectives at the community level, the DHHS has established grant programs to support the efforts of local community organizations. Steps to a Healthier US program, for example, has awarded $13.7 million to communities working to combat diabetes, asthma, or obesity epidemics by promoting prevention and improving access to health care. These three conditions were identified as community targets because they have reached epidemic proportions and are generally responsive to prevention efforts. Another grant program, the Community Implementation Program, administered by the DHHS Office of Disease Prevention and Health Promotion, distributes small grants in support of health promotion pilot projects consistent with Healthy People 2010 goals and objectives in North Carolina and Connecticut.

To further encourage local Healthy People 2010 initiatives, publications were developed to aid state, community, and professional leaders in initiating health promotion programs. The Healthy People 2010 Toolkit provides guidance, technical tools, and other resources for state-specific programs. Community health endeavors are assisted by the *Healthy People in Healthy Communities* planning guide offering information and resources on how to establish and operate **community coalitions.** In addition, the *Healthy Workforce 2010* publication targets professional leaders who are well positioned to initiate health promotion efforts at their work sites. The publication explains preventive efforts (addressing Healthy People 2010 objectives) and their influence on creating a healthier workforce. A list of healthy workforce objectives and strategies is also presented to provide a road map for administering work site health promotion programs.

Private partners have also made formal agreements with federal agencies to work toward achieving the Healthy People 2010 objectives. Private partners include organizations such as the American Medical Association (AMA), the National Recreation and Parks Association, and the Academy of General Dentistry. For example, the American Heart Association and the American Stroke Association have developed a partnership to prevent cardiovascular disease through community-based health education programs, public awareness campaigns, and policy, professional development, and additional collaboration with organizations and agencies. The progress of the joint partnership is being evaluated yearly to assess its future direction.

The Healthy People 2010 Information Access Project is a strategic partnership between federal agencies, public health organizations, and health sciences libraries. The collaboration, Partners in Information Access for the Public Health Workforce, provides easy access to published research relevant to the Healthy People 2010 objectives. The National Library of Medicine and the Public Health Foundation designed a program simplifying the search engine of the Pub Med database, which offers 11 million research citations through MEDLINE and other life science journals. The open door to abundant evidence-based research allows the benefits of this partnership to be realized at every level of the health care workforce.

Tracking Progress in Achieving National Objectives

To achieve the Healthy People initiative national health objectives by 2010, it is essential to monitor improvement regularly to ensure resources are directed appropriately and effectively. A set of ten measurable **leading health indicators** (LHIs) was developed to facilitate the monitoring of progress toward achieving

TABLE 6.1. LEADING HEALTH INDICATORS FOR THE UNITED STATES

Indicator	Priority Health Topics
1	Physical activity
2	Overweight and obesity
3	Tobacco use
4	Substance abuse
5	Responsible sexual behavior
6	Mental health
7	Injury and violence
8	Environmental quality
9	Immunization
10	Access to health care

Source: U.S. Department of Health and Human Services (2002).

Healthy People 2010 objectives. The LHIs (Table 6.1) were selected from the national health objectives, emphasize high-priority public health issues, and were included based on the availability of data to measure their progress. Each LHI is tracked and reported throughout the decade.

Each of the 467 Healthy People 2010 objectives is also tracked through 190 data sources to ensure that progress assessment can be made at multiple levels of the public health workforce. The National Center for Health Statistics (NCHS) has established a data surveillance system for these objectives with quarterly updates available on NCHS's DATA2010 Web site. Annual updated assessments of the nation's health are also published by the secretary of Health and Human Services in the *Health, United States* reports. And finally, as each initiative comes to a close, NCHS prepares a concluding review of progress made toward meeting the national objectives. The next report is due in 2010.

Framework to Resolve Disparities

In support of the Healthy People initiative and other calls to arms for eliminating disparities, we propose a single unifying solutions-focused framework (based on models presented in Chapters One and Two) to improve the nation's health and

resolve disparities for vulnerable populations. The framework focuses on both social and medical points of intervention to create a multifaceted approach to
reducing disparities in health and health care by race/ethnicity, SES, and health
insurance coverage. The framework is built on the ballasts of both social and medical care determinants, because the combination of these factors ultimately shapes
health and well-being (see Figure 6.3). It should be noted that health in this model
includes the positive concept of well-being and encompasses its physical, mental, and social components (Institute of Medicine, 2001).

FIGURE 6.3. CONCEPTUAL MODEL OF POINTS OF INTERVENTION FOR VULNERABLE POPULATIONS

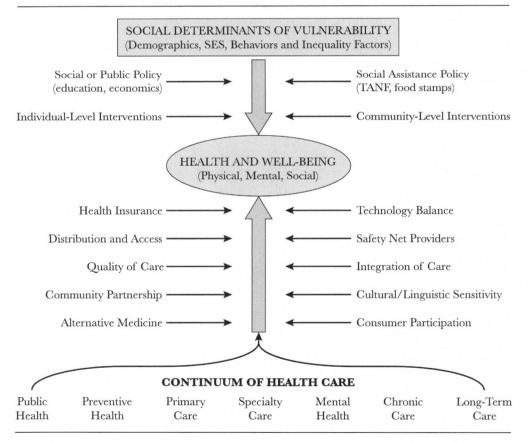

Social and Medical Influences on Vulnerability

The framework synthesizes much of what we have described in previous chapters. In this model, social determinants of vulnerability reflect personal and community-level influences, including demographics, SES factors, and aspects of social interactions. More specifically, these factors include race/ethnicity, SES (such as income, education, and occupation), behavioral factors, and social interactions (such as social networks at the individual level and social cohesion at the community level) that influence health care access and health. Behavior, it should be noted, should not be isolated from the social and environmental contexts that influence what choices are available and made.

While social determinants influence the health and resources that patients bring to the health care system, the medical care system focuses primarily on treating poor health. The framework includes a broad range of medical services and interventions to improve health. While public health, preventive care, and primary care will contribute to general health status, other services, such as specialty and long-term care, will be more influential in end-of-life care services and mortality. Without access to medical care, individuals will have difficulty treating health problems. For patients who gain access and move across the spectrum of care, they will contend with continuity and coordination of care.

In considering solutions for health disparities, policymakers should examine the balance of social and medical influences on vulnerability. While social factors are likely to have stronger influences on health than medical care (since medical care typically intervenes only when a problem is identified), there are extremely important roles for medical care in improving health, promoting well-being, enhancing quality of life, and ultimately lengthening life expectancy. In trying to solve health disparities, one should consider the respective contributions and likely effectiveness of social and medical interventions.

Since medical care absorbs such a large proportion of national spending, special consideration should be given to where resources are directed. Should equal investments be made in all health services, or are some investments better than others? Increasing resources for primary care, for example, may make basic health services available to more individuals but would reduce the availability of specialty care. Directing resources toward specialty care (such as higher-technology services) may enhance care and extend life for people with more severe health conditions but would draw away resources from basic primary care services for all. Other considerations, such as the quality of care and access to alternative therapies, may also have an impact on health care experiences and health outcomes.

Social and Medical Points of Intervention

Considering that both social and medical determinants are responsive to numerous outside forces, our framework highlights many important intervention points. Reductions in health and health care disparities are obtainable through interventions at four levels: (1) policy interventions, (2) community-based interventions, (3) health care interventions, and (4) individual interventions. These general approaches are described below and then used to organize our discussion of intervention strategies to address vulnerability.

Policy Interventions. Social or public policy influences the health and health care of the population in many ways. Product safety regulations, screening food and water sources, and enforcing safe work environments are a few of the ways in which public policy directly guards the welfare of the nation. With fewer resources at their disposal, however, vulnerable populations are uniquely dependent on social and public policy to develop and implement programs that address basic nutritional, safety, social, and health care needs. Many of the mechanisms relating vulnerable status to poor health are amenable to policy intervention, and policy initiatives can be primary prevention strategies to alter the fundamental dynamics linking social factors to poor health.

Community-Based Interventions. Disparities in health vary substantially at the community level, suggesting that some sources of health disparities may be addressed at the community level. Neighborhood poverty, the presence of local social resources, and societal cohesion and support are all likely to contribute to the level of health inequalities in a community. Intervention strategies have to be tailored to address these community health risks. Because community partnerships reflect the priorities of a local population and are managed by members of the community, they minimize cultural barriers and improve community buy-in to the program.

Community-based strategies have the particular benefit of mobilizing resources at the local level to address these problems. Community resources can be applied directly to community members, providing businesses and other local organizations with greater incentives to contribute to local health causes. Community approaches also benefit from **community participatory decision making,** where local researchers, practitioners, social services, businesses, and community members are invited to contribute to the process of designing, implementing, evaluating, and sustaining interventions. Many community programs are operated by nonprofit organizations and, in exchange for providing services, receive subsidies through federal, state, or local funds and receive tax exemptions.

Thus, they are able to offer health services at lower cost than private organizations obligated to shareholders to earn a profit.

Health Care Interventions. Billions of dollars are spent annually to monitor and improve facets of health care in the United States. Interventions have been designed for systems of care (such as designing integrated electronic medical record systems to better coordinate care for populations with multiple chronic and acute conditions), health care providers (such as continuing education for pediatricians to better target developmental services to children most in need), and consumers of health services (such as educating pregnant women to attend regular prenatal care visits). Health care monitoring initiatives in national, state, and local surveys have been designed to monitor the quality of care provided in health plans and can be used to examine and reduce disparities across demographic groups.

Individual-Level Interventions. While less comprehensive in scale and scope, individual-level initiatives intervene and minimize the effects of negative health-related behaviors. Altering individual behaviors that influence health, such as reducing smoking and encouraging exercise, is the focus of these individual-targeted interventions, and there are numerous theories that identify the complex pathways and barriers to elicit improvements in behavior. The integration of behavioral science into the public health field has been a valuable contribution, providing a toolbox of health-related behavior change strategies.

One of the most prominent models integrating behavioral science and public health is social action theory. Behavior in this model is described as the interaction of biology, environment, and social context, which is critical in determining the success of any health-related behavior intervention (Institute of Medicine, 2001). Behavioral change programs can be implemented at the community level, such as in neighborhoods or in community groups, but the focus of behavior change is nonetheless on each individual.

Resolving Disparities in Health and Health Care

In this section, we summarize comprehensive and progressive strategies (not necessarily programs) that address racial/ethnic, SES, and health insurance disparities in health and health care. Many of the strategies stem from basic principles of epidemiology, including surveillance of the problem, examining modes of transmission, modifying or halting the process of transmission, and monitoring the problem to prevent recurrence. These concepts, which have been the foundation for many of the successes of public health (such as the displacement in the twentieth century of communicable diseases from the leading causes of morbidity and mortality), are now serving as tools for the elimination of more socially rooted health disparities. We present potential strategies for resolving disparities that focus on both individual and more integrative frameworks that address the cumulative effects of these vulnerabilities.

Strategies to Resolve Racial/Ethnic Disparities

Many promising and progressive strategies have been proposed to reduce racial/ethnic disparities in health and health care. These strategies generally target specific social or cultural factors, and many approaches overlap with those designed to address SES disparities. Examples targeting racial/ethnic disparities at the policy, community, health care, and individual levels are discussed below.

Policy Interventions. Beginning with civil rights legislation in the 1940s through the 1960s, equality has been hard won for racial/ethnic minorities in the United States. Laws mandating equal access to education and employment (such as the creation of the Equal Employment Opportunity Commission to regulate equity in employment) and prohibiting racial discrimination in public places are the foundation for major improvements in the health and health care access of minorities. Affirmative action laws were also implemented to enhance education and employment opportunities for minorities (and women and the disabled) who had suffered from discrimination.

The term *affirmative action* was first used by President John F. Kennedy in 1961 in a federal order requiring businesses with government contracts to hire employees without regard to race, ethnic origin, religion, or gender. Later, government contracts were awarded based on race and gender to ensure that the workforce reflected the population, and a fixed portion of contracts were set aside for minority- or women-owned businesses. Many states, communities, businesses, and schools also created their own affirmative action programs.

In 1995, the U.S. Supreme Court held that federal affirmative action programs were not constitutional unless particular programs were designed to make up for specific past instances of discrimination. This ruling opened the door widely to critics of affirmative action, and in 1996, California voters banned racial/ethnic and gender preferences in public hiring, contracting, and education. In 1998, Washington State followed suit. Rescinding affirmative action programs has caused substantial national upset, particularly with regard to opportunities for higher education in the University of California system, and recent Supreme Court decisions have ruled again for the constitutional inclusion of minority and gender status in higher education admissions.

While affirmative action policies have increased higher education enrollment rates for minorities, these rates are still not comparable to those of whites. Considering that these lower education levels lead to severe long-term financial, social, and health deficits and that affirmative action policies are constantly on the political chopping block, efforts should be made to bolster the stability of these programs. Some institutions have implemented alternate diversity programs (to replace affirmative action), but additional resources and attention should be devoted to ensuring that all vulnerable populations enter higher education at high levels. Moreover, social policies seeking to reduce broader institutionalized discrimination in higher education, the workplace, and clinical settings are helping to level the playing field for minorities and should be continued.

Social and health policies have been designed to address cultural barriers among minority populations influencing access to and quality of medical care. In response to research illustrating negative health and health care quality for minorities associated with patient-provider language or cultural discordance, policymakers have established subsidy programs to financially support minorities entering provider-training programs. These initiatives support a racially and ethnically diverse health care workforce, mirroring the diverse American population.

The Health Careers Opportunity Program of the Health Resources and Services Administration (HRSA), for example, provides financial support and supplemental training, counseling, and stipends to help minority or underprivileged students complete a broad range of healthcare professions degrees. Other agencies such as the National Institutes of Health (NIH), the Agency for Healthcare Research and Quality, and the National Science Foundation are working also to promote the entry of minorities in health care provider training programs (Reede, 2003).

Community-Based Interventions. An example of a successful community-based program to address racial/ethnic disparities was a Racial and Ethnic Approaches to Community Health (REACH) 2010-funded initiative in Chicago targeting diabetes outcomes (Giachello, Arrom, et al., 2003). The Latino Health Research Center at the University of Illinois at Chicago developed the program through a series of town meetings with interested parties and devised a new coalition of African American and Latino organizations from Chicago's diverse Southeast Side to address the well-documented disparities in diabetes outcomes. Both groups are characterized by large population size, low levels of education, high levels of poverty, and poor access to care. The coalition used a process referred to as participatory action research to design the initiative, including gathering data, building community capacity, and raising the local awareness of the problem. For a comparison of community participatory action research with traditional research, see Table 6.2.

TABLE 6.2. DIFFERENCES BETWEEN TRADITIONAL RESEARCH AND PARTICIPATORY ACTION RESEARCH

Traditional Research	Participatory Action Research
Rigid	**Flexible**
Limited application to community problems	Aimed at solving specific community problems
Seeks limited community representation when funding	Seeks community participation representation at all stages of the research project
Uses mainly quantitative methods	Uses both qualitative and quantitative methods
	Tends to include women and racial/ethnic minority groups Maximizes efforts to include groups affected by the problems
Stresses deficits and "victim" ideology	Stresses community assets and community empowerment
Research is "on" populations	Research is "with" and "by" populations
Principal investigators are in control	Shared control among principal investigator, community, and participants
Project ends when data are collected and analyzed	Real action starts when data are analyzed
Partnership is limited	Partnership is maximized
Researcher is the "expert"	Researcher is a "resource"

Source: Giachello, Arrom, et al. (2003).

A number of factors contributed to the community's focus on diabetes, including high diabetes mortality, high diabetes-related hospitalization rates, and high gestational diabetes rates in the area. The initiative collected additional information using telephone interviews of local community residents, assessed health services capacity by conducting an inventory of all community resources ready to address diabetes, and reviewed local epidemiological health and health care utilization data from both state and national sources. Focus groups were conducted with health care providers and potential clients with diabetes to help determine how best to solve the disparities.

The results of this research were presented at community forums along with a proposed action plan to address these problems. Specifically, the coalitions decided to (1) develop a centralized diabetes patient–tracking information system in hospitals and clinics, (2) create a health system–based diabetes management and control educational program for people with diabetes or at risk for diabetes, and (3) establish diabetes self-care resource centers. The coalition so far has created two resource centers managed by lay community health workers. In addition to regular client diabetes education programs, nutrition classes, and social support, the centers help clients navigate the health care system, access medications and devices such as those for monitoring glucose, and organize community health fairs. Evaluation of the program, required by REACH 2010, is under way and was guided by the community coalitions.

The Urban League is another example of a nonprofit community-based movement with programs in over a hundred cities. The Urban League's mission is to improve the socioeconomic status of African Americans through economic self-sufficiency and educational attainment. Its programs across the country include educational support, money management skills, and professional development.

The NULITES (National Urban League Incentives to Excel and Succeed) program is one of the community-based programs sponsored by the Urban League. The NULITE youth initiative is designed to promote educational, character, and leadership qualities among local youths. Its primary strategy is a structured curriculum including required educational seminars and community service projects. The programs are carried out in forty-nine NULITE chapters across the country. Each chapter is sponsored by a local Urban League affiliate. The Urban League also sponsors several community programs to teach adults how to manage their money. These Financial Literacy and Know Your Money programs are offered by community-based Urban League affiliates across the country. There are also programs for building good credit, home ownership, and professional development.

Afterschool.gov is a federal initiative that has recognized the potential of community-based programs. Among other initiatives, Afterschool.gov provides grants to community-based initiatives seeking to improve minority health. The community organizations eligible for grants explore social determinants of health, including cultural and community norms and pressures, and environmental conditions. Each community organization must demonstrate an innovative strategy to contend with these social challenges that, if successful, could be modified to help other communities. Current strategies include community outreach, improving access to health care for minorities in high-risk, low-income communities, and promoting community health coalitions involving nontraditional partners.

Health Care Interventions. Another approach to resolving racial/ethnic disparities in health and health care is to tailor health care interventions to cultural differences in health beliefs, values, preferences, and behaviors. These differences include variations in perceptions of health symptoms and health care needs, ways of communicating health needs to professionals who understand their meaning, expectations and preferences for health care services, and differences in health behaviors and treatments for illnesses. These factors are thought to influence interpersonal interactions, including discrimination, between individuals and health professionals and to affect health care decision making in ways that contribute to health disparities (Smedley, Stith, et al., 2002).

This process has been termed **cultural competence** and should be distinguished from basic language competence, in which a health care system or provider ensures that its services are available and rendered in the languages spoken by their patient panels. This is infrequently, but most thoroughly, accomplished through the hiring of specialized translators trained in communicating complex medical issues. Cultural competence requires a more complex understanding of social and cultural influences on individual beliefs and expectations about health and health care, and how these may influence health behaviors and influence the delivery of health care at multiple levels of the health care delivery system (Carrillo, Green, et al., 1999).

Betancourt and colleagues have proposed a three-level framework for improving cultural competence in the health care system (Betancourt, Green, et al., 2003). This framework consists of organizational interventions that ensure that the leadership and workforce of a health system is diverse and representative of its patient population; structural interventions to ensure that health services are accessible and of the highest quality for all patients (for example, by offering interpreter services and ensuring that health education interventions and materials are tailored to meet the needs of diverse patients); and clinical interventions that train health professionals to be effective at negotiating different styles of communication, adapting to differences in decision-making preferences, different roles of the family, sexual and gender issues, and broader issues of mistrust, prejudice, stereotyping, and racism. In order to address racial and ethnic disparities in health through mechanisms of cultural competence, strategies should be addressed at each of these levels.

A review by Brach and Fraser (2000) provides substantial conceptual and empirical support for the potential effectiveness of cultural competence strategies at reducing racial and ethnic disparities. The authors discuss how cultural competence is likely to improve the accessibility of health care services for some minority groups, benefit interpersonal patient-provider interactions, increase the effectiveness of health education efforts, and possibly reduce misdiagnoses and improve the overall quality of care. The authors note that most cultural competence strategies have not been evaluated, and the linkages of specific strategies to improving the processes of delivering health care and patient outcomes have yet to be clearly demonstrated. This step is important because addressing cultural competence at all organizational, structural, and clinical levels will require a substantial investment of resources.

Professional development programs in health care teach providers to deliver culturally appropriate care, and recommendations have been made to incorporate more cultural competency programs into graduate medical education (Council on Graduate Medical Education, 1998). The Cross-Cultural Health Care Program, for example, has developed books, resources, and training programs to improve cultural competency among health care providers. Harmony in the patient-provider relationship benefits patients by improving interactions that result in more effective communication about illness symptoms and origins and greater continuity of care.

Another factor to consider in the health care delivery process is the increasing use of **complementary or alternative medicine** (CAM). Complementary medicine is used in conjunction with conventional allopathic medicine, and alternative medicine in place of conventional medicine. According to a recent study, individuals use CAM for its greater compatibility with their personal views on health and illness, in addition to individual dissatisfaction with conventional medicine (Astin, 1998).

With more CAM therapies, such as acupuncture and chiropractic procedures, passing clinical trials, opportunities for accessing this type of care are increasing, in effect broadening the health care market to provide individuals with choices in health care they had not previously had. This addition to the care delivery system benefits that segment of the population skeptical of conventional medicine and those wishing to combine the two types of medicine for disease prevention and treatment. Minorities, particularly immigrants, may find themselves more familiar and comfortable with alternative care than with the conventional care more commonplace in the United States. Again, greater patient satisfaction results in higher rates of continuity with a primary source of care, which ultimately benefits the patient's health.

How accessible is alternative medicine? Interest in CAM therapies has been building during the past decade. The interest was officially acknowledged in 1991 when the NIH established the Office of Alternative Medicine to evaluate and identify effective CAM therapies. In 1998, the office was upgraded to a center and renamed the National Advisory Council on Complementary and Alternative Medicine (NCCAM). Since the OAM's initial budget of $2 million, the NCCAM's budget has grown to an impressive $114 million for fiscal year 2003. The NCCAM's primary focus is still to identify promising alternative therapies using rigorous scientific methods. Despite the federal government's effort to raise the public's awareness of CAM, patient access to CAM is often limited.

Patient access is limited by the restrictions placed on CAM practitioners. Many states do not license CAM practitioners. Naturopaths are licensed in eleven states, acupuncturists in thirty-four, and chiropractors in all fifty states (Miller, 2000). Without a license, practitioners are limited in the types of care they can provide to the public and risk legal action if they practice without licensure. The CAM licensure process has been controversial, pitting allopathic practices against CAM-affiliated organizations that claim allopathic interest groups have purposefully undermined their licensure process to prevent additional competition.

Ironically, there is conflict among CAM-affiliated organizations about whether the industry is better served by state licenses. Many practitioners feel strongly that the licensure process is an expensive burden, particularly when the therapies they provide, such as massage, have little potential for harming patients. Furthermore, because some states do not offer the option for licensure, it prevents practitioners from providing and patients from having access to these therapies in these states. Other CAM practitioners feel that the licenses lend credit to a field of medicine that has defended itself against insinuations of quackery from the very beginning.

A resulting Health Freedom movement has resulted in new legislation in some states that allows CAM therapists to practice without a license. Minnesota's Alternative Health Care Freedom of Access Act, for example, allows massage therapists, body workers, naturopaths, homeopaths, herbalists, and Ayurvedic healers to practice without licenses, certification, or registration in the state. The act, which went into effect in July 2000, established the Office of Unlicensed Complementary Health-Care Practice to oversee the industry. The legislation's goal is to provide patients with ample access to these unconventional health care services (Menehan, 2001).

Patient access to CAM therapies has been improved by other legislation protecting CAM practitioners from charges of professional misconduct. Lawsuits against CAM practitioners for providing unconventional treatment to patients bolstered suspicions of allopathic doctors obstructing the entry of CAM into the marketplace. The lawsuits also included allopathic doctors who had integrated components of CAM therapies into their practices. In response, Alaska, Colorado, and Georgia drafted laws to protect all CAM practitioners from professional misconduct claims.

Patient access to CAM is increasing, albeit slowly. Access has improved due to coverage by progressive insurance companies such as Blue Cross of Washington and Alaska, Kaiser Permanente, Prudential, and Mutual of Omaha (Rauber, 1998). Access to CAM therapies can also be dictated by physician buy-in. Not all physicians feel comfortable educating their patients about alternative medicine or providing referrals to CAM practitioners. However, medical schools are now integrating more alternative medicine content into their curriculums, which should familiarize future generations of doctors with the benefits and risks of CAM (Eisenburg, Davis, et al., 1998). In fact, a survey of 117 medical schools found that 64 percent offered courses in CAM or courses with CAM content (Wetzel, Eisenberg, et al., 1998).

Numerous professional organizations such as the Complementary Alternative Medical Association, the National Center for Homeopathy, and the Coalition for Natural Health are doing their best to educate consumers, practitioners, and policymakers on the benefits of CAM therapies.

Individual-Level Interventions. Many approaches have been developed to improve health at the individual level through interventions to change behaviors that influence health and well-being. While most of these initiatives have been focused on the general population, growing recognition of the importance of cultural differences in health-related behavior has encouraged the adoption of these programs to specific populations.

Many national organizations aim to improve the health of minorities by providing education, information, training, and support for the adoption of healthier life choices. The National Rural Health Association (NRHA), for example, champions the health of rural minorities through educational interventions. NRHA has created the Contextual Community Health Profile, an intervention development tool that assists local programs in identifying demographic-specific needs of minority groups often omitted from interventions intended for the general population. This tool assists programs in constructing culturally appropriate interventions for the specific target population.

An innovative Internet-based program developed by the Black Women's Health Imperative (BWHI) is another example of an organization targeting a specific racial/ethnic population's health behaviors to address their unique health needs. The BWHI developed an educational intervention in response to data showing that heart disease was the leading cause of death among black woman and that black women have particularly high levels of risk factors (such as obesity) compared to other women. The BWHI created the Walking to Wellness program, which educates black women about the risks of heart disease, develops personalized training plans, and motivates women to take steps (literally ten thousand walking steps per day) to prevent heart disease.

Smoking cigarettes and abusing alcohol are two other negative health behaviors that are more prevalent among certain minority and low-income populations. For example Native Americans have higher rates of alcohol use than other racial/ethnic groups, and African American men are more likely to smoke than white men (National Center for Health Statistics, 2003). Cigarette makers continue to target blacks and Hispanics for promotional efforts in niche magazine advertising, strategically located billboards, and sponsorship of athletic, cultural, and entertainment events.

Interventions to reduce these disparities in smoking include mass media antismoking campaigns geared toward these populations using a culturally appropriate message or language. The campaigns seek to raise public awareness of the addictive nature of cigarettes and the harmful long-term effects of smoking. Multifaceted cessation programs have also incorporated tax increases on cigarette products and aggressive enforcement of the 1992 law restricting tobacco sales to minors. Using these methods in statewide cessation programs in the 1990s, California, Massachusetts, and Oregon have reduced cigarette consumption.

There are also numerous resources published on the Internet to motivate individuals and guide them throughout a cessation program. The Centers for Disease Control (CDC) has published several cessation programs for individuals, such as Pathways to Freedom: Winning the Fight Against Tobacco, the You Can Quit Smoking Consumer Guide, and Don't Let Another Year Go Up in Smoke. Other available resources and programs include the American Legacy Foundation's Quit Plan and Smokefree.gov.

A well-known behavior change program targeting alcohol abuse is Alcoholics Anonymous. The foundation of the program is a twelve-step process that leads alcohol abusers from admitting they have a problem to acknowledging they need help for the problem and seeking that help from the fellowship of recovered alcoholics participating in the program. The intervention has been relatively successful in changing behavior. For this success, the organization credits the twelve-step process and the unique ability of recovered alcohol abusers to reach out to the community and encourage alcoholics to seek help. The abuse of alcohol is also controlled by federal laws mandating the sale and consumption of alcoholic beverages.

Racial/ethnic minorities suffer disproportionately from AIDS. Hispanics have nearly four times and African Americans nearly ten times the prevalence rates of AIDS than whites: 14 cases per 100,000 population for whites, compared to 39 cases per 100,000 among Hispanics and 112 cases per 100,000 among African Americans (National Center for Health Statistics, 2003). With AIDS and other sexually transmitted diseases (STDs) spreading with epidemic efficiency, particularly chlamydia in teen populations, educating adolescents about healthy sexual decision making is essential to stemming the spread of disease as well as reducing rates of teen pregnancy. Advocates for Youth, a nonprofit organization, aims to educate adolescents about sexual health using state and community action teams, partnerships with national organizations, and community and family involvement.

The action teams promote sexual health programs focusing on the specific challenges faced by the community. Many Advocates for Youth programs target minority and gay or lesbian populations aggressively to reduce disparities. When partnering with state or national initiatives, Advocates for Youth provides technical assistance, resources, and training. Family involvement projects educate parents about their role in communicating with their children, a proven strategy to reduce unhealthy sexual behavior.

Strategies to Resolve SES Disparities

Strategies to address SES disparities in health and health care became particularly prevalent in the 1960s and have since evolved extensively. Strategies have generally focused on income, but more progressive efforts have focused on ensuring equal access to high-quality education and employment to preempt future disparities in income. One **income redistribution** program, the U.S. welfare systems (now known as Temporary Assistance to Needy Families, or TANF), has been reformed to limit the amount of time families can receive benefits while remaining unemployed. These changes, which are intended to encourage self-sufficiency, have had some negative impact on insurance coverage and possibly health (Wood, Smith, et al., 2002; Wise, Wampler, et al., 2002).

Policy Interventions. To reduce the rates of low SES, it is necessary to intervene in each of its antecedents: income, education, and occupation. Well-enforced social policies protect low-income families from exploitation. The Fair Labor Standards Act, for example, is a federal policy requiring employers to pay employees at least a set minimum wage. Some states have set higher minimum wage standards that companies within the state must comply with.

The act also protects vulnerable populations by regulating child labor. Children of low-income, often minority families are more likely to be employed out of necessity to contribute to the family's income. Regulations specify the maximum daily and weekly work hours for children during a school year, a minimum wage, and nonhazardous work environment. The act further ensures that education and safety are prioritized. Employers can be heavily fined if their employees do not comply with the federal and state regulations.

Public policies also reduce poverty rates. The Earned Income Tax Credit (EITC) reduces the amount of federal tax required of lower-income families. Similar to wage regulations, some states have their own EITC programs that combine with the benefits of the federal program to offer greater tax savings to low-income families. Tax credit legislation was first passed in 1975 and has succeeded in reducing poverty

(Neumark and Wascher, 2001). The Center on Budget and Policy Priorities published a study in 1998 reporting poverty decreases attributed to the EITC (Neumark and Wascher, 2002). The study found an 8 percent decrease for all Americans and a 14.5 percent decrease for children. The policy has succeeded in reducing poverty by helping workers increase their earnings from below-poverty level to above poverty, thereby allowing more opportunity for social and economic mobility (Smeeding, Phillips, et al., 2000; Greenstein, 2002; Alegria, Perez, et al., 2003).

Public policy can also influence education levels in the population. As mentioned in Chapter Three, educational opportunities are not equal for all Americans. Studies have shown public schools to be of lower quality in areas of concentrated poverty. Consequently, low-income students struggle to receive adequate education to prepare themselves for college or employment. The No Child Left Behind Act of 2001 works to give parents and students more of a choice in where students receive their education. This program allows students to transfer to another school in the district if their assigned school does not meet federal quality standards. If unable to transfer to a higher-performing school, students are entitled to supplemental educational services such as tutoring or remedial classes. The act empowers educational consumers by motivating schools to achieve federal quality standards and offering alternatives to students to avoid the consequences of receiving inadequate education from low quality schools.

While in theory the program aims to improve educational quality, it places extensive and undue additional administrative pressures on schools, teachers, and students and orients teachers to train students to achieve on performance tests (without additional funds to help prepare children adequately) so that schools can maintain their already tragically low levels of funding. Moreover, recent federal testing results have produced inconsistent and confusing messages. For example, in Florida, nearly 75 percent of all schools failed to meet the federal testing standards despite most being lauded by the governor for their achievements in meeting state standards. These inconsistencies suggest trouble within the No Child Left Behind program and create difficulties with ensuring that the 75 percent of all state children who now have the option to move to "achieving" schools can be adequately accommodated. Finally, with ongoing reductions in federal funding for education, carrying out the act as intended will be difficult at best.

The federal **Head Start** program is another public policy program working to equalize the educational experience. The program is designed to prepare students from low-SES families for the school year. Summer classes improve school readiness for students without the same educational guidance and support as higher-income families. For example, illiterate or immigrant parents not fluent in English have difficulty helping their children develop reading, writing, and language skills, placing these children at a disadvantage before the school year begins. Head Start's services are provided outside the school curriculum and deliver additional academic support to improve learning skills. The program also offers medical, dental, and mental health services for children to ensure healthy development and reduce health disadvantages that can interfere with school readiness.

Additional policy efforts have been made to equalize the health effects of employment disparities. As discussed in Chapter Three, vulnerable populations are more likely to hold lower-status jobs that have higher rates of injury and exposure to toxic substances. The federal government's Occupational Safety and Health Administration (OSHA), for example, ensures a certain standard of safety for every employee in the United States. In this way, employees not educated, organized, or powerful enough to advocate for themselves can be unconditionally protected by government regulations. The standards, which are numerous and differ by work environments, are enforced through substantial fines levied to noncompliant employers.

While these policies address root causes of vulnerable characteristics associated with low SES, the policies discussed next aim to minimize negative health behaviors, some of them associated with lower SES. Although public policy can be very effective at protecting individuals by limiting behaviors, policymakers cannot control the individual responses to the laws and are limited in their influence. Personal safety regulations enforced by state or federal authorities, for example, include mandatory seat belt and car seat use and the regulation of alcohol use at an inappropriate age or while driving. The use and sale of drugs and prostitution are outlawed in most states in order to protect individuals from the potentially harmful side effects of these behaviors. Policies also modify behavior through disincentives. For example, alcohol and cigarette products are highly taxed to increase their retail price and discourage their purchase. Policymakers use public education to improve population health. By increasing awareness of risks and promoting healthy behaviors, public policy can instruct the general population to make healthier life choices (Warshaw, Gugenheim, et al., 2001).

Community-Based Interventions. One of the most progressive methods for resolving SES disparities in health has been to strengthen neighborhood resources through community building. Similar to participatory action research, **community building** refers to the strategic process of engaging community residents and leaders in the process of making change, building relationships, and ultimately enhancing the capacity of communities or neighborhoods to analyze and solve local problems. Prior to addressing specific racial and ethnic disparities, for example, community building strengthens the organizational assets and abilities of a community in order to identify and develop remedies for health and health care disparities. Essential to the practice of community building is a belief that communities are the foundation for the improvement of health and well-being for individuals and families (Bell, Bell, et al., 2002).

Even groups of people that are not defined by neighborhoods or other geographical boundaries are nonetheless affected by community factors in other ways. For example, some populations, such as migrant and rural populations, may live in a dispersed network of communities, but travel to obtain health care in select villages or neighborhoods. Community building in such cases involves linking them with much larger centralized resources, as well as increasing the ability of even the smallest neighborhoods to address their health issues. Community building is not limited to direct medical care issues, but also involves issues of transportation, food security, social supports, and leadership development that enhance the ability to address health issues.

One example of community building is the Harlem Children's Zone, a community-based organization that works to enhance the quality of life for children and families in a very low-income area in Harlem in New York City. The program, which was founded in the 1970s, focuses not just on education, health care, and social service initiatives but also on rebuilding community life. The design of the community work was established by the community itself and includes asthma screening programs and fitness and nutrition programs; most important, it includes community-building actions such as after-school programs for children, recreational activities for families, homework assistance programs, computer training, and leadership development. These latter aspects of the program are critical to the development of future social improvements that would be expected to contribute to future capacity to address socioeconomic health disparities (Bell, Bell, et al., 2002).

Vocational Foundation, Inc. (VFI) is another community-oriented nonprofit initiative providing professional development training to economically and educationally disadvantaged young adults in New York City. The initiative's goal of economic self-sufficiency is similar to that of the Urban League, though VFI does not target any minority group in particular. The VFI program integrates academic and occupational training with counseling to address job placement and retention challenges. Since it was established in 1936, the VFI has helped 150,000 of New York City's most economically and educationally challenged residents find employment.

The Turning Point program takes a broader approach to building community partnerships. The program, supported by the Robert Wood Johnson and W. K. Kellogg foundations, is a nationwide initiative encouraging community-based and collaborative health care partnerships as a means of strengthening the country's public health infrastructure. Based on the theory that current interventions do not adequately address destructive social determinants, Turning Point hopes that uniting sectors such as education, criminal justice, and faith communities with health delivery systems will address essential needs outside the clinical domain. Nebraska, Virginia, Oklahoma, and several other states are working with Turning Point to build these partnerships among their communities.

Health Care Interventions. As shown in Chapter Three, individuals living in medically underserved areas (MUAs) have poor access to health care. Federal and state governments have been trying for years to develop effective strategies to recruit more physicians to MUAs. Several states use financial incentives to attract physician practices to these areas. Maine's financial incentive strategy requires all physicians who purchase malpractice insurance to pay an additional fee that is redistributed to rural obstetricians providing care in federally designated MUAs. Alabama and Louisiana reward physicians moving to rural areas with a $5,000 state income tax credit, and Oregon's rural recruitment strategy is similar and extends to other health professionals, including nurse practitioners and physician assistants. Several states also sponsor *locum tenens* programs that allow physicians working in MUAs temporary relief from their demanding and understaffed practices. These programs use medical school faculty and residents to rotate through designated underserved areas to relieve doctors. *Locum tenens* programs reduce physician burnout and improve retention rates for medically underserved areas.

The Domestic Violence and Mental Health Policy Initiative (DVMHPI) is an impressive example of integrating fragmented services to provide better-quality care to vulnerable populations. Advocates for domestically abused women identified a glaring omission in their treatment programs. The traumatic effects of abuse render these women in dire need of significant mental health care. However, among the seventeen hundred domestic abuse agencies in the United States supported by public and private funds, none were redirecting resources to offer the necessary mental health support. The public mental health system could not bridge the gap because their funds were earmarked for more severe cases.

Securing additional funds from private and public sources, the DVMPHI completed a needs assessment to gauge the paucity of mental health services for domestically abused women and searched nationwide for promising models to build upon. With an initial focus on Chicago, the initiative built collaboration between fragmented providers with the help of large-scale training sessions, interagency working groups, cross-consultation, and service provider awareness campaigns to inform providers of the link between abuse and mental health (Warshaw, Gugenheim, et al., 2003).

New telecommunication and computer technologies have made telemedicine a successful method for increasing MUA access to health care services. States are promoting telemedicine programs that use real-time, video-imaging communication between geographically distant doctors and patients. Georgia has an extensive telemedicine network, with over sixty sites. The network includes rural community hospitals, an ambulatory center, a public health facility, and correctional institutions (Tymann and Orloff, 1996). The programs also provide continuing medical education and training to doctors in rural areas.

Safety net providers offer a broad spectrum of care or services at low or no cost to patients who are underinsured or unable to afford out-of-pocket payments and private insurance premiums. Safety net programs are designed to care for the underserved in unique ways that include recruiting providers who will volunteer their services, establishing accessible and local care sites such as school clinics and mobile health vans, and reaching out to specific populations to educate them about health needs and available services. (Chapter Five offers an in-depth review of diverse national and community-level safety net programs.)

The fact remains that over 40 million Americans, including about 14 percent of children, are uninsured ("Health Care for Children and Youth," 2002). One of the more recent strategies to broaden the nation's safety net is to expand current public programs. The State Children's Health Insurance Program (SCHIP) has expanded the eligible population since the program's inception in 1997. Initially, children's uninsurance rates did not decrease, largely due to problems with enrollment. Since then, however, there have been dramatic increases in enrollment, with the greatest results seen in areas with high rates of uninsurance. In addition to programs such as SCHIP and Medicaid, states often expand their safety net services beyond the federal requirements (Cunningham, 2003).

There are also numerous publicly funded safety net programs offering prenatal and well-baby services to care for the young. For example, the CDC sponsors the Vaccines for Children program, which places a price cap on all vaccines used in federal contracts prior to 1993. As a result, providers can better afford to administer vaccines to uninsured children. Before the program's inception, vaccine prices often forced providers to refer uninsured children to public health department clinics for vaccines, resulting in lower immunization rates. Buying vaccines for participating providers affords the program enough collective purchasing power to keep vaccine costs low. In addition, the program provides free vaccines to all children who are uninsured, Medicaid recipients, Native Americans, or Alaska Natives at their doctors' offices.

Individual-Level Interventions. Based on a 1992 recommendation from the American Academy of Pediatrics (AAP), the U.S. Public Health Service, the AAP, the SIDS Alliance, and the Association of SIDS and Infant Mortality Program initiated a national public education campaign in 1994 to reduce the incidence of sudden infant death syndrome (SIDS), which occurs more frequently among lower-income populations. The AAP's recommendation stated that the back and side are the safest sleeping positions for infants to avoid death from SIDS. The original AAP recommendation was revised in 1996 to state that the back, not the side, is the safest sleeping position. The campaign sought to educate physicians and caregivers by distributing information to hospital nurseries, day care centers, and clinics. A public media campaign targeted parents through television commercials and other media. The campaign was a success, and by 1998, 95 percent of those surveyed had received information recommending the back or side sleeping position. From 1992 to 1998, the percentage of infants put to sleep on their stomachs declined from 70 to 17 percent. Concurrently, the incidence of SIDS decreased by about 40 percent (National Institute of Child Health and Human Development, 2001).

Strategies to Resolve Disparities by Health Insurance

Several innovative strategies have been proposed to ensure that all individuals are financially capable of accessing health care. While the main strategies to reducing health and health care disparities according to health insurance status are typically variations on expanding coverage to the uninsured, there are several new approaches that are being proposed to ensure that everyone has financial access to medical care. Strategies include encouraging enrollment in public health insurance programs for those who are already eligible, incrementally expanding public insurance coverage eligibility, and unique state- or locally based initiatives to provide universal coverage.

Policy Interventions. There are many policy approaches for addressing disparities in health insurance coverage.

Encouraging Enrollment for Eligible Individuals. Proposals to expand health insurance coverage continue to cross the minds and desks of public health leaders; medical societies and associations; and national, state, and local legislators. While this is a critically important and valid solution to the problem of the uninsured, this is frequently a tough political sell, particularly in the U.S. environment of economic tightness and a continuing disinterest in government control of health care. Given the continuing political challenge of legislating substantial expansions of coverage, one often overlooked solution is addressing the large number of people who are eligible for, but not yet enrolled in, government-sponsored health insurance programs.

According to the most recent estimates, approximately 74 percent of uninsured children (6.8 million children) and 5 percent of uninsured adults (1.7 million people) across the United States are eligible for, but not enrolled in, Medicaid or SCHIP (Davidoff, Garrett, et al., 2001; Holohan, Dubay, et al., 2003). These estimates suggest that the government is already prepared to provide financial access to health care for the majority of the uninsured. But there are substantial barriers preventing the uninsured from enrolling in these programs. Research suggests that the main barriers to enrolling are lengthy and complicated administrative procedures, lack of knowledge of the availability of the programs, and not actually wanting or needing the coverage (Holohan, Dubay, et al., 2003).

Many program and administrative requirements that create these barriers were established for legitimate reasons, including ensuring that the programs serve only the children they were intended to serve (Lewit, Bennett, et al., 2003). Most public assistance programs are **means tested** and require extensive documentation of income, but for many applicants, this slows the process substantially, requiring that individuals make multiple visits, complete in-person interviews, and reapply annually, if not more frequently. In some cases, potential applicants never return for a second visit, and this contributes to being eligible but still uninsured.

While a process of presumptive eligibility is already in place for SCHIP (individuals who appear to be eligible for either SCHIP or Medicaid are presumed to be eligible in order to allow them to receive needed health care), this approach only temporarily covers individuals until a full eligibility determination can be made (Rissman, 1998; Manos, Leyden, et al., 2001; Klein, 2003). This grace period typically lasts only one month; in order to maintain coverage, an individual must participate in the regular application process. This does not eliminate the barriers created by requiring people to enroll in public assistance programs separately.

An exceptional example of the efforts to improve enrollment in public health insurance programs is a process that encourages streamlining and the elimination of duplicative processes of enrolling individuals in public aid programs. Recent work has found that nearly 63 percent of children who are uninsured and eligible for public insurance programs are already receiving aid or benefits through programs such as food stamps, the National School Lunch Program, or the Special Supplemental Nutrition Program for Women, Infants, and Children (WIC; Horner, Morrow, et al., 2000). Since these programs frequently have tougher eligibility criteria than SCHIP and Medicaid, many eligible children could be enrolled in public health insurance programs by conducting outreach to families who are enrolled in other aid programs, allowing automatic enrollment of children in health insurance programs if they are already enrolled in other aid programs, or combining enrollment processes for separate programs into a single application (Horner, Lazarus, et al., 2003).

While there are substantial challenges to coordinating enrollments across aid programs, several states have initiated creative forms of "express lane eligibility"

(Horner, Lazarus, et al., 2003). Ohio, for example, has implemented a process in its public schools to allow parents to submit a form along with their school lunch applications to obtain low-cost health care. Schools then mail these forms to the state, and application packages are mailed to interested parents for Healthy Start and the state's Medicaid and SCHIP programs. In Vermont, a family submits an application to WIC, Medicaid, or SCHIP programs, and the family is automatically considered for each program. In Los Angeles, the Department of Public Social Services conducted a computerized search to locate families enrolled in the school lunch program but not yet enrolled in Medicaid. These families were sent notices of their potential eligibility, and interested families returned cards that allowed food stamp information to be used to determine eligibility for Medicaid and SCHIP.

Incrementally Expanding Public Insurance Coverage. In addition to enrolling individuals who are already eligible for public insurance programs, advocacy groups and politicians interested in health disparities have continued to push for the passage of legislation to expand coverage to individuals and families at even higher income levels. While attempts to pass universal health insurance coverage have consistently failed in the United States, more incremental approaches to providing insurance coverage for specific, targeted groups have been much more successful. The most recent example has been the passage of SCHIP, but now some states are beginning to use funds from SCHIP to cover low-income pregnant women and parents of children who are already enrolled in the program.

As of early 2003, five states had obtained approval from DHHS to provide health insurance coverage to pregnant women of potentially SCHIP-eligible children. This sets a precedent for states to offer coverage for children from conception until age nineteen, the cut-off for the SCHIP program (National Governors Association, 2003). While Medicaid requires states to cover pregnant women up to 133 percent of poverty, these incremental expansions provide coverage for women who do not qualify for Medicaid but earn too little to obtain coverage through employment or through private purchase.

The most prominent incremental insurance expansion has been focused on parents of children who are enrolled in SCHIP. Remarkable estimates reveal that about one-third of all children who are in Medicaid or SCHIP have at least one parent who is uninsured (Davidoff, Kenney, et al., 2001). There is some evidence that parents who do not have insurance coverage may be less able to manage the health care needs of their children (Hanson, 1998; Gifford, Weech-Maldonado, et al., 2001) and that increasing parent coverage may also help enroll more children (Selden, Banthin, et al., 1999). Synthesis of these findings has encouraged some states to consider the use of SCHIP funds to expand coverage to parents of children as well (Dubay and Kenney, 2001).

Many states have expanded coverage to low-income parents of children through Medicaid, but this allows coverage only of parents up to 100 percent of the federal poverty level (Howell, Almeida, et al., 2002). As of July 2002 only twenty states covered parents up to the federal poverty line. In 2000, however, states were given the option of using SCHIP funds to cover parents (Ross and Cox, 2002). This required that a special **1115 waiver** be obtained from the secretary of Health and Human Services, but as of June 2002, ten states had used this process to cover parents at 200 percent of poverty or more, thus matching the eligibility levels for children in their states (Lewit, Bennett, et al., 2003).

Wisconsin, for example, has used SCHIP funds to expand coverage to parents. At the time that the program was enacted, 25 percent of all parents with income less than 200 percent of poverty were uninsured. In 1999, the state decided to expand coverage for parents up to 100 percent of poverty using Medicaid dollars to fund an expansion program called BadgerCare (using an 1115 waiver). This expansion began the process of ensuring coverage for parents who were not eligible for the traditional Medicaid program, and the state further used SCHIP funds (with another 1115 waiver) to cover parents up to 200 percent of poverty. The program actually enrolls only parents with incomes up to 185 percent of poverty, but allows them to remain eligible until their income exceeds 200 percent of FPL. BadgerCare, and its extensive outreach and advertising campaigns, has proven to be very successful at providing families with insurance coverage; the current enrollment is at 108,100 people, 73,000 of whom are parents.

Because many innovations in health policy begin at the state level, this approach to incremental expansions of health insurance is likely to become an attractive model for many states to provide insurance to many of their uninsured. Economic considerations, tightening fiscal budgets, and SCHIP funds that diminish over time may discourage the use of these incremental approaches by states. Changes at the federal level to fund these expansions to parents in a more stable and permanent manner are likely required to keep parents enrolled for more than a few years. With federal level funds for such coverage at least a few years away, some states have developed their own programs to cover parents; in other words, instead of waiting for the ship to come in, they are building the ship themselves.

Unique State Approaches to Providing Universal Coverage. To the chagrin of many medical, public health, and health policy professionals, the United States has not managed to implement any form of universal health coverage for its citizens, despite literally hundreds of legislative proposals. While universal health coverage currently remains an unlikely national political feat, some states and localities have taken it on themselves to attempt to provide universal coverage for their specific, smaller populations.

States have played a remarkable role in pioneering health policies, new programs, and proposals to reduce disparities in health and health care through universal health insurance coverage at the state and local levels because of their greater **political feasibility,** relatively easier implementation, and ability to tailor innovative programs. Advocates of these more state- and community-focused approaches are convinced that proving that universal insurance strategies can be successful will one day influence federal initiatives or become model programs for national policies.

One recent example is the passage of legislation in Maine that helps ensure that every resident in the state is covered by health insurance. In June 2003 the state enacted the Dirigo Health program that helps residents pay their health insurance premiums. Quite different from many national proposals for universal coverage, Dirigo Health acts as the sole liaison to private health insurers for low-income individuals, families, small and large employers, and the self-employed in order to obtain affordable coverage. The state pools available federal and state dollars and negotiates health insurance premiums with private plans. It then offers uninsured individuals the ability to purchase health insurance on a sliding scale, with very low payments for those with low income and slightly higher payments for those with higher incomes. Individuals and employers can all make use of this program, and providers have been asked to voluntarily limit any annual price increases to less than 3 percent, with the assurance that they will have to provide much less uncompensated care (one of the driving forces behind price increases).

While Maine is not a very large or extremely diverse state, it had the eleventh highest health care expenditures in the country and more than 180,000 uninsured individuals. The relatively homogeneous political will of Maine legislators to act as political leaders in the national health policy arena is a critical component to the passage of this program. Evaluations are under way to study the success or failure of this program, but regardless of the results, the political wheels have been set in motion again for more changes at the state, and eventually the federal, level.

California also received substantial media attention in 2003 for a number of health care proposals that were targeted at ensuring universal or near-universal health insurance coverage for all state residents. Proposals ranged from establishing the state as the **single payer** (acting as the insurance provider for all residents) to a new health plan called Healthy California, to which employers that do not provide health benefits to their employees would contribute in order to cover the uninsured (Sanders, 2002). Perhaps the most interesting proposal, which has gathered some national attention, is one proposed by Bruce Bodaken, the CEO of Blue Shield of California.

The proposal is one of only a few ever to be proposed by a health insurance plan. The plan was announced at the end of 2002 to provide universal coverage to residents of California. It uses a combination of approaches, including a mandate that all large employers offer a basic package of health benefits to its employees (preventive care, physician services, hospital care, and prescription drug coverage), an exemption for small businesses, no changes to the Medicaid or SCHIP program, and a sliding scale for other individuals to purchase subsidized insurance coverage. According to the CEO, the plan would generate savings for the state by expanding preventive care, promoting earlier treatment, and offering a more secure financing system for all groups involved: patients, physicians, hospitals, and insurers ("Blue Shield of California CEO," 2002).

The proposal sparked interest not only in California; it has also garnered national media attention. The plan has drawn so much interest, in fact, that research studies have been conducted to assess the costs and impact of implementing the plan nationally. The findings suggest that the costs of ensuring health insurance coverage for everyone in the nation would require a $75 billion increase in federal spending, but could be balanced by decreases in spending by businesses and individuals of more than $43 billion (Thorpe, 2003). There are many critics of this plan, who are challenging the ability to mandate that individuals must purchase subsidized coverage. Nevertheless, many have lauded the focus on ensuring a basic level of health coverage for everyone without requiring a complete restructuring of the health system. While adoption of this plan at either the state or national level may be unlikely (given the current unstable financial and political climate), it opens the door for players other than politicians and advocates to propose ways of reducing disparities in health.

Community-Based Interventions. A significant challenge to these insurance programs is raising public awareness of their availability. Many underprivileged individuals do not have the resources, ability, or opportunity to research safety net options for themselves or their families. Programs such as Washington's Children's Alliance, a nonprofit organization, help to educate the public about state-sponsored health insurance eligibility through community outreach. The alliance works closely with school districts to identify and enroll eligible children in the state's SCHIP plan. Similarly, New York's Hispanic Federation works with Latino families to boost their enrollment in health insurance programs. Providing essential translation services and assistance navigating the complex enrollment process, the Hispanic Foundation helped five hundred Latino families enroll in public health insurance programs in 2002.

Integrative Approaches to Resolving Disparities

While many of the potential strategies for addressing disparities in health and health care focus on single racial/ethnic, socioeconomic, or health insurance pathways, this book has highlighted the importance of addressing multiple vulnerabilities factors simultaneously. Without addressing the larger package of population risks, strategies to deal effectively with these disparities may be partially effective at best and undermining at worst. Because of their relative simplicity, narrowly focused strategies and programs have the potential to direct resources away from programs, agendas, and social strategies that could more comprehensively and fundamentally address disparities. To refocus national attention on solving disparities using a broader approach, several integrative and unifying models of solving disparities are helpful. These models provide a broader view of health disparities and could serve to align and synchronize the aims of the fragmented strategies in place. In many cases, these integrative models are based on common wisdom, but they are substantiated and enlightened with modern scientific evidence.

Benzeval U.K. Framework for Addressing Disparities

One of the most useful approaches to addressing health and health care disparities has been proposed in the United Kingdom. In a report released by the King's Fund in the United Kingdom in 1995, Benzeval and colleagues proposed a framework for tackling inequalities in health. The framework proposed four strategies for intervention: (1) make changes to the physical environment, including ensuring adequate housing and living space, improving working conditions, and reducing pollution levels; (2) address social and economic factors, including ensuring adequate income and personal wealth, reducing unemployment, and affording individuals time and resources to develop social support systems; (3) improve access to health care and social services; and (4) reduce barriers to adopting healthy lifestyles and changing behavioral risk factors. Used as a whole, this framework can be adapted to address the combined influences of racial/ethnic disparities, disparities in SES, or health insurance status.

Enhancing Education

Education is an important contributor to health. As shown extensively in earlier chapters, educational level is strongly predictive of health status, morbidity, and mortality. Education not only influences health behaviors (for example, higher education is linked to fewer health risk behaviors), but more important, it contributes to social position, which has profound influences on health through subtle but powerful forces such as stress, life control, and political power. These nonmaterial influences of educational level have few points of intervention. Even health behaviors, which are modifiable, are harder to change among individuals with less education, who experience high levels of stressors.

Education is also an important resource for upward mobility. Chapter Two highlights the essential role of education in granting access to employment in higher-level professions. Employment in these professions helps to generate higher income and also provides access to employment-based health insurance coverage. Higher education, higher-level employment, and higher income are defining features of social position, such that individuals who attain these resources benefit not only from material improvements in life but also from the health-related benefits of higher social class. In short, education continues to be the main door opener to social and economic mobility, as well as optimal health.

Education is one of the few social resources that is nearly universally available in the United States. Both primary and secondary education are required by law for all children and adolescents. Public education is financed through taxation and is available to all families, although an increasing number of families have sought education from private schools and other alternate means, such as home schooling (Gerald and Hussar, 2003). Disparities in school resources and quality have developed based on differences in local tax bases (schools in higher-income areas derive more financial support than schools in lower-income areas), leading to concerns about the education quality provided in many public schools.

Tightening state and national budgets have also forced public schools to serve an increasing number of students with decreasing funds. Despite this, schools that have the fewest resources are being required to have their students undergo more frequent testing, which directly influences the funding the schools receive. In effect, schools that are the most financially strapped, and therefore have the fewest resources to hire high-quality teachers and provide students with good learning environments, are performing poorly on such tests and are receiving even less public funding as a result. This cycle is disproportionately influencing the lowest-SES schools, schools in geographical areas with more racial/ethnic minorities, and schools serving families where other vulnerabilities are particularly concentrated, such as in medically underserved and rural areas.

These differences in school resources and school quality contribute to disparities in educational attainment among vulnerable populations. Higher dropout rates among African Americans and Hispanics are evidence of the disproportionate struggles of these schools, which are compounded by other barriers to student achievement in vulnerable communities. For example, single-parent families, parents working in multiple jobs, and community violence are much more common in some of these communities and create a number of barriers to educational achievement.

Moreover, early poor educational performance in school reduces the chances that a student will choose to pursue and be admitted to higher education. These levels of education provide the most opportunity for upward social and economic mobility, and vulnerable populations still do not obtain higher education at the same rate as nonvulnerable populations. For example, only 17.0 percent of African Americans and 11.0 percent of Hispanics have a college degree compared to 27.2 percent of whites. While programs such as affirmative action have greatly helped to improve enrollment in higher education for vulnerable groups, current rollbacks in affirmative action programs have put future college admittance for these groups on shaky ground.

Fundamentally altering how resources are allocated to primary and secondary public schools so that each school has adequate, equitable, and stable funding may be one of the most important ways to ensure equitable educational opportunities for all children. Because early success in school predicts future educational achievement, this may give vulnerable children more equal footing in obtaining higher education. While there are many other social barriers to ensuring that children succeed academically, having greater funding available for all public schools may improve the chances that children will graduate from high school, obtain higher education, and enter a world of higher social position that affords many health benefits.

Community Social Cohesion

Instead of waging separate, independent battles to overcome negative social risks to individual and community health, individuals can work together in community teams to change the circumstances influencing health. Social cohesion is defined by a community's social fabric, such as the forming of associations, church groups, and advocacy organizations, as well as more subtle characteristics of social interaction, such as interpersonal trust and community norms. Research has shown that strengthening social support and cohesion helps to buffer individuals from the stress of challenging social environments and other risk factors (Institute of Medicine, 2001).

Community partnerships have particular promise for improving social cohesion by using the strengths and resources of community members to participate in and manage the initiative. Because the key players have a vested and long-term interest in the initiative's outcome and goals, there is a greater chance at sustainable success. Furthermore, a community-oriented approach sets priorities that reflect the needs of the local population. And the process of building these community partnerships, by definition, increases social cohesion.

Many American communities have realized the value of social cohesion and designed interventions to bolster it. For example, in the Bronx borough of

New York City, East Side House Settlement project has established a family and community-building initiative to discourage adolescents from using alcohol or illegal drugs. The project's expectation is that by strengthening social bonds, the community will have more success in preventing negative health behaviors among community residents.

The strategies for strengthening social cohesion in this Bronx neighborhood include involving more community members in local plans and decision making, as well as creating partnerships between local agencies and organizations that share compatible community-building goals. The project reaches out to the community through its community centers, early childhood services, school-based programs, technology services, and senior citizen programs.

A similar community organization seeks to strengthen social cohesion among the Latino population in Boston. The Sociedad Latina aims to reinforce the minority community's bonds through programs promoting community leadership, educational attainment, cultural identity, and the preservation of Latino traditions. To establish a relationship with the Latino population, the organization offers services to minority-related challenges such as immigration issues and translation assistance, as well as short-term crisis intervention, family counseling, and referrals for food and homeless shelters.

Sociedad Latina's community-strengthening strategies include establishing the Viva La Cultura Club, which promotes and celebrates cultural pride. The Sociedad Latina sponsors a parents' support group and leadership development program, Latinos in Leadership Action and Change. In addition, there are several professional development and educational support projects offered to the local Hispanic population to enrich their individual lives and make a stronger contribution to their community.

The greatest health achievements of social cohesion are likely to be obtained when social cohesion is not limited to specific racial/ethnic groups or socioeconomic tiers. As suggested in Chapter Two, social cohesion efforts that cross these boundaries and cultivate cohesion among distinct groups are likely to have the greatest impacts on health and well-being. Interrelationships among these groups will help to direct resources to needed areas, improve strategic efforts to address cross-cutting health issues, and potentially reduce relative deprivation.

Balancing Primary Care and Specialty Care

Technology has broadened the range of medical treatment options. Rapidly developing medical technology has significantly reduced the specter of infectious disease using vaccinations and antibiotics, thereby increasing the U.S. life expectancy. The current focus of technological innovation is on chronic, genetic, and acute disease. Technology's curative potential has become a powerful force in health care delivery, and the resulting cultural shift among patients and providers embracing technology has established its use as the standardized norm (Patton, 2001).

Although technology has proven to be a worthwhile investment in health care (Cutler and McClellan, 2001), the overuse of technology can create negative outcomes. Given the limited resources to invest in the American health care system, it is essential to think carefully before assuming that the best solution involves often expensive, technological innovation. Considering the broad benefits of primary care in preventing acute conditions requiring technological intervention, it seems essential to strive for a balanced investment in both high- and low-technology medicine. It is also important to keep in mind the greater risks associated with technological intervention, particularly when compared to less risky preventive interventions.

Disparity in health status could also be improved with a better-balanced investment in both high- and low-technology medicine. Recent studies have shown that minorities are more likely than nonminorities to experience preventable hospitalizations, which could be the result of lower-quality care or limited access to care (Gaskin and Hoffman, 2000). A similar effect was found among low-SES populations. One study that compared preventable hospitalization rates of low- and high-income cohorts in the United States and Canada found a much smaller discrepancy among low- and high-income Canadians than Americans (Billings, Anderson, et al., 1996). The likely explanation is that the accessible primary and preventive care available through Canada's universal health coverage provides equitable services regardless of individual wealth. Thus, the American system is more likely to spend a greater proportion of financial resources handling illness that has slipped through the cracks of cost-effective primary care and eventually requiring expensive technological intervention.

In addition, it could be argued that overuse of emergency departments for primary care or preventable care reveals the inadequate investment currently being made in the nation's primary care delivery system. Allocating more resources to provide preventive services, including primary care and chronic disease management, to underserved populations would certainly reduce costs in the health care system.

Managed care organizations have sought to equalize investment in primary and acute technological care as a cost-saving measure. However, their choices to reduce costs through restricted coverage or strategic treatment recommendations have come under scrutiny for patient negligence, as well as retarding the diffusion of medical technologies (Cutler and McClellan, 2001).

Administrators are using utilization management strategies to curb unnecessary visits to the emergency department. The strategies include improving same-day or next-day appointment access for primary care practices, offering telephone consultations with providers, and educating patients on the appropriate use of emergency departments. Some health insurers restricted their coverage for emergency department visits to discourage the behavior. After consumers protested these restrictions, insurers eased off and provided better coverage. Instead of refusing to cover emergency department visits, insurers are now increasing individual co-payments to control the visits (Tufts Managed Care Institute, 2001).

Some public health researchers have identified emergency department visits as primary opportunities to educate a patient population that is less likely to have a regular source of care, and with good reason: studies have shown improved outcomes for patients who have received health education information during these visits (Wei and Camargo, 2000).

Another factor affecting the health care experience of vulnerable patients is service-provider integration. Historically, health care in the United States has been hindered by a fragmented system of delivery. A categorical payment structure by payers, public payers in particular, directs funds to individual populations or individual illnesses, making it difficult for patients to experience continuity of care for a diverse range of health needs (Hughes, Brindis, et al., 1997). Currently, many health care professionals advocate a removal of the restrictions placed on federal and state money that impose a fragmented delivery of care. The hope is that with fewer payment restrictions, the delivery structure can change to provide better, more integrated care (Newacheck, Hughes, et al., 1995).

Furthermore, with the advent of managed care in the 1990s, health care organizations sought to reduce costs by expanding the roles of lower-paid nonphysician providers such as nurse practitioners, psychologists, and physician assistants to include clinical responsibilities previously reserved for physicians. As a result, in the 1990s many more patients were receiving care from nonphysician providers in addition to their physician providers than they had in the 1980s (Druss, Marcus, et al., 2003).

Under the best of circumstances, these additions to the workforce translate into benefits for patients. Recent studies have shown that integrated, multidisciplinary teams provide better preventive services and care for chronic conditions and achieve more successful outcomes for addiction treatment than single-discipline teams (Wagner, 2003; Weisner, Mertens, et al., 2001).

If the multidisciplinary team is not well managed, the increase in nonphysician providers will fragment care among the team members further. Toward this end, administrators have established professional development programs to train multidisciplinary teams to communicate effectively and integrate services efficiently to maximize quality of care (Druss, Marcus, et al., 2003).

In response to these findings and others, clinical groups and public health care programs are working to integrate their services better using nonphysician providers, including community and lay health workers. Hospitals are now beginning to advertise the benefits of their integrated teams of physicians, nurses, community outreach coordinators, and social services staff. Training programs such as Washington D.C.'s Area Health Education Center (AHEC) offers instruction for medical students and health professionals in providing care to underprivileged populations. AHEC discourages an autonomous practice model as incapable of meeting the health care needs of the broader community. As reflected in its curriculum, AHEC's community-oriented model depends largely on interdisciplinary team coordination and communication for success.

Life Course Health Development

A novel, unifying approach to resolving health disparities is based on the simple axiom that what happens early in life influences health and well-being later in life. This model was generated through the synthesis of empirical research from the fields of medicine, psychology, sociology, and public health. The model serves a groundbreaking role in the context of eliminating health disparities in that it provides a model of health as the cumulative result of physical, psychosocial, environmental, and historical experiences. Some of these experiences are protective of health, and others are injurious to health and well-being. It is this tug-of-war between these experiences at critical junctures or periods in life that ultimately sets the trajectory for future health and well-being across the life course (Halfon and Hochstein, 2002).

According to this model, disparities in health are determined to a large extent in the early years of life. Human physiological systems, including nervous, endocrine, and immune systems, are functionally enmeshed with one another and adapt to changes in the external environment. These systems undergo a process of embedding and programming at early ages and are susceptible to insults from environmental causes (Hertzman, 1999). For example, an infectious illness or exposure to allergens during prenatal or postnatal periods can affect the development of lungs and the responsiveness of the immune system, leading to child asthma and significant reductions in adult lung function (Holt and Sly, 1997, 2000).

This early imprinting of the human physiological system is susceptible to more than biological threats. Social factors, interpersonal relationships, and family stress that infants and children experience early in life influence the development of physiological systems and contribute to health in later life. Maternal depression, for example, has been associated with poorer parenting habits, such as expressing more negative affect toward children, being less attentive to and engaged with infants, and failing to respond to the emotional signals of infants and children. These infants develop a shorter attention span, do not flourish in mastering new tasks, have elevated heart rates, and have elevated levels of cortisol (a hormone associated with stress), which have been associated with lower cognitive ability in childhood and poorer mental health in adulthood (Dawson, Ashman, et al., 2000; Ashman, Dawson, et al., 2002).

Extensive evidence now links many experiences at the beginning of life with many health, disease, and functional ability outcomes later in life (Singer and Riff, 2001; Ben-Shlomo and Kuh, 2002). The risk factors include low birth weight, poor weight gain during infancy, low maternal SES, parent divorce, child physical and sexual abuse, and parent smoking. These factors have been linked with poor adult cognitive functioning, diminished physical growth, high blood pressure, teen smoking, prevalence of adult STDs, psychotic illness, and many other health and mental health outcomes (Felitti, Anda, et al., 1998; Anda, Croft, et al., 1999; Hillis, Anda, et al., 2000; Repetti, Taylor, et al., 2002; Lu and Halfon, 2003).

The application of this health development model to addressing health disparities across the life course would suggest that intervention should be targeted to the critical period of early childhood, where lifelong health trajectories are set. Reducing health disparities requires reducing exposure to risk factors and promoting exposure to protective factors in order to aim and launch the life-course health trajectory as high as possible (see Figure 6.4).

Consider, for example, a three-year-old child who comes from a low-income family and experiences many risk factors: having been born prematurely and with low birth weight, poor nutritional status, and a single mother who is working multiple jobs to support the family, smokes, and is depressed. This child may also be uninsured because the mother earns too much to qualify for Medicaid but works jobs that do not offer health insurance. Protective factors are also present for the family, including a grandmother who is available to provide a source of child care, a church program that provides social support for single mothers, and a nearby community health center that provides many free health services for her family.

According to the model, the current child health trajectory can be improved by reducing the risks and increasing the protective factors. For example, when the child reaches school age, he can be enrolled in the free or reduced-price lunch program to help him obtain better nutrition; the minimum wage could be raised to offer greater stability to families working low-wage jobs; and a primary care physician could screen the mother for depression and help her obtain appropriate treatment. Similarly, the number of protective factors could be increased. For example, the local community health center could provide outreach and enrollment services for the SCHIP program to ensure that the child, and perhaps the mother, are cov-

FIGURE 6.4. LIFE COURSE HEALTH DEVELOPMENT TRAJECTORY

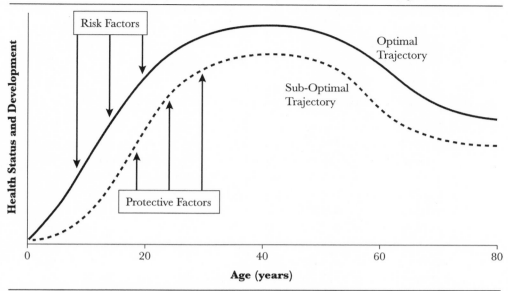

Source: Halfon and Hockstein (2000).

ered by insurance; the child could be enrolled in Head Start and Healthy Start programs to promote child development and early learning; and parenting support groups, such as the one at the church, could provide training sessions and children's books to help both mother and grandmother read to the child (to promote literacy), or literature and support to help the mother cope with stress or even quit smoking.

The life course health development model can be used at individual, community, and health and social policy levels to ensure that health trajectories are maximized early in childhood and are equivalent for all individuals in the United States. The model has implications for redesigning health care systems in a way that would focus on better integrating all necessary care for a population across the life span, while making substantially greater investments in early childhood health and development (Hochstein, Halfon, et al., 1998; Halfon, Inkelas, et al., 2000). Health systems and health plans would be rewarded for providing more thorough developmental services to all families, including pediatric services such as health supervision about parenting, injury prevention, literacy, and other family and psychosocial factors. Developmental surveillance systems (that is, screening children for developmental problems over time) could also be instituted in a standard way across health plans and child-focused organizations, such as health clinics, preschools, and child care centers. Although the model is likely to influence thinking about the creation and persistence of health disparities, actual changes at the policy level to focus more resources on child development may be extremely difficult.

Improving National Monitoring of Disparities

Trying to equalize the quality of care for all Americans is a challenge. The American population tolerates a conspicuously high variation in health care quality—in fact, high enough that that such variation in quality would be considered unacceptable in many other industries, such as travel and technology. One of the greatest obstacles for equalizing quality is the difficult task of establishing standardized methods that effectively measure quality across the health care spectrum. According to a RAND Health study (1999), the resources to measure quality are available, as are the distribution channels to provide clinicians, consumers, and policymakers with the information. The problem is a lack of organization and oversight that prevents a systematic measurement and distribution of health care quality data. The RAND study recommends that the federal government, private sector, or an integrated partnership between the two take on the task.

The federal government does collect and distribute some data on health care quality. In a coordinated effort with other agencies such as the NIH and Food and Drug Administration, and CDC, the Agency for Healthcare Research and Quality (AHRQ) oversees much of the federal government's health quality data collection. AHRQ is a public health service agency in the Department of Health and Human Services. One of its primary goals is to improve the quality of health care by strengthening quality measurement and improvement. The resulting information can empower patients, providers, policymakers, and administrators to make informed decisions about health care. The agency hopes to employ technology in its strategy to achieve these goals with the use of information systems to distribute performance measures and create better communication among health data organizations. In addition to quality measures, the agency conducts research on other health care outcomes, including cost, use, and access.

The Health Plan Employer Data and Information Set (HEDIS) performance measures are another standardized approach to gathering data on health care quality. In addition to measuring clinical performance, HEDIS incorporates a consumer experience component to its assessments. HEDIS guidelines and assessment tools are developed by the National Committee for Quality Assurance (NCQA), an independent, nonprofit organization.

Distributing the information is essential. Only in this way can clinicians understand how their performance rates, how consumers make educated choices about their care, and how policymakers assess the health care systems' success at serving patients. Both the AHRQ and NCQA are working to make their information accessible. Currently, information for consumers is readily accessible over the Internet, though many individuals in vulnerable populations do not have the resources for access. AHRQ Web documents are also available from the DHHS by placing orders over the telephone. While some of the consumer-oriented information is available on the NCQA Web site for free, the quality assessments with information more relevant to providers and administrators must be purchased.

Consumer participation is another avenue for overcoming barriers to access. Patients are increasingly interested in educating themselves about the quality and type of care they receive and have become more assertive about receiving quality care. Recent research suggests that patients would use provider and hospital performance statistics to make health care decisions if the information were available (Kizer, 2001).

Consumer participation also offers a strategy to reduce health care costs through patient-centered improvements in health care quality. Increased communication between provider and patient will help address the broader issues of health, giving providers enough information to understand the origins of a patient's disease, in addition to managing symptoms.

Although providers must learn to encourage such a dialogue and support autonomous decision making, educating patients is the best means of empowering them and enabling a consumer-driven health care system to work. Ostensibly, patients who are educated about health, the health care system, and their choices within it could reduce emergency and acute care costs through self-care or improved personal management of their chronic illnesses (Lansky, 2003).

In an era of rapid information dissemination with the expansion of Internet use, it seems there is no better time than the present to engage health care consumers. However, there are problems with relying on the Internet to educate the nation's populace on health care needs and quality services. First, the digital divide once again draws a sharp contrast between underprivileged and privileged Americans. With greater health needs and less access to care, vulnerable populations could benefit most from the Internet's accessible information but are less likely to have the means or knowledge to use it. Second, the multitude of health information Web sites disperse information ranging in accuracy from detailed and precise to misleading and vague (Baugh, 2003).

Health care consumers across the nation have organized themselves effectively to better promote their empowerment movement. Organizations such as the Consumer Coalition for Quality Health Care represent a diverse patient population: the elderly, children, the disabled, and other vulnerable groups. Health care employees are also active in the organization, which works primarily through advocacy to place health care quality issues on the national agenda.

Another national nonprofit organization, Families USA, works to raise awareness among health care consumers through public information campaigns using multimedia outlets. The organization also considers itself a clearinghouse for information relevant to all consumers. Working on a more local level, Families USA offers training assistance to communities challenged by local health care issues. The Center for Health Care Rights uses similar strategies to empower consumers in the health care marketplace, with a particular focus on quality-of-care regulation in HMOs and other managed care plans.

The health care delivery strategies examined here aim to improve access to care and quality of care for vulnerable populations. We also reviewed interventions to eliminate negative social determinants contributing to poor health outcomes among vulnerable populations. The ultimate goal is to improve population health and reduce disparity in the United States. To achieve the desired benefit, the suggested strategies cannot be implemented in isolation but must be integrated. Only in this way can social determinant characteristics and health care delivery factors come together to create an environment harmonious for our diverse population.

Challenges and Barriers in Implementing the Strategies

Strategies and interventions to reduce disparity can make an impact to improve the health care experience of vulnerable populations. However, the widespread change to the American health care system that many consumers and professionals yearn for is struggling to gain momentum in our current political and cultural climate.

Instigating change in the nation's public health is consistently challenged by the conflict of long- versus short-term gains. Effective interventions may require a decade or generation before revealing a positive and sustainable outcome; however, the public prefers to see benefits in a shorter time frame. Even for policymakers, it is difficult to allocate resources to strategies that may improve health status for the next generation when the current generation still faces unmet health needs (Lurie, 2002). An encouraging exception can be found in the federal Healthy People projects, which specifically identify long-term health goals to complete over a ten-year period.

As the result of political pressure to make visible changes over the short term so candidates can be reelected, investments in public health have not always been made with the population's health as the top priority. Another significant form of political pressure exerted on policymakers is that of interest groups. Buffered by influential campaign contributions and the voting power of the people they represent, interest groups can also compromise the priority of population health. To propel their agendas forward, interest groups hire professional lobbyists able to maneuver strategically through the nation's political labyrinth.

Minnesota witnessed this firsthand while trying to implement its first anti-smoking media campaign in the 1990s. The tobacco industry organized opposition to the campaign by claiming it infringed on individual rights. The industry built alliances with communities throughout the state and targeted industry groups that supported the infringement claims. The tobacco industry destabilized the political setting with influential campaign contributions to key legislators as well as created its own media campaign that publicly questioned the financial solvency of the antismoking program. The industry's integrated strategy was a success, leading to the defeat of the state's antismoking program and serving as a lesson to other states considering a program of their own (Tsoukalas and Glantz, 2003).

American culture also contributes to the nation's sluggish changes in health care policy. While Americans have passionately championed many causes in the past century, a social movement for comprehensive health care benefits for underprivileged groups has not been cultivated by the public so as to motivate revolutionary change (Oldenburg, McGuffog, et al., 2000). Instead, the changes and expansions to government-funded care for the underprivileged have been incremental and fragmented.

In lieu of a national health system, the United States has a fragmented approach in which numerous governmental agencies and congressional committees control the nation's health care budget. Public health care consumers are forced to navigate various sources of care and payment options across the health care spectrum because some services are financed differently from others. Considering that individuals over a lifetime will require most forms of care across that spectrum (preventive health, mental health, and specialty care, to name a few), fragmentation will have a negative effect on the nation's vulnerable populations by restricting access and reducing the quality of their care.

From a social determinants perspective that incorporates education, employment, behavior, and community factors into the health care paradigm, the health care delivery system is even more fragmented, making it difficult to integrate these factors into health care interventions. For example, according to Oldenburg, McGuffog, et. al. (2000), behavior modification interventions are successful if they target more than just individual behavior. Local support in the form of recreational access or designated nonsmoking areas can encourage the sustainability of these interventions.

The economic repercussions of such a fragmented system have made the United States what it is: the member country of the Organization for Economic Cooperation and Development (OECD) that spends the highest percentage of its gross domestic product on health care yet does not offer universal coverage. Such a complex payment system conspicuously increases the administrative needs and costs of the health care system, creating expenditures that do not translate into benefits for patients. Our costs are also higher as a result of salaries paid to health care providers that are higher than those paid to providers in other OECD countries (Anderson, Reinhardt, et al., 2003).

Would expanding the role of the federal government simplify the system? Possibly, but public disdain for governmental intervention makes significant federal expansion an unlikely option. Although health care concerns are at the center of presidential debates every four years, Americans appear to be much more comfortable with state and local autonomy, perhaps a cultural remnant from the early days of the nation's history.

Another barrier to garnering support for strategies to reduce disparities is the focus of federal health policy on **cost containment.** With a growing deficit, policymakers are concerned by the nation's consistent increase in health care costs. Consequently, policies conveyed in terms of cost containment are favored over those addressing access and quality of health care, which creates a challenging political climate in which to address health disparities (Shi and Singh, 2004).

Given the nation's relative comfort with state and local intervention, could an expanded state role encourage strategies to improve health and reduce disparity? According to a 2000 RAND Health Report, expanding the public safety net to cover the uninsured using a state-financed plan would not work. Because states vary significantly in the number of uninsured residents they have, the financial burden per state would be unequal. In fact, the states with the most uninsured are the least able to afford expanding services to care for them. A national program would be more likely to distribute funds according to average family incomes in each state, thereby truly identifying and helping the states that need it.

Other arguments have been made against expanded state control over health care. State autonomy would create a nation of fifty unique health care systems, which could pose particular problems for coordinating national public health strategy, a serious consideration in the light of ongoing threats of terrorism. Furthermore, conspicuous differences in state health policies could lead to population redistribution as residents relocated to the states offering better health benefits.

Another challenge faced by the numerous programs and interventions reviewed is the difficult task of measuring outcomes. Particularly where social determinants are concerned, it is challenging to tease out the effects caused by the intervention and not by other economic, social, or health care influences. However, to reap the full benefit of an intervention's investment, it is essential to distribute the program's results to create an integrated, collective foundation building toward a better understanding of the mechanisms linking poor health outcomes to vulnerable populations.

Furthermore, communities feel they have been taken advantage of when they participate in research but never receive feedback or see benefits from their participation. Considering the value that community participation and partnership contribute to public health initiatives, it would be wise to strengthen the relationship through open communication.

Course of Action for Resolving Disparities

The idea that underprivileged populations in the United States have poorer health status is not recent; however, Americans have not reacted strongly by advocating aggressively in a unified voice on behalf of these populations. It is not particularly difficult to explain the public's response. Americans have been known to tolerate high levels of inequality because they have a great faith in the nation's opportunities for individual upward mobility (Graham and Oswald, 2003). While many Americans may acknowledge these vast disparities, they may also believe that social programs such as providing universal health insurance coverage cannot be done without lapsing into socialism. Many Americans fear that having a government bureaucracy control the health care system would reduce personal freedoms in seeking health care or create large waiting lists for care (Navarro, 2003). Americans likely have a similarly resigned attitude toward the persistence of disparities in health as well as the likelihood that a truly integrated local and federal effort could eliminate them.

By examining social shifts in other developed countries that have successfully motivated an unresponsive public to take action, we can identify a course of action to move us toward our goal of changing the political and social climate to benefit vulnerable populations. In seeking to provide an agenda for placing public health issues higher on the public's agenda, we suggest the following course of action that consists of ten steps in four evolving stages.

In the *preparation stage,* efforts are made to enhance awareness, demonstrate severity, and establish the relevance of the issues. In the *design stage,* programs and initiatives are developed that focus on multiple major determinants of the problem, are integrated in nature, and are feasible. In the *implementation stage,* attention is given to applying effective implementation strategies, persevering, and making sure that incremental progress is guided by and built on efforts that have already proven successful and credible. In the *postimplementation* stage, programs and initiatives are evaluated.

Step 1: Enhance Awareness

Given the great number of articles in the medical and social science literature on health care disparities in the United States and recent government reports addressing the problem of health disparities, one might be surprised to find that experts still consistently cite lack of problem recognition as a barrier to eliminating health disparities. Many individuals, including some policymakers, still think that Americans enjoy the best health care in the world and that our health status leads that of all other nations. The vast disparities presented in this book are not fully known or acknowledged. It is critical that the public and policymakers understand the true state of our health and disparities among us.

Education can be used as a tool to raise awareness about health care disparities and to promote a climate of outrage and support for programmatic changes to eliminate such disparities. Education-based approaches generally fall into one of three categories: educating policymakers and the general public about health care disparities, educating vulnerable groups, and promoting better educational attainment in general as a strategy to eliminate health care barriers.

One way to draw attention to a public health issue such as disparity is to illustrate the issue's pervasiveness using local, state, and national data. There have been some efforts to bring the issue of health disparities to greater community and public attention. Healthy People 2010, which has as one of its top two goals the elimination of health disparities among different segments of the population, and the brochure *Healthy People in Healthy Communities: A Community Planning Guide Using Healthy People 2010* (U.S. Department of Health and Human Services, 2001), which highlights the problem of health disparities and offers strategies for communities to build coalitions and alliances in order to address the issue, are two noteworthy examples. However, even more such efforts are needed.

Statistics can often make the issue more compelling to a public unaware that vulnerability is so widespread. Socioeconomic data are recorded at the local, state, and national levels, but they are not always analyzed (Krieger, Williams, et al., 1997). Examining untapped data resources for valuable metric contributions to the field of study will promote a public health cause further. The use of data can also be advanced by improving the way in which disparity is measured. It is challenging to establish clear and precise methods to measure complex and qualitative factors such as stress and discrimination; however, continued development of statistical methods to measure such factors could make a tremendous positive impact on disparity research. Improved metrics would also enable progress to be better tracked over time.

To go a step further, policy alternatives and quantitative goals need to be widely publicized. Technology has provided innumerable means for distributing information. A media campaign incorporating Internet, television, radio, and print ad channels with a simple, readable, and galvanizing message could reach and motivate a broad segment of the population. Policy alternatives, goals, and research, in particular, should also be well published in highly regarded academic publications in order to ensure consistent political pressure on policymakers.

Step 2: Demonstrate Severity

It is critical that the public and policymakers understand the severity of the problem. Policymakers are more likely to act when there is a clear public demand and a perceived crisis. One way to demonstrate severity is the publication of international rankings on key health and health care indicators. Taking advantage of national pride by highlighting a public health issue for which the United States performs poorly compared to other countries may motivate the public to take steps to improve their national ranking. This strategy has often been invoked to garner support for infant mortality interventions. The dismal ranking of the United States among OECD countries as the seventh highest in infant mortality continues to inspire outrage that a country with so many resources does not ensure adequate care for vulnerable citizens.

Step 3: Establish Relevance

Although most Americans are concerned about the plights of the vulnerable populations, relatively few have considered these to be their own problems. Fewer have the understanding that it is actually to their economic advantage to address the plights of vulnerable populations. A rational review of the costs and benefits associated with improving the health of vulnerable populations reveals the advantage of making such an investment. The consideration of costs to the nation resulting from poor health status among the vulnerable cannot evade the public's attention much longer.

Numerous studies have explored the costs of limited access to care and inadequate quality to the underserved populations and the cost to the general public as well. The American public does not seem to relate the suffering of vulnerable populations to the suffering of the nation or to associate wasted human potential with poor health status among vulnerable populations. Missed workdays, social and interpersonal violence, inefficient use of health care dollars, and compromised educational attainment are just a few of the factors putting America at a competitive disadvantage as a result of an insufficient health care system (Miller, 1995).

For example, depression, a condition that is much more common among vulnerable populations, costs employers $44 billion each year in lost labor time.

Studies have also estimated that about 3 to 5 percent of hospital days used by the uninsured could have been prevented if the patients had been insured and received appropriate ambulatory or primary care (Stewart, Ricci, et al., 2003; Hadley, 2002). Taking all these and other factors into account, if vulnerable population groups had health status levels equivalent to nonvulnerable groups, our national earnings could improve by 10 to 30 percent (Hadley, 2002).

Every taxpayer is affected by the health status of vulnerable populations. The total cost of health care services used by the uninsured was estimated to be $98.9 billion for 2001. Uninsured individuals receive about $35 billion in uncompensated care each year, the majority of it provided by federal, state, and local governments (Institute of Medicine Committee on the Consequences of Uninsurance, 2003). The Institute of Medicine's Committee on the Consequences of Uninsurance concluded that the aggregate cost of the poor health status and high mortality rate of uninsured Americans is between $65 and $130 billion for each year of health insurance forgone.

Communities are also affected by the health status of vulnerable populations as they shoulder a disproportionate amount of the subsidized care that uninsured individuals receive. As a result, other health care services such as infectious disease control, immunization programs, and emergency preparedness that are dependent on the local tax revenue may be shortchanged to provide basic health needs to a community with many underprivileged residents. It is also important to consider the liability these communities face when service providers such as hospitals and clinics become financially insolvent as a result of providing uncompensated care. These service providers can no longer afford to offer services to anyone in the community (Institute of Medicine Committee on the Consequences of Uninsurance, 2003).

Current data strongly suggest that the nation's health care system does not function cost-efficiently (Hadley and Holahan, 2003). While spending more money than any other OECD country, more than 40 million residents in the United States have no dependable means to pay for their health care, and the nation's health system financing is deteriorating as a consequence. Does the nation have the resources to fix itself? And if so, how can the public and their policymakers be motivated to redistribute those resources?

In the conclusion of a lengthy analysis on the hidden costs of uninsurance in the United States, a 2003 Institute of Medicine report determined that the benefits of providing health insurance to residents currently uninsured would substantially outweigh the costs to be incurred. In fact, as Democratic Senator John Breaux from Louisiana has pointed out, the estimated cost of extending the safety net to all ($600 to $700 billion over ten years) is less than the expected average annual revenue loss from the federal tax cuts since 2001 ("Breaux Proposes Universal Care—American Style," 2003).

Step 4: Expand the Focus to Multiple Risk Factors

The United States needs to begin to develop a health policy agenda that reflects not just the impact of medical care services on health, but also, more important, the impact of social and environmental factors. An examination of current health policy debates reveals that most debates center primarily on the financing of health care rather than health outcomes or social determinants of health. The United States should expand this focus on financing and issues of cost containment to include **health impact assessment,** which would estimate the influence of social, economic, and health care policies on population health, not just cost savings.

Based on our solutions-focused framework (Figure 6.3), interventions may not have a significant and long-lasting impact if they focus on only immediate determinants of health (such as quality of care) while neglecting more fundamental determinants of health such as personal and community levels of SES. While it is much more difficult to change social and economic policies than pass new regulations to monitor health care quality, it is necessary to examine and intervene, when possible, much earlier in the process of poor health development. Since many of these social factors are the root causes of poor health tackling them will be paramount to resolving health disparities. As this book has repeated continually, most interventions used today are not comprehensive and focus on a single narrowly defined problem or population segment. For example, programs have been developed to serve specifically individuals with HIV, natives of Hawaii or the Pacific Islands, those who are disabled, and those who are homeless, among others. These programs no doubt have had an important role in improving health for these groups, but they have a very limited focus and often have to compete among each other (even within government health departments) for the funding to sustain their efforts.

These programs often address only one aspect of what makes a group vulnerable. For example, homeless individuals have many vulnerable risk factors, including being low income, not having a stable social support system, and lacking stable housing, and frequently they are unemployed and lack health insurance. They may be dealing with mental health and physical health issues that complicate and exacerbate these social problems. But programs serving homeless individuals are generally not sufficiently coordinated to affect substantial long-lasting and comprehensive changes.

Homeless shelters, for example, are generally funded through a network of local public and private partners and charities. The very best of these shelters offer referrals to health care and psychological counselors, and have support programs for educating, training, and case management for these individuals in finding stable sources of social assistance, employment, and housing. More commonly, these shelters simply provide a roof for the night and have little influence on any of these other risk factors. Even the federal Health Care for the Homeless Program, which provides exceptional physical and mental health services on-site to many homeless individuals, has limitations in its mandate and cannot address the full range of risk factors that are present for homeless individuals.

What has evolved is an elaborate patchwork of local, state, and national programs and policies that have varying comprehensiveness and sustainability in serving vulnerable populations. If these programs could be synthesized or national efforts could be developed to provide more overarching guidance and direction to address these multiple risks simultaneously, these programs would have better chances of success in intervening in the creation of vulnerability. For example, addressing mental health issues among the homeless would bolster the successes of other areas, such as helping individuals develop social support networks and make use of education, training, and employment assistance. Combining these efforts would allow these more effective and comprehensive services to be touted to funding agencies as packages and could help to reduce levels of competition among programs serving these vulnerable populations.

Step 5: Stress the Multilevel Integration of Interventions

Invariably, for some vulnerable groups there are gaps in service provision, and for others there are major duplications. Building on the focus on multiple risk factors, efforts could be made toward unifying services across agencies and organizations with common goals. Domestic and foreign public health initiatives have shown greater promise when using the collective resources of public and private advocates. Recognizing common goals encourages multisector alliances and minimizes partisan or other political barriers.

Participation and empowerment at many political and community levels is another critical component of acceptance, success, and continuation of any set of interventions. For example, the National Commission to Prevent Infant Mortality is a successful joint public, private, and congressional effort to combat infant mortality in the United States. It is not a coincidence that this consortium, based on collaboration among organizations at many levels, has made substantially greater progress in reducing infant mortality than the United States has made in other areas.

Improving the health of vulnerable populations will require the participation of traditional health agencies and involvement from education, housing, environmental, criminal justice, and economic agencies. To achieve cross-agency collaboration, these agencies should create standing mechanisms for policy development among sectors, promote interdepartmental collaboration, and create networks among public and private agencies and particularly with advocates to study, evaluate, and disseminate policy options. These efforts should also include greater community involvement and leadership in priority setting and policy development.

Perhaps one of the best ways to include communities in decision making is to focus on community strengths and resources rather than community deficits or problems. Communities should be seen as action centers for development, progress, and change. Community members and community leaders should have a central role in planning and managing initiatives. Through community mobilization, skill building, and resource sharing, communities can be empowered to identify and meet their own needs, making them stronger advocates in supporting the vulnerable populations within and across their community boundaries.

Step 6: Ensure Feasibility

Making sure intervention is feasible is also critical to its success. Areas of feasibility to be considered include **technical feasibility** (whether the intervention can plausibly solve or reduce the problem as defined), **economic feasibility** (the costs and benefits of a given intervention from an economic standpoint), political feasibility (a proposed intervention must survive the test of political acceptability, which depends on support from key officials, other stakeholders inside and outside of government, and ultimately voters.), and administrative feasibility (assessing how possible it would be to implement an intervention given a variety of social, political, and administrative constraints).

Step 7: Apply Effective Implementation Strategies

In the implementation stage, proper use of strategies is critical to success. An approach that has been successful in Europe, restating the public health issue using different language, may attract new attention to an issue not previously compelling to the public or policymakers. In the past, advocates have used the **social justice** argument to persuade the public that inequality in the United States needs to be eliminated. Politicians in the Netherlands were more impressed by a discussion centering on "lost human potential" than inequality, and perhaps the same effect would be seen among Americans if the national conversation focused less on social justice. Furthermore, Moss (2000) recommends that the discussion not target special populations but include the whole spectrum of socioeconomic status, broadening the appeal of the policy issue.

Another strategy is to work on realistic intervention. This strategy is a call to action for academics, advocates, and associated organizations to investigate and construct policy options. Presenting the public with choices they can mobilize around reduces the frustration and resulting resignation brought about by a system of limited alternatives. Quantitative targets, like the ones established by Healthy People 2010, also help the public focus their efforts toward specific goals.

To ensure that public health issues remain on the policy agenda, it is essential for the public to be able to gauge an initiative's progress, or lack thereof. Promoting action steps using media channels will help keep the public engaged.

Foundations may be mobilized in shaping public opinion. Foundations provide a unique avenue for promoting scientific and policy discussion of a public health issue. In addition to providing the necessary financial resources to explore issues such as disparity, foundations can influence public opinion through publications and media and the discourse it inspires.

Behavior and lifestyle have been shown to have great contributions to health. Studies estimate that roughly one-quarter of socioeconomic differences in mortality are attributable to variations in lifestyle (Syme, 1989). One important strategy is to target health promotion campaigns to vulnerable populations (Adler, Boyce, et al., 1993). In doing so, there are important caveats to consider. Oldenburg cautions that "traditional health promotion and disease prevention efforts are not as effective in people from lower SES groups" (Oldenburg, McGuffog, et al., 2000, p. 490). One way to address this is to have more community involvement in development of messages, more culturally appropriate materials, and media campaigns using local community groups and faith-based organizations.

However, there are other important factors to consider. "During the past 25 years, US government intervention to improve health has come almost entirely through initiatives aimed at changing individual behavior. . . . Individual behaviors are, to a large extent, shaped by social class position and the material environment" (Moss, 2000, p. 1631). In other words, it will take more than a focus on individual behavior modification campaigns in order to change individuals' behaviors. Interventions with a behavioral focus are more successful if the information and education are complemented by support and structural change (Oldenburg, McGuffog, et al., 2000). Through safe play and park areas, urban renewal projects to build safe and affordable housing, tax incentives to attract grocery stores to urban areas, and enforcement of existing legislation to promote cleaner air (to name just a few examples), urban planning, housing, and environmental policies can provide the structural support for healthy behaviors.

Step 8: Persevere

The vast disparities in health and health care that we experience today are the result of social, economic, and health policies, or the lack of, in the past several decades. It is naive to believe these disparities can be eliminated quickly, especially when some of our current policies and programs contribute toward widening the disparities. Although politicians like quick fixes and slogans (as stating eliminating disparities in Healthy People 2010), we have to be prepared for a long-term, sustained campaign.

Step 9: Use Guided Incrementalism

Given the nature of social and health policies in the United States, more success may be expected if we use guided **incrementalism** and build on initiatives that already have credibility. A new intervention is more likely to be taken seriously if its objective is integrated with an older initiative that has already achieved credibility. The Healthy Schools, Healthy Communities initiative provides an illustrative example. This national program funded by the Bureau of Primary Health Care began as a school-based initiative to provide primary care to vulnerable children. Over time, additional services have been integrated into the program to address other public health needs of this population. As a result, Healthy Schools, Healthy Communities has expanded beyond primary care to include violence prevention, fitness, parenting groups, and self-esteem enhancement programs. It is likely that the integrity established early on by the Healthy Schools program encouraged participants to take advantage of new services of the program.

Step 10: Evaluate and Refine Programs and Initiatives

In the postimplementation stage, programs and initiatives should be thoroughly evaluated, modified, and continually improved. Evaluation, feedback, and refinement processes should be built into the funding of every intervention or policy, and the results of these analyses should guide future program and policy development. While a culture of continual process improvement should be developed, it will be important to judge the progress made by these interventions in a realistic way. Programs that are comprehensive in scope (addressing multiple risks) should be evaluated along multiple dimensions, but should be appropriately evaluated against criteria that are feasible to obtain. In too many circumstances, health and social programs are judged on whether they have a direct impact on the health of their consumers, even though the program is funded for short-term cycles (just two or three years). If these results are possible over a longer period, programs must be held accountable to meeting their goals to improve health.

Conclusion

Our hope is that considering these ten steps in any course of action will help to promote health disparities to a more prominent position on the public agenda. It is essential to keep the public engaged and educated. Health disparities among vulnerable populations are not unavoidable. Interventions to eliminate socioeconomic and racial and ethnic disparities have been successful in the United States through health care delivery interventions (Fiscella, Franks, et al., 2000). Integrated efforts in Canada and Australia have made progress outside the medical realm toward reducing health inequalities associated with the more socially based determinants of health (Dixon, Douglas, et al., 2000). Using these action steps and adapting them to the needs of the U.S. population are the requisite next steps to prevent the occurrence of and reduce the consequences of health vulnerability.

Review Questions

1. Healthy People 2010 calls for the elimination of disparities. What are the strategies to achieve this goal?
2. Describe how one might resolve the nation's disparities using the framework presented in Figure 6.3.
3. What are the challenges and barriers in implementing strategies to resolve disparities?

Essay Questions

1. Healthy People 2010 calls for the elimination of health and health care disparities. What progress, if any, has been made toward reducing disparities in one of the following: infant mortality, cardiovascular disease, or adult mortality? To what can this progress, if any, be attributed, and what strategies could be implemented to improve on the successes achieved so far?
2. Based on the book and your own research, what do you think are critical next steps to take to resolve health disparities in this country? Be specific, and provide the steps or strategies that should be taken for one well-known health disparity (for example, HIV infection rates across racial or ethnic groups). Consider preparation, design, implementation, and postimplementation steps.

GLOSSARY

Affirmative action: A ruling by the Supreme Court in 1978 supported this effort by permitting race to be used as admission criteria under certain circumstances. The intended result was to counter the earlier effects of discrimination in excluding minorities from higher education.

Ambulatory care sensitive conditions: Health conditions such as asthma, diabetes, or high blood pressure that can be relatively easily managed in a primary care (or ambulatory care) setting. These conditions are often used to study inadequate access to primary health care, which would be evidenced by an emergency department visit or hospitalization for these conditions.

Ambulatory visits: Use of same-day (that is, without institutionalization) health care services, typically in a noninstitutional setting, such as a doctor's office or community health center. Patients also use health care services at hospital-based clinics or outpatient departments that provide same-day services.

Ancillary services: Nonessential but supportive services that complement medical care services. Examples are dietetic services, laboratory services, pharmacy services, cardiorespiratory care, and speech therapy.

Anticipatory guidance: The counseling of parents by health providers about developmental changes that will occur in their children. Both the American Academy of Pediatrics and Bright Futures initiative have recommended a range of anticipatory guidance topics that providers should discuss with parents, including child safety and injury prevention, feeding and sleeping routines, reading to children, guidance and discipline, and obtaining high-quality child care.

Capitation: A reimbursement mechanism that health plans (typically managed care organizations) use whereby physicians received a specified monthly payment to provide all the necessary care for a particular patient.

Communicable disease: A disease passed from one human to another, such as a sexually transmitted disease or the flu.

Community building: Enhancing relationships with other community organizations and customers—for example, an alliance of locally driven urban initiatives working to reduce poverty and create social and economic opportunity.

Community coalitions: Partnership among community organizations to promote shared missions, such as serving vulnerable populations.

Community health centers (CHCs): A program established by the federal government in 1969 to improve access to health care services to low-income families. CHCs were created under the Economic Opportunity Act and are currently operated by the Bureau of Primary Health Care. The CHC program provides family-oriented primary and preventive health services for people living in rural and urban underserved communities.

Community linkages: Working together with related organizations in the community to coordinate and integrate services so as to better fulfill organizational mission.

Community participatory decision making: Involving consumers and non–health sector organizations to participate in decisions and policies that affect health care delivery. Community participation is critical for acceptance and adoption.

Complementary or alternative medicine: A group of diverse medical and health care systems, practices, and products that are not considered to be part of conventional or Western medicine.

Continuity of care: A principal attribute of primary care, it refers to longitudinality of care and presupposes the existence of a regular source of care and its use over time. Continuity of care is beneficial to both patients and providers.

Cost containment: Measures that curtail escalating health care cost. Both supply-side (aimed at providers) and demand-side (aimed at patients) cost-containment measures are necessary to sustain health care cost.

Cost sharing: Individual payments for health services that are required by health insurance plans to dissuade the use of unnecessary health services. These payments include insurance premiums, deductibles, and copayments for visits or prescriptions.

Covariates: Related measures or variables based on a conceptual understanding of the concept. To fully understand the concept, known covariates need to be included in the analysis.

Cultural competence: A set of congruent behaviors, attitudes, and policies that come together in a system, agency, or among professionals and enables that system, agency, or those professionals to work effectively in cross-cultural situations. Operationally defined, cultural competence is the integration and transformation of knowledge about individuals and groups of people into specific standards, policies, practices, and attitudes used in appropriate cultural settings to increase the quality of services, thereby producing better outcomes.

Culturally appropriate: Suitable to a particular culture. For example, culturally appropriate care will enable people with different cultural backgrounds to feel comfortable and familiar in the receipt of care. Receiving culturally appropriate care can improve patient-provider relationship and enhance satisfaction with the experience.

Developmental disabilities: Severe disabilities that typically begin in childhood and are lifelong in duration. The federal Developmental Disabilities Act defines a developmental disability as a severe, chronic disability that (1) is attributable to a mental or physical impairment or a combination of mental or physical impairments, (2) is manifested before the individual attains age twenty-two, (3) is likely to continue indefinitely, and (3) results in substantial functional limitations in major life activities. Examples are cerebral palsy, autism, epilepsy, and hearing impairment.

Developmental risk: The rapid and cumulative physical and emotional changes that characterize childhood and the potential impact that illness, injury, or untoward family and social circumstances can have on a child's life course trajectory.

Developmental screening: Preventive health care services typically for children from birth to five years. The health checkup is intended to make sure that children are achieving appropriate developmental milestones on critical indicators such as hearing, cognitive development, and motor skills.

Discrimination: Unfavorable or unfair treatment of a person or class of persons—in comparison to others—based on race, gender, color, religion, national origin, age, physical or mental disability, or sexual orientation.

Diversity: The degree to which environments (such as communities, schools, and workplaces) have heterogeneity (as opposed to homogeneity) in their population, usually in terms of race/ethnicity, gender, religion, or sexual preference. The U.S. census measures racial/ethnic diversity as the percentage of times that two randomly selected people in a given area would be of different racial/ethnic backgrounds.

Economic feasibility: Refers to consideration of a given program or policy from an economic standpoint.

Effectiveness: Whether programs are able to accomplish their objectives.

1115 waiver: A reference to section 1115 of the federal Social Security Act, which allows the secretary of Health and Human Services to waive any provision of Medicaid law for demonstration projects that test a program improvement or develop a new idea of interest to the Health Care Financing Administration (currently centers for Medicare and Medicaid Services or CMS). For example, under a section 1115 waiver, a state may be exempt from compliance with usual requirements or may receive federal matching funds for expenditures not ordinarily eligible under Medicaid. All 1115 waiver demonstration projects must be budget neutral, that is, they cannot result in greater federal expenditures than would have otherwise been spent in the absence of the waiver.

Entitlement program: A federal program that guarantees a certain level of benefits to persons or other entities who meet requirements set by law, such as Social Security or unemployment benefits. It thus leaves no discretion with Congress on how much money to appropriate, and some entitlements carry permanent appropriations.

Equity: The absence of potentially remediable, systematic differences in one or more aspects of health or health care across socially, economically, demographically, or geographically defined population groups or subgroups.

Evaluation: Evaluation is the systematic application of scientific research methods for assessing the conceptualization, design, implementation, impact, and/or generalizability of organizational or social (including health services) programs.

Family-centered care: The way that health care practitioners relate to the families and patients that they serve. Patients receive care (that is, diagnosis and treatment) that incorporates gathering knowledge about the context of the family. For example, in caring for children with asthma, it is important that the health care provider ask about the home situation, whether other members of the family have asthma, and what barriers may exist at home to preventing asthma-attacks (for example, lack of finances to procure appropriate allergen-free bedding or a poor housing situation and how this can be rectified). Asking about family history with regard to a particular disease is perhaps the most common and obvious form of family-centered care.

Fee for service: A mechanism by which insurance companies reimburse health care providers for each particular service that is delivered to a patient. This was the traditional reimbursement mechanism until the emergence of managed care organizations, which reimburse providers using capitation.

Foundations: Nonprofit organizations that provide support and funds to a particular stated cause. In the United States, private support through foundations is a major approach to expanding care to the uninsured and vulnerable.

Framework: A simplified, often graphical, description of a complex process or theory.

Gatekeeping: An organizational arrangement in some health insurance plans whereby a patient must see a primary care provider before additional specialty care services can be obtained. In these arrangements, the primary care provider is informally and critically referred to as a gatekeeper of access to these services.

Gini index: A measure that is frequently used to describe the degree to which income is distributed unequally in a population. This measure has consistently been found to be strongly related to the level of health in a population. The measure is a single statistic (ranging from 0 to 1) to summarize the degree of income dispersion across a population. A score of 0 indicates perfect equality, where everyone receives an equal share of income; and a score of 1 indicates complete inequality, where all of the income is received by a single person.

Gradients: Different levels of a particular measure. For example, gradients of income status refers to individuals with low, medium, and high income status.

Head Start: Head Start and Early Head Start are comprehensive child development programs that serve children from birth to age five, pregnant women, and their families. They are child-focused programs and have the overall goal of increasing the school readiness of young children in low-income families.

Health: Defined by the World Health Organization as a "state of complete physical, mental, and social well-being and not merely the absence of disease or infirmity." This definition recognizes that health is influenced by a combination of biological, social, individual, community, and economic factors. In addition to its intrinsic value, health is a means for personal and collective advancement. It is not only an indicator of an individual's well-being, but a sign of success achieved by a society and its institutions of government in promoting well-being and human development.

Health disparities: Differences in the incidence, prevalence, mortality, burden of disease, or other adverse health conditions that exist among specific population groups.

Health impact assessment: A data-driven decision-making tool that is designed to take account of the wide range of potential effects that a given proposal may have on the health of its target population. Such analyses help to make informed decisions about health programs or policies to maximize positive and minimize negative health impacts.

Health maintenance organization (HMO): A health care system that assumes or shares the financial risks associated with providing comprehensive medical services to a voluntarily enrolled population in a particular geographical area, usually in return for a fixed, prepaid fee. There are many variations in types of HMOs, but they are nearly all characterized by at least some use of capitation and restrictions on care seeking, such as seeking care only from providers who work for the HMO or are in the HMO's provider network.

Health outcomes: The effects of health care services. Mostly these are effects on health, but they also often include experiences in care or patient satisfaction.

They may refer to the outcome for an individual such as the relief of pain after treatment for an injury. Or they may refer to outcomes for the local community (for example, the prevention of measles in children by introducing an immunization program) or the wider population (for example, reduction of deaths from breast cancer after the introduction of a national screening program).

Health-risk behaviors: Personal behaviors such as smoking or driving without wearing a seat belt that put an individual at risk for poor health.

Health trajectories: How health evolves over one's lifetime. People with different socioeconomic status have different health trajectories.

Healthy People Initiative: A set of health objectives for the nation to achieve over a ten-year period. It can be used by many different people, states, communities, professional organizations, and others to help them develop programs to improve health. Healthy People 2010 builds on initiatives pursued over the past two decades. The 1979 Surgeon General's Report, *Healthy People,* and *Healthy People 2000: National Health Promotion and Disease Prevention Objectives,* established national health objectives and served as the basis for the development of state and community plans.

incidence: The number of new cases of a health problem or disease that occur during a specified period of time in a population at risk for developing the disease. An example would be the number of new breast cancer cases during the year 2005 among all women. This would be referred to as the incidence of breast cancer among women in 2005.

Income redistribution: The presence of a wide disparity in income that can be observed in the personal income distribution. The wealthiest 20 percent of the families in the United States receive 41 percent of the total income. Income redistribution or income maintenance programs such as Social Security, welfare, and unemployment benefits aim at remedying hardship of the destitute while still preserving the incentive to work hard for higher income.

Incrementalism: Gradual movement toward a final goal while taking into account social and contextual limitations.

Inequalities: Unacceptable difference in health care access, quality of care, and health outcomes among population segments (for example, those with difference socioeconomic status and racial/ethnic background).

Infant mortality rate: Death rates of children under age one, often measured per 1,000 live births. High infant mortality rates may indicate poor maternal health, inadequate prenatal care, infant malnutrition, or limited access to adequate health care.

Integration of care: The provision of comprehensive health care services and their coordination. Particularly important where there are multiple funding sources and services.

Leading health indicators: Indicators that reflect the major public health concerns in the United States. They were chosen based on their ability to motivate action, the availability of data to measure their progress, and their relevance as broad public health issues.

Linguistically appropriate: A term applied to medical literature and information when the material is produced in the language and format that is most appropriate to the racial/ethnic or cultural group to which it is targeted. To make sure that health-related materials and information are linguistically appropriate, materials must be carefully reviewed for relevance, tone, and dialect and should not simply rely upon literal translation. Service providers may also aim to be linguistically appropriate by becoming familiar with the language and dialect in use within any given community to avoid miscommunication and misunderstanding.

Logistic regression: A statistical analysis where the dependent variable is binary and independent variables are continuous or dichotomous.

Managed care organization: A general term that refers to a broad range of health plans that use managed care arrangements and have a defined system of selected providers that contract with the plan. A health maintenance organization is generally considered the purest form of a managed care organization because it employs managed methods for managing the services and costs of care.

Material deprivation: The lack of material resources that enable the protection or promotion of health. These resources also enable a person to obtain adequate health care when faced with ill health. For example, a steady income is fundamental to obtaining clean water and adequate housing, proper nutrition, electricity for warmth, and a safe environment.

Means tested: Programs that restrict eligibility for benefits to persons with nonwelfare income below a certain level. Individuals with nonwelfare income above a specified cutoff level may not receive aid. Temporary Assistance to Needy Families benefits are means-tested and constitute welfare, but Social Security benefits are not.

Medicaid: A combined federal and state initiative to provide health insurance for the poor. It was initially tied to state welfare programs (to simplify administration of the program), but this was undone recently, so that being poor no longer automatically makes a person eligible for Medicaid. In fact, most people become eligible for the program by meeting a specific criterion: advanced age, blindness, disability, or membership in a single-parent family with dependent children. Within this rubric, states may set very different eligibility criteria.

Medically underserved areas (MUAs): Established under the U.S. Public Health Service Act, MUAs are federal designations of a geographical area (usually a county or a collection of townships or census tracts) that meet the criteria as needing additional primary health care services. Designation as an MUA is based on the availability of health professional resources within a rational service area. The definition of a rational service area is usually based on a thirty-minute travel time. Other factors considered in the designation process are the availability of primary care resources in contiguous areas and the presence of unusually high need, such as a high infant mortality rate or a high poverty rate.

Medicare: The nation's single largest payer for medical care services, covering about 40 million beneficiaries. Most of the recipients of these government-sponsored health insurance benefits are over sixty-five years of age, but the architects of the program included eligibility for two smaller categorical groups: those who are permanently disabled and those with end-stage renal disease. Medicare is financed through a form of social insurance that requires employers and employees to contribute to a fund that finances the coverage for those who are currently enrolled in the program. Medicare offers two major benefit categories: Part A, which covers hospital and limited long-term care costs, and Part B, which covers physician services and most other ambulatory care services. Those who are eligible for Medicare are automatically enrolled in Part A and are offered the opportunity to purchase Part B through monthly premiums.

Mental distress: Acute mental health problems such as depression or the expression of symptoms of these problems.

Migrant and seasonal farm workers: Farm workers who typically work from place to place and during the farm season. They have a history of many problems: uncertain jobs and problematic transportation, mistreatment on farms and in communities, too little money to support them between jobs, inadequate housing, poor health, and too little schooling. These problems are especially acute for migrants who rely on farm work as their principal employment, not the part-timers who work on farms during vacation from school.

Minority: Generally, the smaller of two population groups defined along a particular characteristic, such as race/ethnicity, gender, or religion. More commonly used synonymously with any racial/ethnic group that is not white. This term may not be technically accurate in some geographical areas where certain nonwhite racial/ethnic groups, such as Latinos, are more populous than whites.

Missed opportunities: An event where a health care provider misses the chance to deliver an important health service to a person or family. The most common example is when a provider sees a child who is not fully immunized and does not provide immunizations to this child. This term has been generalized to other health services, such as counseling to encourage physical activity when a patient is overweight or at risk of being overweight.

Modifiable risk: A risk factor for poor health or health care access that can be changed (for example, by expanding public health insurance coverage), as opposed to a risk factor that cannot be changed, such as age.

Multivariate analysis: Complex statistical analysis that has more than two variables a time in the model. Multivariate analysis is performed to examine the influence of hypothesized factors on the dependent variable while controlling for known covariates.

Patient autonomy: The degree to which patients have freedom to choose the health care services they receive, when they are received, and from whom they are received.

Patient-provider relationship: Interaction between patients and their health care providers, which is critical to the quality of care received and rendered in the health care setting.

Political feasibility: A proposed policy must survive the test of political acceptability which depends on support from key officials, other stakeholders inside and outside of government, and ultimately voters. Analysis of political feasibility can be used to determine which alternative can be implemented with the least political opposition. Or it can be used to determine, for any given alternative, the likely sources of support and opposition, as well as the intensity of that support and opposition.

Potential access: The features of the health care system that enable the use of services, such as the number of providers in the community, the number of hospital beds available, and personal factors, such as having health insurance coverage and adequate income to purchase health services.

Predictor: In research, an independent variable (a cause) that is used to predict another variable (the effect) such as lack of health insurance predicting a person's ability to get needed health care. Health insurance would be the predictor in this example.

Preventive care: Health care services designed to promote health and well-being or reduce risks of poor health. Preventive care may include tangible services such as providing immunizations, screening for high blood pressure, or prescribing medication to prevent contracting malaria or some other disease. Other preventive care includes counseling or anticipatory guidance about health promoting or risk-reducing behaviors (such as counseling to quit smoking or encouraging physical activity).

Preventive counseling: Discussions that health care providers have with patients about promoting health and reducing risks of health problems. Examples include discussing quitting smoking, engaging in physical activity more often, and perhaps taking aspirin for adults who are at risk for heart disease.

Primary care: That level of a health service system that provides entry into the system, provides person-focused care over time, provides care for all but very uncommon or unusual conditions, and coordinates or integrates care provided elsewhere or by others.

Primary care experiences: Ratings or reporting of specific experiences, health provider behaviors, and services that are available or received in primary health care. Measures of primary care experiences reflect the key domains of primary health care: accessibility, longitudinality (continuity), comprehensiveness, and coordination. *See* primary care.

Proxy measure: A measure used to represent something else that was not measured. For example, education may sometimes be used as a proxy measure for occupation, since the two measures are so closely related.

Qualitative experiences: In research, the subjective feelings, beliefs, perceptions, and sense of satisfaction of individuals that are assessed through interviews with individuals or focus groups. These data are generally intended to elicit more complex and detailed information about a particular subject, and are distinct from quantitative experiences, such as counts of the number of medical visits, the length of the visit measured in minutes, and costs of that care. Both qualitative and quantitative experiences are integral to informing research studies, though most studies are either primarily qualitative or quantitative.

Quality of care: According to the Institute of Medicine, the degree to which health services for individuals and populations increase the likelihood of desired health outcomes and are consistent with current professional knowledge.

Realized access: The actual use of health care services (for example, visits to a physician or hospitalization).

Regular source of care: Often defined as a health care provider whom a person reports seeing for obtaining health care for a new health care problem. Optimally, this provider would be a source of both preventive and illness care. Having a regular source of care is considered evidence of either good access to care or continuity of care, and is promoted by many health care and physician organizations.

Reinsurance: The transfer of some or all of an insurance risk to another insurer. For example, managed care companies (referred to as *ceding companies*) may purchase insurance to share risks with another company (referred to as the *assuming company* or *reinsurer*).

Relative risk: The measure of association most often used by epidemiologists. It refers to the probability of an event in the active group divided by the probability of the event in the control group. High relative risk indicates that compared with the control group, the active group has a higher risk of developing an outcome (for example, a disease).

Risk profiles: Attributes that predict the likelihood of being in poor health. A risk profile can be developed for each person to describe the number and type of risk factors that person has. The three main risk factors described in this book are minority race/ethnicity, low socioeconomic status, and lack of health insurance coverage.

Safety net insurance: Insurance programs such as Medicaid and State Children's Health Insurance Program that are intended to provide coverage to vulnerable populations (such as lower-income families) that are less likely to be able to obtain private insurance.

School-based clinics: Clinics situated in schools that provide primary care, health education, and mental health care for students. These clinics expand access, provide preventive medicine, and help children stay in school while offering a convenient way for parents to ensure their children get quality physical and mental health attention. School-based clinics could encompass physicians, physician assistants, nurses, nurse practitioners, social workers, mental health therapists, and substance prevention counselors.

Self-efficacy: Belief in one's ability to perform and succeed at a given task or behavior. In health and social research, self-efficacy is often used to describe the belief in one's ability to achieve in life (for example, acquiring resources), change or adopt a particular health-related behavior (for example, quitting smoking), or obtain health care services when needed.

Single payer: A national health care system where there is generally one primary payer, the government. When services are delivered, providers send the bill to an agency of the government that subsequently sends payment to each provider.

Sliding-fee scale: A discount or reduction in cost of services provided to the patient based upon reported or documented income level of the patient.

Social capital: The pattern and intensity of networks among people and the shared values that arise from those networks. The main aspects are citizenship, neighborliness, trust and shared values, community involvement, volunteering, social networks, and civic participation.

Social class: Used interchangeably with *socioeconomic status. Social class* is more commonly used in Europe, where explicit definitions (generally based on occupation) have been written into national census initiatives.

Social cohesion: The degree to which a community shares values, deals with challenges, and provides equal opportunities to its members. This can be evident in a sense of trust, hope, and reciprocity among community members.

Social justice: Social justice emphasizes the well-being of the community over that of the individual; thus, the inability to obtain medical services because of a lack of financial resources would be considered unjust. A just distribution of benefits must be based on need, not simply one's ability to purchase it in the marketplace.

Social participation: Reflects one of the nonmaterial pathways by which socioeconomic status may be related to health. Participation includes having time for leisure activity and group participation, having friends or family around for entertainment and support, receiving chances for professional achievement, and ultimately having sufficient opportunities and life control to lead a fulfilling and satisfying life.

Social Security: A social insurance program started by the U.S. government in 1935 that covers most of the nation's workforce. It is often the basic retirement plan to which other benefits are added. It provides retirement, disability, survivor, and Medicare benefits.

Social support: The various types of support, assistance, or help that people receive from others and generally classified into two major categories: emotional and instrumental (and sometimes informational) support. Emotional support refers to the things that people do that make them feel loved and cared for and that bolster their sense of self-worth. Instrumental support refers to the various types of more tangible help that others may provide, such as help with child care or housekeeping and the provision of transportation or money. Informational support refers to the help that others may offer through the provision of information.

Socioeconomic status: A measure of a person's social or economic position that is often assessed and delineated using income, education, and occupation.

Standardized mortality rates: Death rates adjusted for certain population characteristics. For example, age-standardized mortality rates have taken into account variations in age structure. Standardized rates are needed to compare across different geographical areas with different population structures.

State Children's Health Insurance Program (SCHIP): A program that provides about $40 billion for states to expand coverage to children in low-income families. Within broad federal guidelines, SCHIP, part of the Balanced Budget Act of 1997, allows states the choice of expanding coverage through the Medicaid program, through a new child health insurance program developed by the state, or a combination of both. As of 2001, seventeen states had chosen to expand Medicaid coverage, sixteen created a new child health program, and eighteen chose to implement a combination. By 2002, coverage was available for children in families whose income was 200 percent of the federal poverty level or higher in thirty-nine states.

Technical feasibility: A measure of whether the design of a policy or program will achieve its intention. Technical feasibility refers to the study of the existence of any alternatives that could plausibly solve or reduce the problem as defined.

Telemedicine: The use of telecommunications (such as telephone, television, and satellite technology) to provide medical information and services.

Underprivileged: Typically refers to those with fewer financial resources than the average population. Target of public assistance programs.

Universal health coverage: Ensuring that all individuals living within a country are guaranteed access to health care services. Some developed countries provide these services directly through a national health service, and others provide health insurance coverage to all. Using either mechanism, no individual will go without basic access to health care services. The United States is the only developed country, perhaps besides the Republic of South Africa, without universal health coverage.

Unmet health care needs: A health problem or health need that did not receive adequate or any medical attention. A common measure of unmet health needs is asking individuals whether they ever did not receive health care for a health problem that they believed required medical care. Less subjective measures include assessing the nonuse of physician services for individuals with conditions such as high blood pressure or asthma that require regular physician monitoring.

Utilization rates: Reported or measured rates of the use of health care services. Examples include physician visit utilization rates that are often reported as the annual number of visits per person and emergency department utilization rates that are often reported as annual emergency department visits per 1,000 individuals.

Vulnerability: In this book, vulnerability refers to susceptibility to poor health or poor health care access.

Well-child care: Regularly scheduled (though not necessarily regularly attended) medical checkups for young children. These visits are intended to monitor child development, provide preventive counseling and guidance to parents on child rearing and optimizing child health, and provide immunizations.

REFERENCES

Academy for Health Services Research and Health Policy Annual Conference. 2001. *Building on employer-based coverage*. State Coverage Initiatives Workshop for State Officials. Denver, CO.

Acevedo-Garcia, D., K. A. Lochner, et al. 2003. "Future directions in residential segregation and health research: A multilevel approach." *Am J Public Health* 93(2):215–221.

Adams, E. K., and V. Johnson. 2000. "An elementary school-based health clinic: Can it reduce Medicaid costs?" *Pediatrics* 105:780–788.

Aday, L. A. 1993. "Indicators and predictors of health services utilization." In S. J. Williams and P. R. Torrens (Eds.), *Introduction to health services* (4th ed., pp. 46–70). Albany, NY: Delmar.

Aday, L. A. 1994. "Health status of vulnerable populations." *Annu Rev Public Health* 15:487–509.

Aday, L. A. 1999. "Vulnerable populations: A community-oriented perspective." In J. G. Sebastian and A. Bushy (Eds.), *Special populations in the community* (pp. 313–330). Gaithersburg, MD: Aspen.

Aday, L. A. 2001. *At risk in America: The health and health care needs of vulnerable populations in the United States* (2nd ed.). San Francisco: Jossey-Bass.

Aday, L. A., and R. M. Andersen. 1981. "Equity of access to medical care: A conceptual and empirical overview." *Medical Care* 19(12 Suppl):4–27.

Aday, L., G. Fleming, et al. 1984. *Access to medical care in the US: Who has it, who doesn't?* Chicago: Pluribus Press.

Adler, N. E., W. T. Boyce, et al. 1993. "Socioeconomic inequalities in health: No easy solution." *JAMA* 269(24):3140–3145.

Adler, N. E., and J. M. Ostrove. 1999. "Socioeconomic status and health: What we know and what we don't." *Ann NY Acad Sci* 896:3–15.

Alegria, M., D. J. Perez, et al. 2003. "The role of public policies in reducing mental health status disparities for people of color." *Health Aff (Millwood)* 22(5):51–64.

Almeida, C., P. Braveman, et al. 2001. "Methodological concerns and recommendations on policy consequences of the World Health Report 2000." *Lancet* 357(9269):1692–1697.

AMA Council on Ethical and Judicial Affairs. 1990. "Black-white disparities in health care." *Conn Med* 54(11):625–628.

American Medical Association. 1994. "Portraits of major US racial/ethnic groups." In *Culturally competent health care for adolescents* (pp. 39–68). Chicago: American Medical Association.

AMA Council on Ethical and Judicial Affairs. 1990. "Black-white disparities in health care." *JAMA* 263:2344–2346.

AMA Council on Scientific Affairs. 1991. "Hispanic health in the United States." *JAMA* 265:248–252.

Amick III, B. C., S. Levine, et al. 1995. *Society and health.* New York: Oxford University Press.

Anda, R. F., J. B. Croft, et al. 1999. "Adverse childhood experiences and smoking during adolescence and adulthood." *JAMA* 282(17):1652–1658.

Andersen, R. 1995. "Revisiting the behavioral model and access to medical care: Does it matter?" *J Health Social Behavior* 36:1–10.

Anderson, G., R. Brook, et al. 1991. "A comparison of cost-sharing versus free care in children: Effects on the demand for office-based medical care." *Med Care* 29(9):890–898.

Anderson, G. F., U. E. Reinhardt, et al. 2003. "It's the prices, stupid: Why the United States is so different from other countries." *Health Aff (Millwood)* 22(3):89–105.

Anglin, T. M., K. E. Naylor, et al. 1996. "Comprehensive school-based health care: High school students' use of medical, mental health, and substance abuse services." *Pediatrics* 97:318–330.

Antonovsky, A. 1967. "Social class, life expectancy and overall mortality." *Milbank Mem Fund Q* 45(2):31–73.

Ashman, S. B., G. Dawson, et al. 2002. "Stress hormone levels of children of depressed mothers." *Dev Psychopathol* 14(2):333–349.

Assets for health: Findings from the 2001 survey of new health foundations. 2002. Washington, DC: Grantmakers in Health.

Astin, J. 1998. "Why patients use alternative medicine." *JAMA* 279:1548–1553.

Avchen, R. N., K. G. Scott, et al. 2001. "Birth weight and school-age disabilities: A population-based study." *Am J Epidemiol* 154(10):895–901.

Ayanian, J. Z., B. A. Kohler, et al. 1993. "The relation between health insurance coverage and clinical outcomes among women with breast cancer." *N Engl J Med* 329(5):326–331.

Ayanian, J. Z., J. S. Weissman, et al. 2000. "Unmet health needs of uninsured adults in the United States." *JAMA* 284(16):2061–2069.

Backlund, E., P. D. Sorlie, et al. 1999. "A comparison of the relationships of education and income with mortality: The National Longitudinal Mortality Study." *Soc Sci Med* 49(10):1373–1384.

Barnett, E., D. L. Armstrong, et al. 1999. "Evidence of increasing coronary heart disease mortality among black men of lower social class." *Ann Epidemiol* 9(8):464–471.

Barr, D. A. 1995. "The effects of organizational structure on primary care outcomes under managed care." *Ann Intern Med* 122(5):353–359.

Baugh, R. F. 2003. "Defined contribution: A part of our future." *J Natl Med Assoc* 95(8):718–721.

Baum, A., J. P. Garofalo, et al. 1999. "Socioeconomic status and chronic stress: Does stress account for SES effects on health?" *Ann NY Acad Sci* 896:131–144.

Bell, J., J. Bell, et al. 2002. *Reducing health disparities through a focus on communities.* Oakland, CA: PolicyLink.

Ben-Shlomo, Y., and D. Kuh. 2002. "A life course approach to chronic disease epidemiology: Conceptual models, empirical challenges and interdisciplinary perspectives." *Int J Epidemiol* 31(2):285–293.

Ben-Shlomo, Y., I. R. White, et al. 1996. "Does the variation in the socioeconomic characteristics of an area affect mortality?" *BMJ* 312(7037):1013–1014.

Benzeval, M., K. Judge, et al. (Eds.). 1995. *Tackling inequalities in health: An agenda for action.* London: King's Fund.

Bergner, M. 1985. "Measurement of health status." *Med Care* 23:696–704.

Berkman, L. 1995. "The role of social relations in health promotion." *Psychosom Med* 57:245–254.

Betancourt, J. R., A. R. Green, et al. 2003. "Defining cultural competence: A practical framework for addressing racial/ethnic disparities in health and health care." *Public Health Rep* 118(4):293–302.

Billings, J. 1999. "Access to health care services." In A. Kovner and S. Jonas (Eds.), *Health care delivery in the United States.* New York: Springer.

Billings, J., G. M. Anderson, et al. 1996. "Recent findings on preventable hospitalizations." *Health Aff (Millwood)* 15(3):239–249.

"Blue Shield of California CEO proposes universal care plan to cover all Californians." 2002. *California HealthLine.* Oakland, CA.

Boccuti, C., and M. Moon. 2003. "Comparing Medicare and private insurers: Growth rates in spending over three decades." *Health Aff (Millwood)* 22(2):230–237.

Bodenheimer, T. 2003. "The movement for universal health insurance: Finding common ground." *Am J Public Health* 93(1):112–115.

Brach, C., and I. Fraser. 2000. "Can cultural competency reduce racial and ethnic health disparities? A review and conceptual model." *Med Care Res Rev* 57(Suppl 1):181–217.

Braveman, P., B. Starfield, et al. 2001. "World Health Report 2000: How it removes equity from the agenda for public health monitoring and policy." *BMJ* 323(7314):678–681.

"Breaux proposes universal care—American style." 2003. *Med Health* 57(4):4.

Brown, L. D., and M. S. Sparer. 2003. "Poor program's progress: The unanticipated politics of Medicaid policy." *Health Aff (Millwood)* 22(1):31–44.

Brown, T. N., D. R. Williams, et al. 2000. "Being black and feeling blue: The mental health consequences of racial discrimination." *Race Soc* 2:117–131.

Bullard, R. 1994. "Urban infrastructure: Social, environmental and health risks to African-Americans." In I. Livingston (Ed.), *Handbook of black American health: The mosaic of conditions, issues, policies, and prospects.* Westport, CT: Greenwood Press.

Cable, G. 2002. "Income, race, and preventable hospitalizations: A small area analysis in New Jersey." *J Health Care Poor Underserved* 13(1):66–80.

Calle, E. E., W. D. Flanders, et al. 1993. "Demographic predictors of mammography and Pap smear screening in US women." *Am J Public Health* 83(1):53–60.

Caplan, L. S., and S. G. Haynes. 1996. "Breast cancer screening in older women." *Public Health Rev* 24(2):193–204.

Caplan, R. L., D. W. Light, et al. 1999. "Benchmarks of fairness: A moral framework for assessing equity." *Int J Health Serv* 29(4):853–869.

Carrillo, J. E., A. R. Green, et al. 1999. "Cross-cultural primary care: A patient-based approach." *Ann Intern Med* 130(10):829–834.

Casper, M. L., E. B. Barnett, et al. 1997. "Social class and race disparities in premature stroke mortality among men in North Carolina." *Ann Epidemiol* 7(2):146–153.

Center for Studying Health System Change. 2001. *Community tracking study physician survey, 1998-1999* [United States] [Computer file]. ICPSR version. Washington, DC: Center for Studying Health System Change [producer], 2001.

Centers for Disease Control. 2003. *At a glance: Racial and ethnic approaches to community health (REACH 2010): Addressing disparities in health.* Atlanta, GA: Centers for Disease Control.

Cohen, S., R. C. Kessler, et al. 1995. "Strategies for measuring stress in studies of psychiatric and physical disorders." In S. Cohen, R. C. Kessler, et al. (Eds.), *Measuring stress: A guide for health and social scientists* (pp. 3–26). New York: Oxford University Press.

Cole, R., and D. Deskins Jr. 1988. "Racial factors in site location and employment patterns of Japanese auto firms in America." *Calid Manage Rev* 31:9–22.

Coleman, J. 1990. *Foundations of social theory.* Cambridge, MA: Harvard University Press.

Colhoun, H., Y. Ben-Shlomo, et al. 1997. "Ecological analysis of collectivity of alcohol consumption in England: Importance of average drinker." *BMJ* 314(7088):1164–1168.

Collins, K., D. Hughes, et al. 2002. *Diverse communities, common concerns: Assessing health care quality for minority Americans.* New York: Commonwealth Fund.

Collins, R. 1994. *Four sociological traditions.* New York: Oxford University Press.

Conry, C. M., D. S. Main, et al. 1993. "Factors influencing mammogram ordering at the time of the office visit." *J Fam Pract* 37(4):356–360.

Cooney, E. 2003. "Health care cuts bemoaned." *Telegram and Gazette,* March 15, A3.

Cooper, L., and D. Roter. 2002. "Patient-provider communication: The effect of race and ethnicity on process and outcomes of healthcare." In B. Smedley, A. Stith, et al. (Eds.), *Unequal treatment: Confronting racial and ethnic disparities in health care.* Washington, DC: National Academies Press.

Copper, R. L., R. L. Goldenberg, et al. 1993. "A multicenter study of preterm birth weight and gestational age-specific neonatal mortality." *Am J Obstet Gynecol* 168(1 Pt. 1):78–84.

Council on Graduate Medical Education. 1998. *Twelfth report: Minorities in medicine.* May.

Cooper-Patrick, L., J. Gallo, et al. 1999. "Race, gender, and partnership in the patient-physician relationship." *JAMA* 282(6):583–589.

Cunningham, P. J. 2002. "Mounting pressures: Physicians serving Medicaid patients and the uninsured, 1997–2001." *Track Rep* (6):1–4.

Cunningham, P. J. 2003. "SCHIP making progress: Increased take-up contributes to coverage gains." *Health Aff (Millwood)* 22(4):163–172.

Cunningham, P. J., C. M. Clancy, et al. 1995. "The use of hospital emergency departments for nonurgent health problems: A national perspective." *Med Care Res Rev* 52(4):453–474.

Cunningham, P. J., J. Hadley, et al. 2002. "The effects of SCHIP on children's health insurance coverage: Early evidence from the community tracking study." *Med Care Res Rev* 59:359–383.

Cunningham, P. J., E. S. Schaefer, et al. 1999. *Who declines employer-sponsored health insurance and is uninsured?* Washington, DC: Center for Studying Health System Change.

Cutler, D. M., and M. McClellan. 2001. "Is technological change in medicine worth it?" *Health Aff (Millwood)* 20(5):11–29.

Dalzell, M. D. 2002. "Has capitation weathered the storm?" *Manag Care* 11(7):18–22, 24, 26.

Davidoff, A., B. Garrett, et al. 2001. *Medicaid-eligible adults who are not enrolled: Who are they and do they get the care they need?* Washington, DC: Urban Institute.

Davidoff, A., G. Kenney, et al. 2001. *Patterns of child-parent insurance coverage: Implications for expansion of coverage.* Washington, DC: Urban Institute.

Dawson, G., S. B. Ashman, et al. 2000. "The role of early experience in shaping behavioral and brain development and its implications for social policy." *Dev Psychopathol* 12(4):695–712.

Deal, L. W., and P. H. Shiono. 1998. "Medicaid managed care and children: An overview." *Future of Children* 8(2):93–104.

DeNavas-Walt, C., R. Cleveland, et al. 2001. *Money income in the United States 2000.* Washington, DC: U.S. Census Bureau.

DeNavas-Walt, C., R. Cleveland, et al. 2003. *Income in the United States, 2002.* Washington, DC: U.S. Census Bureau.

Dever, A. 1984. *Epidemiology in health services management.* Rockville, MD: Aspen.

DeVita, C. J., and K. M. Pollard. 1996. "Increasing diversity in the US population." *Stat Bull Metropol Life Insur Co* 77:12–17.

DeVoe, J. E., G. E. Fryer, et al. 2003. "Receipt of preventive care among adults: Insurance status and usual source of care." *Am J Public Health* 93(5):786–791.

Dievler, A., and T. Giovannini. 1998. "Community health centers: Promise and performance." *Med Care Res Rev* 55:405–431.

Diez-Roux, A. V., S. S. Merkin, et al. 2001. "Neighborhood of residence and incidence of coronary heart disease." *N Engl J Med* 345(2):99–106.

Diez-Roux, A. V., F. J. Nieto, et al. 1997. "Neighborhood environments and coronary heart disease: A multilevel analysis." *Am J Epidemiol* 146(1):48–63.

Diez-Roux, A. V., F. J. Nieto, et al. 1999. "Neighbourhood differences in diet: The Atherosclerosis Risk in Communities (ARIC) Study." *J Epidemiol Community Health* 53(1):55–63.

Dixon, J. M., R. M. Douglas, et al. 2000. "Making a difference to socioeconomic determinants of health in Australia: A research and development strategy." *Med J Aust* 172(11):541–544.

Djojonegoro, B. M., L. A. Aday, et al. 2000. "Area income as a predictor of preventable hospitalizations in the Harris County Hospital District, Houston." *Tex Med* 96(1):58–62.

Donelan, K., R. J. Blendon, et al. 1996. "Whatever happened to the health insurance crisis in the United States? Voices from a national survey." *JAMA* 276(16):1346–1350.

Doty, H. E., and R. Weech-Maldonado. 2003. "Racial/ethnic disparities in adult preventive dental care use." *J Health Care Poor Underserved* 14(4):516–534.

Draper, D. A., R. E. Hurley, et al. 2004. "Medicaid managed care: The last bastion of the HMO?" *Health Aff (Millwood)* 23(2):155–167.

Dressler, W. W. 1990. "Lifestyle, stress, and blood pressure in a southern black community." *Psychosom Med* 52(2):182–198.

Druss, B. G., S. C. Marcus, et al. 2003. "Trends in care by nonphysician clinicians in the United States." *N Engl J Med* 348(2):130–137.

Dubay, L., and G. Kenney. 2001. *Covering parents through Medicaid and SCHIP: Potential benefits to low-income parents and children.* Washington, DC: Kaiser Commission on Medicaid and the Uninsured and Urban Institute.

Dwyer, T., L. Blizzard, et al. 2002. "Cutaneous melanin density of Caucasians measured by spectrophotometry and risk of malignant melanoma, basal cell carcinoma, and squamous cell carcinoma of the skin." *Am J Epidemiol* 155(7):614–621.

Dwyer, T., G. Prota, et al. 2000. "Melanin density and melanin type predict melanocytic naevi in 19–20 year olds of northern European ancestry." *Melanoma Res* 10(4):387–394.

Earle, C. C., H. J. Burstein, et al. 2003. "Quality of non-breast cancer health maintenance among elderly breast cancer survivors." *J Clin Oncol* 21(8):1447–1451.

Eisenburg, D., R. Davis, et al. 1998. "Trends in alternative medicine use in the United States, 1990–1997." *JAMA* 280:1569–1575.

Erikson, J. 2003. "Cuts in health, child aid called danger to economy." *Arizona Daily Star,* May 5.

Escobar, G. J., B. Littenberg, et al. 1991. "Outcome among surviving very low birthweight infants: A meta-analysis." *Arch Dis Child* 66(2):204–211.

Ettner, S. L. 1996. "The timing of preventive services for women and children: The effect of having a usual source of care." *AJPH* 86(12):1748–1754.

Evans, G. W., and E. Kantrowitz. 2002. "Socioeconomic status and health: The potential role of environmental risk exposure." *Annu Rev Public Health* 23:303–331.

Evans, R., M. Barer, et al. 1994. *Why are some people healthy and others not?* New York: Walter de Gruyter.

Feinberg, E., K. Swartz, et al. 2002. "Family income and the impact of a children's health insurance program on reported need for health services and unmet health need." *Pediatrics* 109:E29.

Feinstein, J. S. 1993. "The relationship between socioeconomic status and health: A review of the literature." *Milbank Q* 71(2):279–322.

Felitti, V. J., R. F. Anda, et al. 1998. "Relationship of childhood abuse and household dysfunction to many of the leading causes of death in adults: The Adverse Childhood Experiences (ACE) Study." *Am J Prev Med* 14(4):245–258.

Ferguson, W., and L. Candib. 2002. "Culture, language, and the doctor-patient relationship." *Fam Med* 34(5):353–361.

Ferris, T. G., Y. Chang, et al. 2002. "Effects of removing gatekeeping on specialist utilization by children in a health maintenance organization." *Arch Pediatr Adolesc Med* 156(6): 574–579.

Ferris, T. G., J. M. Perrin, et al. 2001. "Switching to gatekeeping: Changes in expenditures and utilization for children." *Pediatrics* 108(2):283–290.

Finch, B., R. Hummer, et al. 2001. "The role of discrimination and acculturative stress in the physical health of Mexican-origin adults." *Hispanic J Behav Sci* 23:399–429.

Fiscella, K., P. Franks, et al. 2000. "Inequality in quality: Addressing socioeconomic, racial, and ethnic disparities in health care." *JAMA* 283(19):2579–2584.

Fiscella, K., P. Franks, et al. 2002. "Disparities in health care by race, ethnicity, and language among the insured: Findings from a national sample." *Med Care* 40(1):52–59.

Flaskerud, J. H., and B. J. Winslow. 1998. "Conceptualizing vulnerable populations health-related research." *Nurs Res* 47:69–78.

Flores, G., M. Abreau, et al. 1998. "Access barriers to health care for Latino children." *Arch Pediatr Adolesc Med* 152(11):1119–1125.

Flores, G., H. Bauchner, et al. 1999. "The impact of ethnicity, family income, and parental education on children's health and use of health services." *AJPH* 89(7):1066–1071.

Flores, G., and L. Vega. 1998. "Barriers to health care access for Latino children: A review." *Fam Med* 30(3):196–205.

Forrest, C., G. Glade, et al. 1999. "Gatekeeping and referral of children and adolescents to specialty care." *Pediatrics* 104(1):28–34.

Forrest, C. B., and B. Starfield. 1998. "Entry into primary care and continuity: The effects of access." *Am J Public Health* 88(9):1330–1336.

Forrest, C. B., and E. M. Whelan. 2000. "Primary care safety-net delivery sites in the United States: A comparison of community health centers, hospital outpatient departments, and physicians' offices." *JAMA* 284:2077–2083.

Fox, H., S. Limb, et al. 2000. *An analysis of states' Medicaid managed care plan arrangements and service requirements affecting children, 1995–1999*. Washington, DC: Maternal and Child Health Policy Research Center.

Franks, P., T. L. Campbell, et al. 1992. "Social relationships and health: The relative roles of family functioning and social support." *Soc Sci Med* 34(7):779–788.

Franks, P., C. Clancy, et al. 1993. "Health insurance and mortality: Evidence from a national cohort." *JAMA* 270(6):737–741.

Freeman, H. E., L. H. Aiken, et al. 1990. "Uninsured working-age adults: Characteristics and consequences." *Health Serv Res* 24(6):811–823.

Freeman, H. E., and C. R. Corey. 1993. "Insurance status and access to health services among poor persons." *Health Serv Res* 28(5):531–541.

Fuller, K. E. 2000. "Low birth-weight infants: The continuing ethnic disparity and the interaction of biology and environment." *Ethn Dis* 10(3):432–445.

Fuller, K. E. 2003. "Health disparities: Reframing the problem." *Med Sci Monit* 9(3):SR9–15.

Furstenberg, F. J., T. Cook, et al. 1999. *Urban families and adolescent success*. Chicago: University of Chicago Press.

Gallo, L. C., and K. A. Matthews. 1999. "Do negative emotions mediate the association between socioeconomic status and health?" *Ann NY Acad Sci* 896:226–245.

Gallo, L. C., and K. A. Matthews. 2003. "Understanding the association between socioeconomic status and physical health: Do negative emotions play a role?" *Psychol Bull* 129(1):10–51.

Gaskin, D. J., and C. Hoffman. 2000. "Racial and ethnic differences in preventable hospitalizations across 10 states." *Med Care Res Rev* 57 Suppl 1:85–107.

Geckova, A., J. P. van Dijk, et al. 2003. "Influence of social support on health among gender and socio-economic groups of adolescents." *Eur J Public Health* 13(1):44–50.

Gerald, D. E., and W. J. Hussar. 2003. *Projections of education statistics to 2013*. Washington, DC: National Center for Education Statistics, U.S. Department of Education.

Geronimus, A. T., J. Bound, et al. 1996. "Excess mortality among blacks and whites in the United States." *N Engl J Med* 335(21):1552–1558.

Giachello, A. L., J. O. Arrom, et al. 2003. "Reducing diabetes health disparities through community-based participatory action research: The Chicago Southeast Diabetes Community Action Coalition." *Public Health Rep* 118(4):309–323.

Gifford, E., R. Weech-Maldonado, et al. 2001. *Encouraging preventive health services for young children: The effect of expanding coverage to parents*. University Park: Academy for Health Services Research and Health Policy, Pennsylvania State University.

Gillum, R. F., B. S. Gillum, et al. 1997. "Coronary revascularization and cardiac catheterization in the United States: Trends in racial differences." *J Am Coll Cardiol* 29(7):1557–1562.

Glascoe, F. P. 2003. "Parents' evaluation of developmental status: How well do parents' concerns identify children with behavioral and emotional problems?" *Clin Pediatr (Phila)* 42(2):133–138.

Glick, S. M. 1999. "Equity in health and health care reforms." *Acta Oncol* 38(4):469–473.

Goel, M. S., C. C. Wee, et al. 2003. "Racial and ethnic disparities in cancer screening: The importance of foreign birth as a barrier to care." *J Gen Intern Med* 18(12):1028–1035.

Gold, M. 2003. "Bay Area counties to provide health coverage for all children." *Los Angeles Times*, Jan. 28, part 2, p. 6.

Gonzales, A. 2002. "Small businesses face 65 percent hike in health premiums." *Business J Phoenix*, Nov. 25.

Gornick, M. E., P. W. Eggers, et al. 1996. "Effects of race and income on mortality and use of services among Medicare beneficiaries." *N Engl J Med* 335(11):791–799.

Grady, K. E., J. P. Lemkau, et al. 1997. "Enhancing mammography referral in primary care." *Prev Med* 26(6):791–800.

Graham, C., and A. Oswald. 2003. *The view from Mars: The missing debate on income inequality in America.* Washington, DC: Brookings Institution.

Grant, E. N., C. S. Lyttle, et al. 2000. "The relation of socioeconomic factors and racial/ethnic differences in US asthma mortality." *Am J Public Health* 90(12):1923–1925.

Gray, B., and J. Stoddard. 1997. "Patient-physician pairing: Does racial and ethnic congruity influence selection of a regular physician?" *J Community Health* 22(4):247–259.

Greenstein, R. 2002. "Welfare reform's hidden ally." *Amer Prospect* 13:A35–A36.

Grumbach, K., D. Osmond, et al. 1998. "Primary care physicians' experience of financial incentives in managed-care systems." *JAMA* 339(21):1516–1521.

Guyll, M., K. A. Matthews, et al. 2001. "Discrimination and unfair treatment: Relationship to cardiovascular reactivity among African American and European American women." *Health Psychol* 20(5):315–325.

Haan, M., G. A. Kaplan, et al. 1987. "Poverty and health: Prospective evidence from the Alameda County Study." *Am J Epidemiol* 125(6):989–998.

Hack, M., N. K. Klein, et al. 1995. "Long-term developmental outcomes of low birth weight infants." *Future Child* 5(1):176–196.

Hadley J. 2002. *Sicker and poorer: The consequences of being uninsured.* Washington, DC: Kaiser Commission on Medicaid and the Uninsured.

Hadley, J., and J. Holahan. 2003. "Covering the uninsured: How much would it cost?" *Health Aff (Millwood)* Suppl:W3–250–265.

Hadley, J., J. M. Mitchell, et al. 1999. "Perceived financial incentives, HMO market penetration, and physicians' practice styles and satisfaction." *Health Serv Res* 34(1 Pt. 2):307–321.

Hadley, J., E. P. Steinberg, et al. 1991. "Comparison of uninsured and privately insured hospital patients: Condition on admission, resource use, and outcome." *JAMA* 265(3):374–379.

Hafner-Eaton, C. 1993. "Physician utilization disparities between the uninsured and insured: Comparisons of the chronically ill, acutely ill, and well nonelderly populations." *JAMA* 269(6):787–792.

Halfon, N., and M. Hochstein. 2002. "Life course health development: An integrated framework for developing health, policy, and research." *Milbank Q* 80(3):433–479.

Halfon, N., M. Inkelas, et al. 1995. "Nonfinancial barriers to care for children and youth." *Annu Rev Public Health* 16:447–472.

Halfon, N., M. Inkelas, et al. 1999a. "Challenges in securing access to care for children." *Health Aff (Millwood)* 18:48–63.

Halfon, N., M. Inkelas, et al. 1999b. "Enrollment in the State Child Health Insurance Program: A conceptual framework for evaluation and continuous quality improvement." *Milbank Q* 77:181–204.

Halfon, N., M. Inkelas, et al. 2000. "The health development organization: An organizational approach to achieving child health development." *Milbank Q* 78(3):447–497.

Halfon, N., L. Olson, et al. 2002. *Summary statistics from the National Survey of Early Childhood Health, 2000.* Washington, DC: National Center for Health Statistics.

Halm, E. A., N. Causino, et al. 1997. "Is gatekeeping better than traditional care? A survey of physicians' attitudes." *JAMA* 278(20):1677–1681.

Hamburg, D. A., G. R. Elliott, et al. 1982. *Health and behavior: Frontiers of research in the biobehavioral sciences.* Washington, DC: National Academies Press.

Han, Y., R. D. Williams, et al. 2000. "Breast cancer screening knowledge, attitudes, and practices among Korean American women." *Oncol Nurs Forum* 27(10):1585–1591.

Hanlon, G., and J. Pickett. 1984. *Public health administration and practice.* New York: Times Mirror/Mosby.

Hannan, E. L., M. van Ryn, et al. 1999. "Access to coronary artery bypass surgery by race/ethnicity and gender among patients who are appropriate for surgery." *Med Care* 37(1):68–77.

Hanson, K. L. 1998. "Is insurance for children enough? The link between parents' and children's health care use revisited." *Inquiry* 35(3):294–302.

Hart, C. L., G. D. Smith, et al. 1998. "Inequalities in mortality by social class measured at 3 stages of the lifecourse." *Am J Public Health* 88:471–474.

Hayward, M. D., and M. Heron. 1999. "Racial inequality in active life among adult Americans." *Demography* 36(1):77–91.

"Health care for children and youth in the United States: 2001 annual report on access, utilization, quality, and expenditures." 2002. *Ambul Pediatr* 2(6):419–437.

Hegarty, V., B. M. Burchett, et al. 2000. "Racial differences in use of cancer prevention services among older Americans." *J Am Geriatr Soc* 48(7):735–740.

Henry J. Kaiser Family Foundation. 2001. *Medicare at a glance.* Washington, DC: Henry J. Kaiser Family Foundation.

Hertzman, C. 1999. "Population health and human experiences." In D. Keating and C. Hertzman (Eds.), *Developmental health and the wealth of nations: Social, biological, and educational dynamics.* New York: Guilford Press.

Hertzman, C., C. Power, et al. 2001. "Using an interactive framework of society and lifecourse to explain self-rated health in early adulthood." *Soc Sci Med* 53(12):1575–1585.

Hillis, S. D., R. F. Anda, et al. 2000. "Adverse childhood experiences and sexually transmitted diseases in men and women: A retrospective study." *Pediatrics* 106(1):E11.

Hochstein, M., N. Halfon, et al. 1998. "Creating systems of developmental health care for children." *J Urban Health* 75(4):751–771.

Holl, J. L., P. G. Szilagyi, et al. 2000. "Evaluation of New York State's Child Health Plus: Access, utilization, quality of health care, and health status." *Pediatrics* 105:711–718.

Holohan, J., L. Dubay, et al. 2003. "Which children are still uninsured and why." *Future Child* 13(1):55–79.

Holt, P. G., and P. D. Sly. 1997. "Allergic respiratory disease: Strategic targets for primary prevention during childhood." *Thorax* 52(1):1–4.

Holt, P. G., and P. D. Sly. 2000. "Prevention of adult asthma by early intervention during childhood: Potential value of new generation immunomodulatory drugs." *Thorax* 55(8):700–703.

Holzman, C., B. Bullen, et al. 2001. "Pregnancy outcomes and community health: The POUCH study of preterm delivery." *Paediatr Perinat Epidemiol* 15 Suppl 2:136–158.

Horbar, J. D., G. J. Badger, et al. 2002. "Trends in mortality and morbidity for very low birth weight infants, 1991–1999." *Pediatrics* 110(1 Pt. 1):143–151.

Horner, D., W. Lazarus, et al. 2003. "Express lane eligibility." *Future Child* 13(1):224–229.

Horner, D., B. Morrow, et al. 2000. *Putting express lane eligibility into practice.* Washington, DC: Children's Partnership and Kaiser Commission on Medicaid and the Uninsured.

House, J. S., K. R. Landis, et al. 1988. "Social relationships and health." *Science* 241(4865):540–545.

House, J. S., C. Robbins, et al. 1982. "The association of social relationships and activities with mortality: Prospective evidence from the Tecumseh Community Health Study." *Am J Epidemiol* 116(1):123–140.

Howell, E. M. 1988. "Low-income persons' access to health care: NMCUES Medicaid data." *Public Health Rep* 103(5):507–514.

Howell, E., R. Almeida, et al. 2002. *Early experience with covering uninsured parents under SCHIP.* Washington, DC: Urban Institute.

Hseih, C., and M. Pugh. 1993. "Poverty, income inequality, and violent crime: A meta-analysis of recent aggregate data studies." *Criminal Justice Rev* 18:182–202.

Hughes, D. C., C. Brindis, et al. 1997. "Integrating children's health services: Evaluation of a national demonstration project." *Matern Child Health J* 1(4):243–252.

Hughes, D. C., and H. S. Luft. 1998. "Managed care and children: An overview." *Future of Children* 8(2):25–38.

Hughes, D., P. Newacheck, et al. 1995. "Medicaid managed care: Can it work for children?" *Pediatrics* 95(4):591–594.

Hurley, R. E., and S. A. Somers. 2003. "Medicaid and managed care: A lasting relationship?" *Health Aff (Millwood)* 22:77–88.

Iglehart, J. K. 1999. "The American health care system—Medicaid." *N Engl J Med* 340:403–408.

Indian Health Service. 2003. www.ihs.gov.

Institute of Medicine. 1988. *The future of public health.* Washington, DC: National Academy Press.

Institute of Medicine. 2001. *Health and behavior: The interplay of biological, behavioral, and societal influences.* Washington, DC: National Academy Press.

Institute of Medicine Committee on the Consequences of Uninsurance. 2002. *Care without coverage: Too little, too late.* Washington, DC: National Academy Press.

Institute of Medicine Committee on the Consequences of Uninsurance. 2003. *Hidden costs, value lost: Uninsurance in America.* Washington, DC: National Academy Press.

Jackson, J. S., T. N. Brown, et al. 1996. "Racism and the physical and mental health status of African Americans: A thirteen year national panel study." *Ethn Dis* 6(1–2):132–147.

James, S. A., A. Z. LaCroix, et al. (1984). "John Henryism and blood pressure differences among black men. II: The role of occupational stressors." *J Behav Med* 7(3):259–275.

Johnson, J., and E. Hall. 1995. "Class, work and health." In B. Amick III, S. Levine, and A. Tarlov (Eds.), *Society and health.* New York: Oxford University Press.

Jones, A. R., L. S. Caplan, et al. 2003. "Racial/ethnic differences in the self-reported use of screening mammography." *J Community Health* 28(5):303–316.

Jones, C. P. 2000. "Levels of racism: A theoretic framework and a gardener's tale." *Am J Public Health* 90(8):1212–1215.

Kaiser Commission on Medicaid and the Uninsured. 2003. *Health insurance coverage in America: 2001 data update.* Washington, DC.

Kaplan, D. W., C. Brindis, et al. 1998. "Elementary school-based health center use." *Pediatrics* 101:E12.

Kaplan, D. W., C. D. Brindis, et al. 1999. "A comparison study of an elementary school-based health center: Effects on health care access and use." *Arch Pediatr Adolesc Med* 153:235–243.

Kaplan, D. W., B. N. Calonge, et al. 1998. "Managed care and school-based health centers: Use of health services." *Arch Pediatr Adolesc Med* 152:25–33.

Kaplan, G. A., E. R. Pamuk, et al. 1996. "Inequality in income and mortality in the United States: Analysis of mortality and potential pathways." *BMJ* 312:999–1003.

Kaplan, J. R., and S. B. Manuck. 1999. "Status, stress, and atherosclerosis: The role of environment and individual behavior." *Ann NY Acad Sci* 896:145–161.

Karasek, R. 1990. *Healthy work: Stress, productivity, and the reconstruction of working life.* New York: Basic Books.

Karlsen, S., and J. Y. Nazroo. 2002a. "Agency and structure: The impact of ethnic identity and racism on the health of ethnic minority people." *Sociol Health Illness* 2002(24):1–20.

Karlsen, S., and J. Y. Nazroo. 2002b. "Relation between racial discrimination, social class, and health among ethnic minority groups." *Am J Public Health* 92(4):624–631.

Kasarda, J. 1989. "Urban industrial transition and the underclass." *Ann Am Acad Political Soc Sci* 501:26–47.

Kaufman, P., M. Alt, et al. 2001. *Dropout rates in the United States: 2000.* Washington, DC: National Center for Education Statistics.

Kawachi, I. 1999. "Social capital and community effects on population and individual health." *Ann NY Acad Sci* 896:120–130.

Kawachi, I., and B. P. Kennedy. 1997. "Health and social cohesion: Why care about income inequality?" *BMJ* 314(7086):1037–1040.

Kennedy, B. P., I. Kawachi, et al. 1998. "Social capital, income inequality, and firearm violent crime." *Soc Sci Med* 47(1):7–17.

Kenney, G., and J. Haley. 2001. *Why aren't more uninsured children enrolled in Medicaid or SCHIP?* Washington, DC: Urban Institute.

Kessler, R. C., K. D. Mickelson, et al. 1999. "The prevalence, distribution, and mental health correlates of perceived discrimination in the United States." *J Health Soc Behav* 40(3):208–330.

Key, J. D., E. C. Washington, et al. 2002. "Reduced emergency department utilization associated with school-based clinic enrollment." *J Adolesc Health* 30:273–278.

King, G., and D. Williams. 1995. "Race and health: A multidimensional approach to African-American health." In B. Amick III, S. Levine, A. Tarlov, and D. Chapman Walsh (Eds.), *Society and health* (pp. 93–130). New York: Oxford University Press.

Kirschenman, J., and K. Neckerman. 1991. "'We'd love to hire them, but . . .': The meaning of race for employers." In C. Jencks and P. Peterson (Eds.), *The urban underclass* (pp. 203–232). Washington, DC: Brookings Institution.

Kizer, K. W. 2001. "Establishing health care performance standards in an era of consumerism." *JAMA* 286(10):1213–1217.

Klag, M. J., P. K. Whelton, et al. 1991. "The association of skin color with blood pressure in US blacks with low socioeconomic status." *JAMA* 265(5):599–602.

Klein, J., K. Wilson, et al. 1999. "Access to medical care for adolescents: Results from the 1997 Commonwealth Fund Survey of the Health of Adolescent Girls." *Journal of Adolescent Health* 25(2):120–130.

Klein, R. 2003. "Presumptive eligibility." *Future Child* 13(1):230–237.

Kramarow, E., H. Lentzner, et al. 1999. *Health, United States, 1999.* Hyattsville, MD: National Center for Health Statistics.

Krieger, N. 1990. "Racial and gender discrimination: Risk factors for high blood pressure?" *Soc Sci Med* 30(12):1273–1281.

Krieger, N., and S. Sidney. 1996. "Racial discrimination and blood pressure: The CARDIA Study of young black and white adults." *Am J Public Health* 86(10):1370–1378.

Krieger, N., D. R. Williams, et al. 1997. "Measuring social class in US public health research: Concepts, methodologies and guidelines." *Annu Rev Public Health* 18:341–378.

Kronebusch, K. 2001. "Children's Medicaid enrollment: The impacts of mandates, welfare reform, and policy delinking." *J Health Polit Policy Law* 26(6):1223–1260.

Kurtzman, L. 2003. "One-tenth of San Mateo County, California's uninsured kids enrolled in new plan." *San Jose Mercury News,* Jan. 28.

Lake, T. 1999. "Do HMOs make a difference? Consumer assessments of health care." *Inquiry* 36(4):411–418.

Lalonde, M. 1974. *A new perspective on the health of Canadians.* Ottawa: Ministry of National Health and Welfare.

Landrine, H., and E. A. Klonoff. 1996. "The Schedule of Racist Events: A measure of racial discrimination and a study of its negative physical and mental health consequences." *J Black Psychol* 22:144–168.

Landrine, H., and E. A. Klonoff. 2000. "Racial discrimination and cigarette smoking among blacks: Findings from two studies." *Ethn Dis* 10(2):195–202.

Lansky, D. 2003. "Creating the new health care consumer: An interview with David Lansky: Interview by Ed Rabinowitz." *Healthplan* 44(4):29–30.

Lantz, P. M., J. S. House, et al. 1998. "Socioeconomic factors, health behaviors, and mortality: Results from a nationally representative prospective study of US adults." *JAMA* 279:1703–1708.

Lave, J. R., C. R. Keane, et al. 1998. "Impact of a children's health insurance program on newly enrolled children." *JAMA* 279:1820–1825.

LaVeist, T. 1994. "Beyond dummy variables and sample selection: What health services researchers ought to know about race as a variable." *Health Serv Res* 29(1):1–16.

LaVeist, T. A., and A. Nuru-Jeter. 2002. "Is doctor-patient race concordance associated with greater satisfaction with care?" *J Health Soc Behav* 43(3):296–306.

LaVeist, T. A., A. Nuru-Jeter, et al. 2003. "The association of doctor-patient race concordance with health services utilization." *J Public Health Policy* 24(3–4):312–323.

LaVeist, T. A., R. Sellers, et al. 2001. "Perceived racism and self and system blame attribution: consequences for longevity." *Ethn Dis* 11(4):711–721.

Lawrence, T. 2002. "Don't dismantle state's outstanding health care coverage." *Telegram and Gazette,* Nov. 21, p. A23.

LeClere, F. B., R. G. Rogers, et al. 1998. "Neighborhood social context and racial differences in women's heart disease mortality." *J Health Soc Behav* 39(2):91–107.

Lee, R. E., and C. Cubbin. 2002. "Neighborhood context and youth cardiovascular health behaviors." *Am J Public Health* 92(3):428–436.

Lefkowitz, B., and J. Todd. 1999. "An overview: Health centers at the crossroads." *J Ambul Care Manage* 22:1–12.

Leibowitz, A., W. Manning, et al. 1985. "Effect of cost-sharing on the use of medical services by children: Interim results from a randomized controlled trial." *Pediatrics* 75(5):942–951.

Levi, L., M. Bartley, et al. 2000. "Stressors at the workplace: Theoretical models." *Occup Med* 15(1):69–106.

Lewin, M., and S. Altman. 2000. *America's health care safety net: Intact but endangered.* Washington, DC: National Academy Press.

Lewit, E., T. Bennett, et al. 2003. "Health insurance for children: Analysis and recommendations." *Future Child* 13(1):5–29.

Lieu, T. A., P. W. Newacheck, et al. 1993. "Race, ethnicity, and access to ambulatory care among U.S. adolescents." *AJPH* 83(7):960–965.

Lillie-Blanton, M., O. Rushing, et al. 2003. *Key facts: Race, ethnicity and medical care.* Menlo Park, CA: Kaiser Family Foundation.

Lobe, J. 2000. "US admits to UN that racism persists." *IPS Daily Journal of the UN,* Sept. 25, p. 175.

Lochner, K. A., I. Kawachi, et al. 2003. "Social capital and neighborhood mortality rates in Chicago." *Soc Sci Med* 56(8):1797–1805.

Lu, M. C., and N. Halfon. 2003. "Racial and ethnic disparities in birth outcomes: A life-course perspective." *Matern Child Health J* 7(1):13–30.

Lundberg, U. 1999. "Stress responses in low-status jobs and their relationship to health risks: Musculoskeletal disorders." *Ann NY Acad Sci* 896:162–172.

Lurie, N. 2002. "What the federal government can do about the nonmedical determinants of health: Taking a 'systems' approach to structuring our government's health investments is an important first step in addressing the many contributors to health and well-being." *Health Aff (Millwood)* 21(2):94–106.

Lurie, N., N. B. Ward, et al. 1984. "Termination from Medi-Cal—Does it affect health?" *N Engl J Med* 311:480–484.

Lurie, N., N. B. Ward, et al. 1986. "Termination of Medi-Cal benefits: A follow-up study one year later." *N Engl J Med* 314:1266–1268.

Lynch, J. W., G. A. Kaplan, et al. 1998. "Income inequality and mortality in metropolitan areas of the United States." *Am J Public Health* 88(7):1074–1080.

Lynch, J. W., G. D. Smith, et al. 2000. "Income inequality and mortality: Importance to health of individual income, psychosocial environment, or material conditions." *BMJ* 320(7243):1200–1204.

Macinko, J., and B. Starfield. 2001. "The utility of social capital in research on health determinants." *Milbank Q* 79(3):387–427.

Malat, J. 2001. "Social distance and patients' rating of healthcare providers." *J Health Soc Behav* 42(4):360–372.

Mann, C. 2002. *Issues facing Medicaid and CHIP: Testimony presented before the Subcommittee on Public Health, US Senate.* Washington, DC: U.S. Senate.

Manos, M. M., W. A. Leyden, et al. 2001. "A community-based collaboration to assess and improve medical insurance status and access to health care of Latino children." *Public Health Rep* 116(6):575–584.

Mark, T. L., and L. C. Paramore. 1996. "Pneumococcal pneumonia and influenza vaccination: Access to and use by US Hispanic Medicare beneficiaries." *Am J Public Health* 86(11):1545–1550.

Marmot, M. G. 1998. "Improvement of social environment to improve health." *Lancet* 351(9095):57–60.

Marmot, M. 2002. "The influence of income on health: Views of an epidemiologist. Does money really matter? Or is it a marker for something else?" *Health Aff (Millwood)* 21(2):31–46.

Marmot, M. G., H. Bosma, et al. 1997. "Contribution of job control and other risk factors to social variations in coronary heart disease incidence." *Lancet* 350(9073):235–239.

Marmot, M. G., G. D. Smith, et al. 1991. "Health inequalities among British civil servants: The Whitehall II study." *Lancet* 337(8754):1387–1393.

Marmot, M., and T. Theorell. 1988. "Social class and cardiovascular disease: The contribution of work." *Int J Health Serv* 18(4):659–674.

Martin, L. M., E. E. Calle, et al. 1996. "Comparison of mammography and Pap test use from the 1987 and 1992 National Health Interview Surveys: Are we closing the gaps?" *Am J Prev Med* 12(2):82–90.

McBean, A. M., and M. Gornick. 1994. "Differences by race in the rates of procedures performed in hospitals for Medicare beneficiaries." *Health Care Financ Rev* 15(4): 77–90.

McCord, C., and H. P. Freeman. 1990. "Excess mortality in Harlem." *N Engl J Med* 322(3):173–177.

McDonough, J. E., C. L. Hager, et al. 1997. "Health care reform stages a comeback in Massachusetts." *N Engl J Med* 336(2):148–151.

McGee, D. L., Y. Liao, et al. 1999. "Self-reported health status and mortality in a multiethnic US cohort." *Am J Epidemiol* 149(1):41–46.

McGinnis, J. M., and W. H. Foege. 1993. "Actual causes of death in the United States." *JAMA* 270:2207–2212.

McKeown, T. 1976. *The role of medicine: Dream, mirage or nemesis.* London: Nuffield Provincial Hospitals Trust.

Mechanic, D., and M. Schlesinger. 1996. "The impact of managed care on patients' trust in medical care and their physicians." *JAMA* 275(21):1693–1697.

Menehan, K. 2001. "Freedom movement picks up steam." *Massage Magazine,* no. 90, Apr.

Merkin, S. S., L. Stevenson, et al. 2002. "Geographic socioeconomic status, race, and advanced-stage breast cancer in New York City." *Am J Public Health* 92(1):64–70.

Miller, J. E. 2000. "The effects of race/ethnicity and income on early childhood asthma prevalence and health care use." *Am J Public Health* 90(3):428–430.

Miller, M. 2000. "CAM Facts compiled for the National Center for Homeopathy, September 2000." http://www.healthlobby.com/camfacts.html.

Miller, R., and H. Luft. 1994. "Managed care plan performance since 1980: A literature analysis." *JAMA* 271(19):1512–1519.

Miller, R., and H. Luft. 1997. "Does managed care lead to better or worse quality of care?" *Health Affairs* 16(5):7–25.

Miller, R., and H. Luft. 2002. "HMO plan performance update: An analysis of the literature, 1997–2001." *Health Affairs* 21(4):63–86.

Miller, S. M. 1995. "Thinking strategically about society and health." In B. C. Amick III, S. Levine, et al. (Eds.), *Society and health* (pp. 342–358). New York: Oxford University Press.

Mills, R., and S. Bhandari. 2003. *Health Insurance Coverage in the United States, 2002.* Rockville, MD: U.S. Census Bureau.

Mitchell, J. M., J. Hadley, et al. 2000. "Measuring the effects of managed care on physicians' perceptions of their personal financial incentives." *Inquiry* 37(2):134–145.

MMWR. 1998. *Self-assessed health status and selected behavioral risk factors among persons with and without health-care coverage—United States, 1994–1995.* Atlanta, GA: Centers for Disease Control.

Montgomery, L. E., J. L. Kiely, et al. 1996. "The effects of poverty, race, and family structure on US children's health: Data from the NHIS, 1978 through 1980 and 1989 through 1991." *AJPH* 86(10):1401–1405.

Morales, L., M. Elliott, et al. 2001. "Differences in CAHPS adult survey reports and ratings by race and ethnicity: An analysis of the national CAHPS Benchmarking Data 1.0." *Health Services Research* 36(3):595–617.

Moss, N. 2000. "Socioeconomic disparities in health in the US: An agenda for action." *Soc Sci Med* 51:1627–1638.

Moy, E., B. A. Bartman, et al. 1995. "Access to hypertensive care: Effects of income, insurance, and source of care." *Arch Intern Med* 155(14):1497–502.

Muntaner, C., J. Lynch, et al. 1999. "The social class determinants of income inequality and social cohesion." *Int J Health Serv* 29(4):699–732.

National Center for Health Statistics. 1998. *Health, United States 1998, with socioeconomic status and health chartbook.* Hyattsville, MD: Centers for Disease Control.

National Center for Health Statistics. 1999. *Health, United States 1999.* Hyattsville, MD: Centers for Disease Control.

National Center for Health Statistics. 2001. *Health, United States, 2001 with urban and rural health chartbook.* Hyattsville, MD: Centers for Disease Control.

National Center for Health Statistics. 2002. *Health, United States 2002, with chartbook on trends in the health of Americans.* Hyattsville, MD: Centers for Disease Control.

National Center for Health Statistics. 2003. *Health, United States 2003.* Hyattsville, MD: Centers for Disease Control.

National Center for Health Statistics. 2004. *Health behaviors of adults: United States, 1999–2001.* Hyattsville, MD: Centers for Disease Control.

National Governors Association. 2003. *MCH update 2002: State health coverage for low-income pregnant women, children, and parents.* Washington, DC: National Governors Association.

National Institute of Child Health and Human Development. 2001. "Targeting sudden infant death syndrome (SIDS): A strategic plan." www.nichd.nih.gov/strategicplan/cells/SIDS_Syndrome.pdf.

Navarro, V. 2000. "Assessment of the World Health Report 2000." *Lancet* 356(9241): 1598–1601.

Navarro, V. 2003. "Policy without politics: The limits of social engineering." *Am J Public Health* 93(1):64–67.

Navarro, V., and L. Shi. 2001. "The political context of social inequalities and health." *Soc Sci Med* 52(3):481–491.

Neckerman, K., and J. Kirschenman. 1991. "Hiring strategies, racial bias, and inner-city workers." *Soc Problems* 38:433–447.

Neumark, D., and Wascher, W. 2001. "Using the EITC to help poor families: New evidence and a comparison with minimum wage." *Natl Tax J* 54(2):281–317.

Neumark, D., and Wascher, W. 2002. "State-level estimates of minimum wage effects: New evidence and interpretations from disequilibrium methods." *J Hum Resour* 37(1):35–62.

Newacheck, P. W. 1994. "Poverty and childhood chronic illness." *Arch Pediatr Adolesc Med* 148:1143–1149.

Newacheck, P. W., D. C. Hughes, et al. 1995. "Decategorizing health services: Interim findings from the Robert Wood Johnson Foundation's Child Health Initiative." *Health Aff (Millwood)* 14(3):232–242.

Newacheck, P. W., D. C. Hughes, et al. 1996. "Children's access to primary care: Differences by race, income and insurance status." *Pediatrics* 97(1):26–32.

Newacheck, P. W., D. C. Hughes, et al. 2000. "The unmet health needs of America's children." *Pediatrics* 105(4 Pt. 2):989–997.

Newacheck, P. W., Y. Hung, et al. 2002. "Access to health care for disadvantaged young children." *Journal of Early Intervention* 25(1):1–11.

Newacheck, P., W. J. Jameson, et al. 1994. "Health status and income: The impact of poverty on child health." *J Sch Health* 64(6):229–233.

Newacheck, P., M. McManus, et al. 2000. "Access to health care for children with special health care needs." *Pediatrics* 105(4 Pt. 1):760–766.

Newacheck, P. W., J. J. Stoddard, et al. 1998. "Health insurance and access to primary care for children." *N Engl J Med* 338(8):513–519.

Norton, S., and S. Zuckerman. 2000. "Trends in Medicaid physician fees, 1993–1998." *Health Aff (Millwood)* 19(4):222–232.

Oakley-Girvan, I., L. N. Kolonel, et al. 2003. "Stage at diagnosis and survival in a multiethnic cohort of prostate cancer patients." *Am J Public Health* 93(10):1753–1759.

Okada, L. M., and T. T. Wan. 1980. "Impact of community health centers and Medicaid on the use of health services." *Public Health Rep* 95:520–534.

Oldenburg, B. F., I. D. McGuffog, et al. 2000. "Making a difference to the socioeconomic determinants of health: Policy responses and intervention options." *Asia Pac J Public Health* 12 (Suppl):S51–54.

O'Malley, M. S., J. A. Earp, et al. 2001. "The association of race/ethnicity, socioeconomic status, and physician recommendation for mammography: Who gets the message about breast cancer screening?" *Am J Public Health* 91(1):49–54.

Orfield, G., and S. Eaton. 1996. *Dismantling desegregation: The quiet reversal of Brown v. Board of Education*. New York: New Press.

Pappas, G., W. C. Hadden, et al. 1997. "Potentially avoidable hospitalizations: Inequalities in rates between US socioeconomic groups." *Am J Public Health* 87(5):811–816.

Pappas, G., S. Queen, et al. 1993. "The increasing disparity in mortality between socioeconomic groups in the United States, 1960 and 1986." *N Engl J Med* 329(2): 103–109.

Park, E., and R. Greenstein. 2002. *Center on Budget and Policy Priorities Report: Congress fails to approve bipartisan legislation to extend expiring funds for children's health insurance*. Washington, DC: Center on Budget and Policy Priorities.

Pastore, D. R., L. Juszczak, et al. 1998. "School-based health center utilization: A survey of users and nonusers." *Arch Pediatr Adolesc Med* 152:763–767.

Patton, G. A. 2001. "The two-edged sword: How technology shapes medical practice." *Physician Exec* 27(2):42–49.

Peacock, D., N. Devlin, et al. 1999. "The horizontal equity of health care in New Zealand." *Aust NZ J Public Health* 23(2):126–130.

Perloff, J. D., P. R. Kletke, et al. 1987. "Physicians' decisions to limit Medicaid participation: Determinants and policy implications." *J Health Polit Policy Law* 12(2):221–235.

Perloff, J. D., P. Kletke, et al. 1995. "Which physicians limit their Medicaid participation, and why." *Health Serv Res* 30(1):7–26.

Peterson, E. D., L. K. Shaw, et al. 1997. "Racial variation in the use of coronary-revascularization procedures: Are the differences real? Do they matter?" *N Engl J Med* 336(7):480–486.

Phillips, K., M. Mayer, et al. 2000. "Barriers to care among racial/ethnic groups under managed care." *Health Aff* 19(4):65–75.

Pincus, T., R. Esther, et al. 1998. "Social conditions and self-management are more powerful determinants of health than access to care." *Ann Intern Med* 129:406–411.

Power, C., and S. Matthews. 1997. "Origins of health inequalities in a national population sample." *Lancet* 350:1584–1589.

Power, C., S. Matthews, et al. 1998. "Inequalities in self-rated health: Explanations from different stages of life." *Lancet* 351:1009–1014.

Proctor, B., and J. Dalaker. 2002. *Poverty in the United States, 2001*. Rockville, MD: U.S. Census Bureau.

Proctor, B., and J. Dalaker. 2003. *Poverty in the United States, 2002.* Rockville, MD: U.S. Census Bureau.

Public Housing Primary Care Program. 2002. www.bphc.hrsa.gov/phpc.

Putnam, R., R. F. Leonardi, et al. 1993. *Making democracy work: Civic traditions in modern Italy.* Princeton, NJ: Princeton University Press.

Rabin, R. 2002. "Paying more for less: Health insurance costs keep rising, forcing change in policies." *Newsday.*

Rahman, S. M., M. B. Dignan, et al. 2003. "Factors influencing adherence to guidelines for screening mammography among women aged 40 years and older." *Ethn Dis* 13(4): 477–484.

RAND Health. 1999. *Taking the pulse of health care in America: Research highlights.* Santa Monica, CA: RAND.

RAND Health. 2000. *Research highlights: Health care coverage for the nation's uninsured: Can we get to universal coverage?* Santa Monica, CA: RAND.

Raphael, S., and M. Stoll. 2002. *Modest progress: The narrowing spatial mismatch between blacks and jobs in the 1990s.* Washington, DC: Brooking Institute Center on Urban and Metropolitan Policy.

Rauber, C. 1998. "Open to alternatives: Pressured by consumer demand, more health plans are embracing nontraditional treatment options." *Mod Healthc,* Sept. 7.

Reede, J. Y. 2003. "A recurring theme: The need for minority physicians." *Health Aff (Millwood)* 22(4):91–93.

Rekindling Reform Steering Committee. 2003. "Rekindling reform: Principles and goals." *Am J Public Health* 93(1):115–117.

Ren, X. S., B. C. Amick, et al. 1999. "Racial/ethnic disparities in health: The interplay between discrimination and socioeconomic status." *Ethn Dis* 9(2):151–165.

Repetti, R. L., S. E. Taylor, et al. 2002. "Risky families: Family social environments and the mental and physical health of offspring." *Psychol Bull* 128(2):330–366.

Reschovsky, J., P. Kemper, et al. 2000. "Does type of health insurance affect health care use and assessments of care among the privately insured?" *Health Services Research* 35(1 Pt. 2): 219–237.

Rice, D. P. 1991. "Health status and national health priorities." *West J Med* 154:294–302.

Riley, T., and B. Yondorf. 2000. *Access for the uninsured: Lessons from 25 years of state initiatives.* Washington, DC: National Academy for State Health Policy.

Rissman, C. 1998. "Children's health insurance programs: Strategies for outreach and enrollment." *States Health* 8(7):1–8.

Rogers, A. C. 1997. "Vulnerability, health and health care." *J Adv Nurs* 26:65–72.

Ronsaville, D. S., and R. B. Hakim. 2000. "Well child care in the United States: Racial differences in compliance with guidelines." *Am J Public Health* 90(9):1436–1443.

Rosenbaum, S. 2002. "Medicaid." *N Engl J Med* 346(8):635–640.

Rosenbaum, S., K. Johnson, et al. 1998. "The children's hour: The State Children's Health Insurance Program." *Health Aff* 17(1):75–89.

Ross, C. E., and J. Mirowsky. 2002. "Family relationships, social support and subjective life expectancy." *J Health Soc Behav* 43(4):469–489.

Ross, D., and L. Cox. 2002. *Enrolling children and families in health coverage: The promise of doing more.* Washington, DC: Kaiser Commission on Medicaid and the Uninsured.

Ross, N. A., M. C. Wolfson, et al. 2000. "Relation between income inequality and mortality in Canada and in the United States: Cross sectional assessment using census data and vital statistics." *BMJ* 320(7239):898–902.

Rowland, D., J. Feder, et al. 1998. "Uninsured in America: The causes and consequences." In S. Altman, U. Reinhardt, et al. (Eds.), *The future U.S. healthcare system: Who will care for the poor and uninsured.* Chicago: Health Administration Press.

Sacks, H., T. Kutyla, et al. 2002. *Toward comprehensive health coverage for all: Summaries of two state planning grants from the US Health Resources and Services Administration.* New York: Commonwealth Fund Economic and Social Research Institute.

Safran, D., J. Montgomery, et al. 2001. "Switching doctors: Predictors of voluntary disenrollment from a primary physician's practice." *J Fam Pract* 50(2):137.

Safran, D., W. Rogers, et al. 2000. "Organizational and financial characteristics of health plans: Are they related to primary care performance?" *Arch Intern Med* 160(1):69–76.

Safran, D. G., A. R. Tarlov, et al. 1994. "Primary care performance in fee-for-service and prepaid health care systems." *JAMA* 271(20):1570–1586.

Saha, S., J. J. Arbelaez, et al. 2003. "Patient-physician relationships and racial disparities in the quality of health care." *Am J Public Health* 93(10):1713–1719.

Saha, S., M. Komaromy, et al. 1999. "Patient-physician racial concordance and the perceived quality and use of health care." *Arch Intern Med* 159(9):997–1004.

Saha, S., S. Taggart, et al. 2000. "Do patients choose physicians of their own race?" *Health Affairs* 19(4):76–83.

Sambamoorthi, U., and D. D. McAlpine. 2003. "Racial, ethnic, socioeconomic, and access disparities in the use of preventive services among women." *Prev Med* 37(5):475–484.

Sameroff, A. J., R. Seifer, et al. 1987. "Intelligence quotient scores of 4-year-old children: Social-environmental risk factors." *Pediatrics* 79(3):343–50.

Sanders, J. 2002. "State health care bind: Fixing inequities can be expensive." *Sacramento Bee,* Dec. 22.

Satcher, D. 2000. "Eliminating racial and ethnic disparities in health: The role of the ten leading health indicators." *J Natl Med Assoc* 92(7):315–318.

Schneider, E. C., A. M. Zaslavsky, et al. 2002. "Racial disparities in the quality of care for enrollees in Medicare managed care." *JAMA* 287(10):1288–1294.

Schoen, C., B. Lyons, et al. 1997. "Insurance matters for low-income adults: Results from a five-state survey." *Health Aff (Millwood)* 16(5):163–171.

Schulman, K., L. Rubenstein, et al. 1995. "The roles of race and socioeconomic factors in health services research." *Health Services Research* 30(1 Part 2):179–195.

Schulz, A., B. Israel, et al. 2000. "Social inequalities, stressors and self reported health status among African American and white women in the Detroit metropolitan area." *Soc Sci Med* 51(11):1639–1653.

Schulz, A. J., D. R. Williams, et al. 2002. "Racial and spatial relations as fundamental determinants of health in Detroit." *Milbank Q* 80(4):677–707.

Seeman, M., and S. Lewis. 1995. "Powerlessness, health and mortality: A longitudinal study of older men and mature women." *Soc Sci Med* 41(4):517–525.

Seeman, T. E., and E. Crimmins. 2001. "Social environment effects on health and aging: Integrating epidemiologic and demographic approaches and perspectives." *Ann NY Acad Sci* 954:88–117.

Selden, T., J. Banthin, et al. 1999. "Waiting in the wings: Eligibility and enrollment in the State Children's Health Insurance Program." *Health Affairs* 18(2):126–133.

Shea, S., D. Misra, et al. 1992. "Predisposing factors for severe, uncontrolled hypertension in an inner-city minority population." *N Eng J Med* 327(11):776–781.

Shi, L. 1992. "The relationship between primary care and life chances." *J Health Care Poor Underserved* 3(2):321–325.

Shi, L. 1994. "Primary care, specialty care, and life chances." *Int J Health Serv* 24(3):431–458.

Shi, L. 1995. "Balancing primary versus specialty care." *J Roy Soc Med* 88(8):428–432.

Shi, L. 2000. "Type of health insurance and the quality of primary care experience." *Am J Public Health* 90(12):1848–1855.

Shi, L., C. B. Forrest, et al. 2003. "Vulnerability and the patient-practitioner relationship: The roles of gatekeeping and primary care performance." *Am J Public Health* 93(1):138–144.

Shi, L., J. Macinko, et al. 2003. "Primary care, income inequality, and stroke mortality in the United States: A longitudinal analysis, 1985–1995." *Stroke* 34:1958–1964.

Shi, L., T. R. Oliver, et al. 2000. "The Children's Health Insurance Program: Expanding the framework to evaluate state goals and performance." *Milbank Q* 78:403–446, 340–401.

Shi, L., and D. A. Singh. 2004. *Delivering health care in America: A systems approach* (3rd ed.). Sudbury, MA: Jones and Bartlett.

Shi, L., and B. Starfield. 2000. "Primary care, income inequality, and self-rated health in the United States: a mixed-level analysis." *Int J Health Serv* 30(3):541–555.

Shi, L., and B. Starfield. 2001. "The effect of primary care physician supply and income inequality on mortality among blacks and whites in US metropolitan areas." *AJPH* 91(8):1246–1250.

Shi, L., B. Starfield, et al. 1999. "Income inequality, primary care, and health indicators." *J Fam Pract* 48(4):275–284.

Shi, L., and G. D. Stevens. In press a. "Vulnerability and unmet health care needs: The influence of multiple risk factors." *J Gen Intern Med.*

Shi, L., and G. D. Stevens. In press b. "Vulnerability and the receipt of recommended preventive services: The influence of multiple risk factors." *Med Care.*

Shihadeh, E., and N. Flynn. 1996. "Segregation and crime: The effect of black social isolation on the rates of black urban violence." *Soc Forces* 74:1325–1352.

Silow-Carroll, S., S. Anthony, et al. 2000. *State and local initiatives to enhance health coverage for the working uninsured.* New York: Commonwealth Fund.

Silow-Carroll, S., E. Waldman, et al. 2001. *Expanding employment-based health coverage: Lessons from six state and local programs.* New York: Commonwealth Fund.

Simpson, L., and I. Fraser. 1999. "Children and managed care: What research can, can't, and should tell us about impact." *Medical Care Research and Review* 56(Suppl 2):13–36.

Singer, B., and B. Riff (Eds.). 2001. *New horizons in health: An integrative approach.* Washington, DC: National Academy Press.

Smedley, B., A. Stith, et al. (Eds.). 2002. *Unequal treatment: Confronting racial and ethnic disparities in health care.* Washington, DC: National Academy Press.

Smeeding, T. M., K. R. Phillips, et al. 2000. "The EITC: Expectation, knowledge, use, and economic and social mobility." *National Tax J* 53:1187–1219.

Smith, G. D., C. Hart, et al. 1998. "Individual social class, area-based deprivation, cardiovascular disease risk factors, and mortality: The Renfrew and Paisley Study." *J Epidemiol Community Health* 52(6):399–405.

Sorlie, P., N. Johnson, et al. 1994. "Mortality in the uninsured compared with that in persons with public and private health insurance." *Arch Inter Med* 154:2409–2416.

South Carolina Commun-I-Care Program. 2002. www.commun-i-care.org.

Starfield, B. 1994. "Primary care: Is it essential?" *Lancet* 344(8930):1129–1133.

Starfield, B. 1998. *Primary care: Balancing health needs, services, and technology.* New York: Oxford University Press.

Starfield, B. 2000. "Evaluating the State Children's Health Insurance Program: Critical considerations." *Annu Rev Public Health* 21:569–585.

Starfield, B., C. Cassady, et al. 1998. "Consumer experiences and provider perceptions of the quality of primary care: Implications for managed care." *J Fam Pract* 46(3):216–226.

Starfield, B., N. R. Powe, et al. 1994. "Costs vs quality in different types of primary care settings." *JAMA* 272:1903–1908.

Starfield, B., A. W. Riley, et al. 2002. "Social class gradients in health during adolescence." *J Epidemiol Community Health* 56(5):354–361.

Starfield, B., J. Robertson, et al. 2002. "Social class gradients and health in childhood." *Ambul Pediatr* 2(4):238–246.

Starfield, B., and L. Shi. 1999. "Determinants of health: Testing of a conceptual model." *Ann NY Acad Sci* 896:344–346.

Staveteig, S., and A. Wigton. 2000. *Racial and ethnic disparities: Key findings from the National Survey of America's Families.* Washington, DC: Urban Institute.

Steenland, K., L. Fine, et al. 2000. "Research findings linking workplace factors to CVD outcomes." *Occup Med* 15(1):7–68.

Steptoe, A., and A. Appels. 1989. *Stress, personal control, and health.* New York: Wiley.

Stevens, G. D., and L. Shi. 2002a. "Effect of managed care on children's relationships with their primary care physicians: Differences by race." *Arch Pediatr Adolesc Med* 156(4):369–377.

Stevens, G. D., and L. Shi. 2002b. "Racial and ethnic disparities in the quality of primary care for children." *J Fam Pract* 51(6):573.

Stevens, G. D., and L. Shi. 2003. "Racial and ethnic disparities in the primary care experiences of children: A review of the literature." *Med Care Res Rev* 60(1):3–30.

Stevens, G. D., L. Shi, et al. 2003. "Patient-provider racial and ethnic concordance and parent reports of the primary care experiences of children." *Ann Fam Med* 1(2):105–112.

Stewart, S. H., and M. D. Silverstein. 2002. "Racial and ethnic disparity in blood pressure and cholesterol measurement." *J Gen Intern Med* 17(6):405–411.

Stewart, W. F., J. A. Ricci, et al. 2003. "Cost of lost productive work time among US workers with depression." *JAMA* 289(23):3135–3144.

Stoddard, J., R. St. Peter, et al. 1994. "Health insurance status and ambulatory care for children." *N Engl J Med* 330(20):1421–1425.

Stoop, N. 2004. *Educational Attainment in the United States, 2003.* Rockville, MD: U.S. Census Bureau.

Strunk, B. C., and P. J. Cunningham. 2001. *Treading water: Americans' access to needed medical care, 1997–2001.* Washington, DC: Center for Studying Health System Change.

Subramanian, S. V., K. A. Lochner, et al. 2003. "Neighborhood differences in social capital: A compositional artifact or a contextual construct?" *Health Place* 9(1):33–44.

Syme, S. 1989. "Control and health: A personal perspective." In A. Steptoe and A. Appels (Eds.), *Stress, personal control and health.* New York: Wiley.

Syme, S. L., and L. F. Berkman. 1976. "Social class, susceptibility and sickness." *Am J Epidemiol* 104(1):1–8.

Szilagyi, P. G. 1998. "Managed care for children: Effect on access to care and utilization of health services." *Future Child* 8(2):39–59.

Szilagyi, P. G., J. L. Holl, et al. 2000. "Evaluation of children's health insurance: From New York State's Child Health Plus to SCHIP." *Pediatrics* 105:687–691.

Szilagyi, P., L. Rodewald, et al. 1993. "Managed health care for children." *J Ambul Care Manage* 16(1):57–70.

Szilagyi, P., and E. Schor. 1998. "The health of children." *Health Serv Res* 33(4 Pt. 2): 1001–1039.

Taira, D., D. Safran, et al. 1997. "Asian-American patient ratings of physician primary care performance." *J Gen Intern Med* 12(4):237–242.

Taira, D. A., D. G. Safran, et al. 2001. "Do patient assessments of primary care differ by patient ethnicity?" *Health Serv Res* 36(6 Pt. 1):1059–1071.

Tang, T. S., L. J. Solomon, et al. 2000. "Cultural barriers to mammography, clinical breast exam, and breast self-exam among Chinese-American women 60 and older." *Prev Med* 31(5):575–583.

Task Force on Black and Minority Health. 1985. *Report of the Secretary's Task Force on Black and Minority Health.* Washington, DC: Department of Health and Human Services.

Taylor, S. E., R. L. Repetti, et al. 1997. "Health psychology: What is an unhealthy environment and how does it get under the skin?" *Annu Rev Psychol* 48:411–447.

Taylor, S. E., and T. E. Seeman. 1999. "Psychosocial resources and the SES-health relationship." *Ann NY Acad Sci* 896:210–225.

Terwilliger, S. H. 1994. "Early access to health care services through a rural school-based health center." *J Sch Health* 64:284–289.

Thompson, J. R., R. L. Carter, et al. 2003. "A population-based study of the effects of birth weight on early developmental delay or disability in children." *Am J Perinatol* 20(6):321–332.

Thorpe, K. 2003. *An analysis of the costs and coverage associated with Blue Shield of California's universal health insurance plan for all Americans.* Atlanta, GA: Emory University.

Tooker, J. 2003. "Affordable health insurance for all is possible by means of a pragmatic approach." *Am J Public Health* 93(1):106–109.

Tsoukalas, T. H., and S. A. Glantz. 2003. "Development and destruction of the first state funded anti-smoking campaign in the USA." *Tob Control* 12(2):214–220.

Tu, S. P., S. H. Taplin, et al. 1999. "Breast cancer screening by Asian-American women in a managed care environment." *Am J Prev Med* 17(1):55–61.

Tufts Managed Care Institute. 2001. *Emergency department utilization: Trends and management.* Medford, MA: Tufts Managed Care Institute.

Tymann, B., and T. Orloff. 1996. *The National Governors Association issue brief: Rural health care access and delivery in the context of a changing environment.* Washington DC: National Governor's Association Center for Best Practices.

Ubel, P. A., J. Baron, et al. 2000. "Are preferences for equity over efficiency in health care allocation 'all or nothing'?" *Med Care* 38(4):366–373.

United Nations Development Program. 2002. *Human development report 2002: Deepening democracy in a fragmented world.* New York: Oxford University Press.

U.S. Census Bureau. 2001a. *Resident population estimates of the United States by sex, race, and Hispanic origin: April 1, 1990 to July 1, 1999, with short-term projection to November 1, 2000.* Washington, DC: U.S. Government Printing Office.

U.S. Census Bureau. 2001b. *Mapping Census, 2000: The geography of U.S. diversity.* Washington, DC: U.S. Government Printing Office.

U.S. Census Bureau. 2001c. *Overview of race and Hispanic origin 2000.* Washington, DC: U.S. Government Printing Office.

U.S. Census Bureau, Population Division, Education & Social Stratification Branch. March 2002. *Educational attainment of the population 25 years and over, by state, including confidence intervals of estimates* (Table 13). Washington, DC: U.S. Government Printing Office.

U.S. Department of Health and Human Services. 1979. *Healthy people.* Washington, DC: U.S. Government Printing Office.

U.S. Department of Health and Human Services. 1991. *Healthy People 2000: National health promotion and disease prevention objectives.* Washington, DC: U.S. Government Printing Office.

U.S. Department of Health and Human Services. 1998. *Health, United States, 1998 with socio-economic status and health chartbook.* Washington, DC: U.S. Government Printing Office.

U.S. Department of Health and Human Services. 1999. *The initiative to eliminate racial and ethnic disparities in health.* http://raceandhealth.hhs.gov.

U.S. Department of Health and Human Services. 2000. *Healthy People 2010: Understanding and improving health.* Washington, DC: U.S. Government Printing Office.

U.S. Department of Health and Human Services. 2001. *Healthy people in healthy communities.* Washington, DC: U.S. Government Printing Office, Feb.

U.S. Department of Health and Human Services. 2002. "HHS awards $16.1 million to 28 health centers to improve access to health care services." *HHS News,* May 16.

U.S. Department of Labor, Bureau of Labor Statistics. 2002. *Employment status of the civilian noninstitutional population 16 Years and over by educational attainment, sex, race, and Hispanic or Latino ethnicity.* http://www.bls.gov/cps/.

U.S. Office of Management and Budget. 1978. "Statistical directive no. 15: Race and ethnic standards for federal agencies and administrative reporting." *Federal Register* 43:19269–19270.

University of California Regents v. Bakke. 1978. 76 U.S. 265.

Urban, N., G. L. Anderson, et al. 1994. "Mammography screening: How important is cost as a barrier to use?" *Am J Public Health* 84(1):50–55.

Valdez, R., R. Brook, et al. 1985. "Consequences of cost-sharing for children's health." *Pediatrics* 75(5):952–961.

van Ryn, M. 2002. "Research on the provider contribution to race/ethnicity disparities in medical care." *Med Care* 40(1 Suppl):140–151.

van Ryn, M., and J. Burke. 2000. "The effect of patient race and socio-economic status on physicians' perceptions of patients." *Social Science and Medicine* 50:813–828.

van Ryn, M., and S. Fu. 2003. "Paved with good intentions: Do public health and human service providers contribute to racial/ethnic disparities in health?" *AJPH* 93(2):248–255.

Wagner, E. H. 2000. "The role of patient care teams in chronic disease management." *BMJ* 320(7234):569–572.

Wallace, R. 1990. "Urban desertification, public health and public order: 'Planned shrinkage,' violent death, substance abuse and AIDS in the Bronx." *Soc Sci Med* 31(7):801–813.

Wallace, R. 1991. "Expanding coupled shock fronts of urban decay and criminal behavior." *J Quantitative Criminology* 7:333–356.

Warshaw, C., A. M. Gugenheim, et al. 2003. "Fragmented services, unmet needs: Building collaboration between the mental health and domestic violence communities." *Health Aff (Millwood)* 22(5):230–234.

Weech-Maldonado, R., L. Morales, et al. 2001. "Racial and ethnic differences in parents' assessments of pediatric care in Medicaid managed care." *Health Serv Res* 36(3): 575–594.

Weech-Maldonado, R., L. S. Morales, et al. 2003. "Race/ethnicity, language, and patients' assessments of care in Medicaid managed care." *Health Serv Res* 38(3):789–808.

Wei, H. G., and C. A. Camargo. 2000. "Patient education in the emergency department." *Acad Emer Med* 7:710–717.

Weigers, M., R. Weinick, et al. 1998. *Children's health, 1996.* Rockville, MD: Agency for Health Care Policy and Research.

Weinick, R. M., and S. K. Drilea. 1998. "Usual sources of health care and barriers to care, 1996." *Stat Bull Metrop Insur Co* 79(1):11–17.

Weinick, R., and N. Krauss. 2000. "Racial and ethnic differences in children's access to care." *AJPH* 90(11):1771–1774.

Weinick, R. M., M. E. Weigers, et al. 1998. "Children's health insurance, access to care, and health status: New findings." *Health Affairs* 17(2):127–136.

Weisner, C., J. Mertens, et al. 2001. "Integrating primary medical care with addiction treatment: A randomized controlled trial." *JAMA* 286(14):1715–1723.

Weissman, J., and A. M. Epstein. 1989. "Case mix and resource utilization by uninsured hospital patients in the Boston metropolitan area." *JAMA* 261(24):3572–3576.

Weissman, J. S., C. Gatsonis, et al. 1992. "Rates of avoidable hospitalization by insurance status in Massachusetts and Maryland." *JAMA* 268(17):2388–2394.

Wetzel, M. S., D. M. Eisenberg, et al. 1998. "Courses involving complementary and alternative medicine at US medical schools." *JAMA* 280(9):784.

Wilkinson, R. 1996. *Unhealthy societies: The afflictions of inequality.* London: Routledge.

Wilkinson, R. G. 1997. "Comment: Income, inequality, and social cohesion." *Am J Public Health* 87(9):1504–1506.

Wilkinson, R. G. 1999. "Health, hierarchy, and social anxiety." *Ann NY Acad Sci* 896:48–63.

Williams, D. R. 1999. "Race, socioeconomic status, and health: The added effects of racism and discrimination." *Ann NY Acad Sci* 896:173–188.

Williams, D. R., and C. Collins. 1995. "US socioeconomic and racial differences in health: Patterns and explanations." *Annu Rev Sociology* 21:349–386.

Williams, D. R., and C. Collins. 2001. "Racial residential segregation: A fundamental cause of racial disparities in health." *Public Health Rep* 116(5):404–416.

Williams, D. R., Y. Yu, et al. 1997. "Racial differences in physical and mental health: Socioeconomic status, stress, and discrimination." *J Health Psychol* 2:335–351.

Williams, R., J. Feaganes, et al. 1995. "Hostility and death rates in 10 US cities." *Psychosom Med* 57(1):94.

Williams, R. L., S. A. Flocke, et al. 2001. "Race and preventive services delivery among black patients and white patients seen in primary care." *Med Care* 39(11):1260–1267.

Williams, T. V., A. M. Zaslavsky, et al. 1999. "Physician experiences with, and ratings of, managed care organizations in Massachusetts." *Med Care* 37(6):589–600.

Willms, J. D. 1999. *Inequalities in literacy skills among youth in Canada and the United States.* Ontario: Canada, National Literacy Secretariat/Human Resources Development.

Wilson, R. W., and T. F. Drury. 1984. "Interpreting trends in illness and disability: Health statistics and health status." *Annu Rev Public Health* 5:83–106.

Wilson, W. 1987. *The truly disadvantaged.* Chicago: University of Chicago Press.

Wilson, W. 1996. *When work disappears: The world of the new urban poor.* New York: Knopf.

Winkleby, M. A., C. Cubbin, et al. 1999. "Pathways by which SES and ethnicity influence cardiovascular disease risk factors." *Ann NY Acad Sci* 896:191–209.

Wise, P. H., N. S. Wampler, et al. 2002. "Chronic illness among poor children enrolled in the temporary assistance for needy families program." *Am J Public Health* 92:1458–1461.

Wood, P. R., L. A. Smith, et al. 2002. "Relationships between welfare status, health insurance status, and health and medical care among children with asthma." *Am J Public Health* 92:1446–1452.

World Health Organization. 1948. "Constitution of the World Health Organization." In World Health Organization, *Basic documents.* Geneva: World Health Organization.

World Health Organization. 2000. *World Health Report 2000: Health system performance.* Geneva, Switzerland: World Health Organization.

World Health Organization. 2001. *World Conference Against Racism, Racial Discrimination, Xenophobia and Related Intolerance: Health and Freedom from Discrimination.* Geneva, Switzerland: World Health Organization.

Wright, R. A., T. L. Andres, et al. 1996. "Finding the medically underserved: A need to revise the federal definition." *J Health Care Poor Underserved* 7:296–307.

Yarcheski, A., N. E. Mahon, et al. 2001. "Social support and well-being in early adolescents: The role of mediating variables." *Clin Nurs Res* 10(2):163–181.

Yarcheski, T. J., N. E. Mahon, et al. 2003. "Social support, self-esteem, and positive health practices of early adolescents." *Psychol Rep* 92(1):99–103.

Yen, I. H., and G. A. Kaplan. 1998. "Poverty area residence and changes in physical activity level: Evidence from the Alameda County Study." *Am J Public Health* 88(11):1709–1712.

Yen, I. H., D. R. Ragland, et al. 1999a. "Racial discrimination and alcohol-related behavior in urban transit operators: Findings from the San Francisco Muni Health and Safety Study." *Public Health Rep* 114(5):448–458.

Yen, I. H., D. R. Ragland, et al. 1999b. "Workplace discrimination and alcohol consumption: Findings from the San Francisco Muni Health and Safety Study." *Ethn Dis* 9(1):70–80.

Young, T. L., S. L. D'Angelo, et al. 2001. "Impact of a school-based health center on emergency department use by elementary school students." *J Sch Health* 71:196–198.

Yu, M. Y., O. S. Hong, et al. 2003. "Uncovering factors contributing to under-utilization of breast cancer screening by Chinese and Korean women living in the United States." *Ethn Dis* 13(2):213–219.

Zuvekas, A. 1990. "Community and migrant health centers: An overview." *J Ambul Care Manage* 13:1–12.

Zuvekas, A. 2002. *Measuring farmworker and homeless patients' experiences in community health centers.* Bethesda, MD: National Association of Community Health Centers.

Zuvekas, S. H., and R. M. Weinick. 1999. "Changes in access to care, 1977–1996: The role of health insurance." *Health Serv Res* 34(1 Pt. 2):271–279.

Name Index

Subject Index

A

Academy of General Dentistry, 208

Access to care: by complementary or alternative medicine (CAM) practitioners, 219–220; equity in, 85; health insurance coverage disparities in, 118–121; measures of, 24; multiple risk factors' influence on, 135–147; as personal right, 68; potential vs. realized, 90; racial/ethnic disparities in, 86–92; socioeconomic (SES) disparities in, 107–109

Adolescents, and individual determinants model, 8

Advocates for Youth, 222–223

Affirmative action, 33–34, 214–215, 237

African Americans. *See* Blacks

Afterschool.gov, 217

Agency for Healthcare Research and Quality (AHRQ), 151, 215, 244, 245

AIDS, 222

Alcohol use/abuse: racial/ethnic disparity in, 221; socioeconomic (SES) disparity in, 116

Alcoholics Anonymous, 222

Alternative Health Care Freedom of Access Act (Minnesota), 220

Alternative medicine. *See* Complementary or alternative medicine (CAM)

Ambulatory care sensitive conditions (ACS), 111

Ambulatory visits, by Medicaid recipients, 137

American Academy of Pediatrics (AAP), 139, 228, 229

American Heart Association, 208

American Medical Association (AMA), 41, 208; Council on Ethical and Judicial Affairs, 2, 42; Council on Scientific Affairs, 2

American Stroke Association, 208

Ancillary services, 186

Anticipatory guidance, 110–111

Area Health Education Center (AHEC) (Washington, D.C.), 241

Arizona, Healthcare Group (HCG), 195, 199

Asians, increasing population of, 36. *See also* Racial/ethnic groups

Assets for Health, 190

Association of SIDS and Infant Mortality Program, 228

Association of State and Territorial Health Officials, 179

B

BadgerCare (Wisconsin), 232

Bakke, University of California Regents v., 33

Behavioral change programs, 213, 256

Benzeval framework (United Kingdom), 235

Bilingual and Bicultural Service Demonstration Grants, 176

Black Women's Health Imperative (BWHI), 221

Blacks: cigarette smoking by, 221; as portion of total population, 36–37. *See also* Racial/ethnic groups

DATE DUE

AUG 0 4 2008			